Lessons from the ICU
Under the Auspices of the European Society
of Intensive Care Medicine

Series Editors
Maurizio Cecconi, Head Dept Anesthesia and ICU
Humanitas Research Hospital Head Dept Anesthesia
and ICU, Rozzano, Milano, Milano, Italy

Daniel De Backer, Dept Intensive Care, Université Libre de
Bruxelles Dept Intensive Care Erasme University
Bruxelles, Brussels Hoofdst.ge., Belgium

Series Editors: M. Cecconi, D. De Backer
Lessons from the ICU is a Book Series published by Springer under the auspices of the *European Society of Intensive Care Medicine* (ESICM). The aim of the Series is to provide focused and state-of-the-art reviews of central topics in Intensive Care. Ultimately, its mission is to transfer the latest knowledge to the bedside in order to improve patient outcomes. Accordingly, the ESICM has also developed *Lessons from the ICU* with the vision or providing the best resources for everyone working in Intensive Care.

Each volume presents a comprehensive review of topical issues in Intensive Care. The volumes are intended to cover the majority of aspects that intensive care professionals are likely to encounter in the course of their career. Books offer an excellent guide for residents who are new to the ICU, and for allied professionals, senior consultants as well as nurses and allied healthcare professionals.

The chapters are organized in a way that allows the reader to quickly familiarize or reacquaint themselves with the pathophysiological background before moving on to diagnosis and treatment. Each chapter includes a list of Take Home Messages, as well as practical examples that apply theoretical knowledge in real clinical scenarios. Each volume in the Series is edited by international Key Opinion Leaders in Intensive Care, and each chapter is written by experts in the field.

In summary, this Series represents a valuable contribution to fill the gap in the current Intensive Care literature by providing top-quality literature reviews that can be easily digested and used at the bedside to improve patient outcomes.

Corresponding Series Editors and responsible for new book proposals :
Maurizio Cecconi @ maurizio.cecconi@hunimed.eu, Daniel De Backer @ ddebacke@ulb.ac.be

Zsolt Molnar · Marlies Ostermann · Manu Shankar-Hari
Editors

Management of Dysregulated Immune Response in the Critically Ill

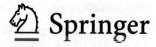

Editors
Zsolt Molnar
Department of Anaesthesiology
and Intensive Therapy
Semmelweis University
Budapest, Hungary

Marlies Ostermann
Department of Critical Care
King's College London, Guy's & St Thomas'
NHS Foundation Trust
London, UK

Manu Shankar-Hari
The Queen's Medical Research Institute
Edinburgh BioQuarter, Centre for
Inflammation Research
University of Edinburgh
Edinburgh, UK

ISSN 2522-5928   ISSN 2522-5936 (electronic)
Lessons from the ICU
ISBN 978-3-031-17574-9   ISBN 978-3-031-17572-5 (eBook)
https://doi.org/10.1007/978-3-031-17572-5

This Springer imprint is published by the registered company Springer Nature Switzerland AG
The registered company address is: Gewerbestrasse 11, 6330 Cham, Switzerland

Foreword

Ferdinand Waldo Demara, whose story is told in the book "The Great Impostor," was a man of enormous ingenuity and guile. After running away from home at the age of 16, he created a series of forged identities, variously becoming a Trappist monk, a prison warden, a psychologist, and the dean of a college. But his most daring role was as a military surgeon who, using a combination of penicillin and a textbook of general surgery, successfully treated 19 badly wounded Korean soldiers on a military hospital ship [1]. Two forces seem to have driven the success of his remarkable story—the need to adapt quickly to survive and the willingness of those he duped to accept, even if only briefly, his fantastic claims of legitimacy.

These same forces are a metaphor for sepsis. The innate immune system that drives sepsis is the product of many hundreds of millions of years of responses to complex forces on the planet that threaten survival. Of necessity, those multicellular creatures who now populate the earth have succeeded because the capacity to evolve has enabled them to pass their genetic material on to the next generation. The array of hostile factors that drove this process is broad and the evolutionary response complex, chaotic, and driven not by some grand design, but by the blunt reality that only survivors reproduce. Viewed from the evolutionary perspective that birthed it, sepsis is the legacy of half a billion years of having the genetic good fortune of surviving to reproduce. Its function was to survive the immediate threat—to limit bleeding by causing blood to coagulate, to kill and eliminate invading microorganisms, to direct blood flow to vital organs when homeostasis was threatened, and to provide the metabolic support needed to ensure cellular survival while supporting the response to threat. Viewed in retrospect, the result of that evolutionary process is a complex and elegant network of cellular and molecular effectors that provide a rapid and effective initial response, based on the recognition of patterns that signify danger, and a nuanced and highly specific response to the particular threat through the activation of an adaptive immune response. We understand it only in the most general of terms, and there is still much to unravel.

All of this complexity evolved in the absence of even the most rudimentary means of external support. Evolution could not anticipate antibiotics, surgical source control, or restoration of intravascular volume through the administration of exogenous fluids. It was blind to the effects of blood transfusion or mechanical ventilatory support—interventions that sustained life but brought new injury. Innate immunity succeeded in limiting damage in the absence of support. The corollary is that for those whose condition was sufficiently severe that support was needed to sustain life, the immune response itself became a part of the problem. Sepsis, as we manage it in the twenty-first century, is a condition that develops only in those who in previous eras would have died quietly of natural causes. It is a disease without biologic precedent.

This brings us to the second insight of the great impostor. The human mind is trusting, and its perceptions are shaped not only by our immediate observations, but also by the expectations we have, based on external authority, of what we think must be. Demara was able to convince the crew of a naval destroyer that he was a skilled surgeon because they accepted the premise that he was a surgeon, based on forged papers and diplomas. He acquired a rudimentary knowledge of medicine through reading and had an innate confidence that the principles could not be that complex. The fact that he struggled to tie a knot or to hold a scalpel was attributed to the rocking of the boat, not his lack of experience. And he did manage to save all 19 patients, including one with the fragment of a shell in the pericardial sac. As a trauma surgeon, I am in equal parts impressed by his skill and chastened by the realization of how basic the principles are.

The same presumption of authority confounds the study of sepsis. Four decades ago, we defined sepsis as the host response to infection; the implication was that any putative therapy for sepsis would only be effective in patients in whom infection was present. As we have learned more about the biology of innate immunity, we have learned that it can be activated by a host of noninfectious molecules, collectively known as danger-associated molecular patterns (DAMPs). Yet, such is the influence of a consensus definition that we have been unable to divest ourselves of the notion that the clinical syndrome we recognize as sepsis may be present in many patients who are not infected. We rely on clinical diagnostic criteria—fever, tachycardia, tachypnea, and leukocytosis—because they were given the professional imprimatur of sepsis syndrome [2] or systemic inflammatory response syndrome [3], not because they have been shown to be manifestations of a common biologic process. Even though a majority of patients with sepsis have significant respiratory insufficiency and infection is the most common risk factor for the acute respiratory distress syndrome, we think of these as separate entities, because we have given them separate names. Conversely, we think of sepsis as a single entity because it is described by a single word.

Demara's exploits provide a fascinating insight into human credulity. As will be apparent in the pages of this book, sepsis evokes strongly held views and convictions. At the same time, it challenges us to think more critically about how these convictions may be misleading us. Are concepts integral to thinking about sepsis—immune suppression, cytokine storm, and hyperinflammation—credible biologic constructs or impostors rooted in tradition and the veneer of authority? We do not know, which makes the story all the more fascinating.

It has been more than 100 years since Sir William Osler observed that his patients admitted with infection seemed to die not because of the infection *per se* but due to the body's response to infection. A few decades later, Hans (Janos) Selye discovered a similar phenomenon by exposing animals to different injuries that resulted in a typical syndrome—which he named "stress"—that was independent of the nature of the injury but represented a response to it.

In the era of modern intensive care medicine, sepsis has become on the one hand the biggest challenge at the bedside but on the other hand the greatest driving force in research activity. It was soon acknowledged that sepsis cannot be solved by administering the right antibiotics; that is, simply controlling the pathogen is not enough. The importance of the host response to infection was already taken into account by Roger Bone and co-workers on the legendary Consensus Conference in 1991, when they invented a new terminology and separated systematic inflammatory response (SIRS) from sepsis, severe sepsis and septic shock and also identified multiple system organ failure.

However, it took another more than two decades to realise that SIRS is a necessity for our immune system to tackle pathogen invasion; in fact, it should be regarded as a normal, i.e., healthy, response to an injury, let it be infectious or non-infectious. The latter occurred when we realised that clinical and biochemical features of septic shock can occur in a number of non-infection-related aetiologies, such as trauma, major surgery and acute pancreatitis, and the driving force behind the pathological consequences irrespective of the aetiology is inflammation.

Since Sepsis-3 was published in 2016, the concept that sepsis is a "life-threatening organ dysfunction due to dysregulated host response" has become more and more accepted worldwide. Although the term "dysregulated immune/host response" appears frequently in manuscripts and scientific presentations, the editors and the authors of this volume felt that a comprehensive summary on this extremely diverse and colourful topic could be of high interest and a nice learning tool for all interested.

We separated the book into four chapters starting with the host immune response (Part I). Part II addresses a few aspects of the assessment of dysregulated host response at the bedside. Part III elucidates that basically all vital organ dysfunctions are the result of and/or driven by inflammatory processes. Finally, Part IV discusses some alternative measures of immunomodulation. There is one common feature in all parts: every chapter was written by well-known, internationally highly acclaimed experts of the field.

By ending this preface, the editors of this book would like to thank all authors who contributed their high-quality work to this volume; the senior editors of this series, initiated by the European Society of Intensive Care Medicine (ESICM); and last but not least, the publisher, Springer, for the great support throughout the development and the publishing phases to enable the completion of this important mission to come true.

References

1. Crichton R. The great impostor. New York: Random House; 1959.
2. Bone RC, Fisher CJ, Clemmer TP, et al. Sepsis syndrome: a valid clinical entity. Crit Care Med 1989; 17: 389–93.
3. Bone RC, Balk RA, Cerra FB, et al. Definitions for sepsis and organ failure and guidelines for the use of innovative therapies in sepsis. Chest 1992; 101: 1644–55.

John C. Marshall
Department of Surgery, University of Toronto,
Toronto, Ontario, Canada

Preface

It has been more than 100 years since Sir William Osler observed that his patients admitted with infection seemed to die not because of the infection *per se* but due to the body's response to infection. A few decades later, Hans (Janos) Selye discovered a similar phenomenon by exposing animals to different injuries that resulted in a typical syndrome—which he named "stress"—that was independent of the nature of the injury but represented a response to it.

In the era of modern intensive care medicine, sepsis has become on the one hand the biggest challenge at the bedside but on the other hand the greatest driving force in research activity. It was soon acknowledged that sepsis cannot be solved by administering the right antibiotics; that is, simply controlling the pathogen is not enough. The importance of the host response to infection was already taken into account by Roger Bone and co-workers on the legendary Consensus Conference in 1991, when they invented a new terminology and separated systematic inflammatory response (SIRS) from sepsis, severe sepsis and septic shock and also identified multiple system organ failure.

However, it took another more than two decades to realise that SIRS is a necessity for our immune system to tackle pathogen invasion; in fact, it should be regarded as a normal, i.e., healthy, response to an injury, let it be infectious or non-infectious. The latter occurred when we realised that clinical and biochemical features of septic shock can occur in a number of non-infection-related aetiologies, such as trauma, major surgery and acute pancreatitis, and the driving force behind the pathological consequences irrespective of the aetiology is inflammation.

Since Sepsis-3 was published in 2016, the concept that sepsis is a "life-threatening organ dysfunction due to dysregulated host response" has become more and more accepted worldwide. Although the term "dysregulated immune/host response" appears frequently in manuscripts and scientific presentations, the editors and the authors of this volume felt that a comprehensive summary on this extremely diverse and colourful topic could be of high interest and a nice learning tool for all interested.

We separated the book into four chapters starting with the host immune response (Part I). Part II addresses a few aspects of the assessment of dysregulated host response at the bedside. Part III elucidates that basically all vital organ dysfunctions are the result of and/or driven by inflammatory processes. Finally, Part IV discusses some alternative measures of immunomodulation. There is one common feature in all parts: every chapter was written by well-known, internationally highly acclaimed experts of the field.

By ending this preface, the editors of this book would like to thank all authors who contributed their high-quality work to this volume; the senior editors of this series, initiated by the European Society of Intensive Care Medicine (ESICM); and last but not least, the publisher, Springer, for the great support the development and the publishing phases to enable the completion of this important mission to come true.

Zsolt Molnar
Budapest, Hungary

Marlies Ostermann
London, UK

Manu Shankar-Hari
Edinburgh, UK

Contents

II   Assessing Dysregulated Immune Response at the Bedside

III   Dysregulated Immune Response and Organ Dysfunction

*Benjamin Deniau, Charles de Roquetaillade, Alexandre Mebazaa,
and Benjamin Chousterman*
Annemieke M. Peters van Ton, Fabio Silvio Taccone, and Peter Pickkers

Contributors

Djillali Annane   Department of Intensive Care, Raymond Poincaré Hospital, APHP Université Paris Saclay, Paris, France

Laboratory of Infection and Inflammation—U1173, School of Medicine Simone Veil, University Paris Saclay Campus UVSQ, Paris, France

FHU SEPSIS, RHU RECORDS, APHP, Université Paris Saclay Campus UVSQ, INSERM, Paris, France

djillali.annane@aphp.fr

Jan Bakker   NYU School of Medicine, NYU Langone Medical Center, New York, NY, USA

Department of Pulmonology and Critical Care, Columbia University College of Physicians and Surgeons, Columbia University Irving Medical Center, New York, NY, USA

Department of Intensive Care Adults, Erasmus MC University Medical Center, Rotterdam, The Netherlands

Facultad de Medicina, Department of Intensive Care, Pontificia Universidad Católica de Chile, Santiago, Chile

jan.bakker@erasmusmc.nl

Michael Bauer   Department of Anesthesiology and Intensive Care Medicine, Jena University Hospital, Jena, Germany

Medical Faculty, Friedrich Schiller University, Jena, Germany

Michael.Bauer@med.uni-jena.de

Lieuwe D. J. Bos   Department of Intensive Care Medicine, Amsterdam University Medical Centers, Academic Medical Center, University of Amsterdam, Amsterdam, The Netherlands

l.d.bos@amsterdamumc.nl

Frank Brunkhorst   Center for Clinical Studies, Department of Anesthesiology and Intensive Care Medicine, Universitätsklinikum Jena, Jena, Germany

frank.brunkhorst@med.uni-jena.de

Carolyn S. Calfee   Division of Pulmonary, Critical Care, Allergy and Sleep Medicine, Department of Medicine, University of California, San Francisco, CA, USA

carolyn.calfee@ucsf.edu

M. Carles   CHU de Nice, France and INSERM U1065, C3M, Université Côte d'Azur, Nice, France

carles.m@chu-nice.fr

Maurizio Cecconi   Department of Anesthesia and Intensive Care Medicine, IRCCS Humanitas Research Hospital—IRCCS, Milan, Italy

Department of Biomedical Sciences, Humanitas University, Milan, Italy

maurizio.cecconi@hunimed.eu

Benjamin Chousterman   Université de Paris, INSERM, Paris, France

Department of Anesthesia and Critical Care Medicine, AP-HP Hôpital Lariboisière, Paris, France

Benjamin.chousterman@aphp.fr

Daniel De Backer   Department of Intensive Care, CHIREC Hospitals, Université Libre de Bruxelles, Brussels, Belgium

ddebacke@ulb.ac.be

Benjamin Deniau   Université de Paris, INSERM, ParisFrance

Department of Anesthesia and Critical Care Medicine, AP-HP Hôpital Lariboisière, Paris, France

Charles de Roquetaillade   Université de Paris, INSERM, Paris, France

Department of Anesthesia and Critical Care Medicine, AP-HP, Hôpital Lariboisière, Paris, France

Romein W. G. Dujardin   Laboratory of Experimental Intensive Care and Anesthesiology, Amsterdam University Medical Center, Amsterdam, The Netherlands

Department of Intensive Care, OLVG Hospital, Amsterdam, The Netherlands

r.w.dujardin@amsterdamumc.nl

Luke Flower   William Harvey Research Institute, Queen Mary University of London, London, UK

luke.flower@doctors.org.uk

John F. Fraser   Critical Care Research Group, The Prince Charles Hospital, Brisbane, QLD, Australia

Faculty of Medicine, University of Queensland, Brisbane, QLD, Australia

Nanon F. L. Heijnen   Department of Intensive Care Medicine, Maastricht University Medical Center, Maastricht, The Netherlands

nanon.heijnen@mumc.nl

Silver Heinsar   Critical Care Research Group, The Prince Charles Hospital, Brisbane, QLD, Australia

Faculty of Medicine, University of Queensland, Brisbane, QLD, Australia

Nicholas Heming   Department of Intensive Care, Raymond Poincaré Hospital, APHP Université Paris Saclay, Paris, France

Laboratory of Infection and Inflammation—U1173, School of Medicine Simone Veil, University Paris Saclay Campus UVSQ, Paris, France

FHU SEPSIS, RHU RECORDS, APHP, Université Paris Saclay Campus UVSQ, INSERM, Paris, France

nicholas.heming@aphp.fr

Dominik Jarczak   Department of Intensive Care Medicine, University Medical Center Hamburg-Eppendorf, Hamburg, Germany

d.jarczak@uke.de

Nicole P. Juffermans   Laboratory of Experimental Intensive Care and Anesthesiology, Amsterdam University Medical Center, Amsterdam, The Netherlands

Department of Intensive Care, OLVG Hospital, Amsterdam, The Netherlands

n.p.juffermans@amsterdamumc.nl

Katrina K. Ki   Critical Care Research Group, The Prince Charles Hospital, Brisbane, QLD, Australia

Faculty of Medicine, University of Queensland, Brisbane, QLD, Australia

k.ki@uq.edu.au

Derek J. B. Kleinveld   Laboratory of Experimental Intensive Care and Anesthesiology, Amsterdam University Medical Center, Amsterdam, The Netherlands

Department of Intensive Care, Erasmus University Medical Center, Rotterdam, The Netherlands

d.j.kleinveld@amsterdamumc.nl

Gunnar Lachmann   Department of Anesthesiology and Operative Intensive Care Medicine (CCM, CVK), Charité—Universitätsmedizin Berlin, Berlin, Germany

Freie Universität Berlin, Humboldt-Universität zu Berlin, Berlin, Germany

Berlin Institute of Health, Berlin, Germany

gunnar.lachmann@charite.de

Daman Lngguth   Clinical Immunology and Allergy, and Sullivan Nicolaides Pathology, Wesley Hospital, Brisbane, QLD, Australia

Daman_Langguth@snp.com.au

Nuttha Lumlertgul   Department of Critical Care, King's College London, Guy's & St Thomas' NHS Foundation Trust, London, UK

Division of Nephrology, Department of Internal Medicine and Excellence, Center in Critical Care Nephrology, King Chulalongkorn Memorial Hospital, Bangkok, Thailand

nuttha.lumlertgul@gstt.nhs.uk

John C. Marshall   St. Michael's Hospital, Toronto, ON, Canada
John.Marshall@unityhealth.to

Alexandre Mebazaa   Université de Paris, INSERM, Paris, France
Department of Anesthesia and Critical Care Medicine, AP-HP, Hôpital Lariboisière, Paris, France

Antonio Messina   Department of Anesthesia and Intensive Care Medicine, IRCCS Humanitas Research Hospital—IRCCS, Milan, Italy
Department of Biomedical Sciences, Humanitas University, Milan, Italy
antonio.messina@hunimed.eu

Zsolt Molnar   Department of Anaesthesiology and Intensive Therapy, Semmelweis University, Budapest, Hungary
Department of Anaesthesiology and Intensive Therapy, Poznan University of Medical Sciences, Poznan, Poland

Axel Nierhaus   Department of Intensive Care Medicine, University Medical Center Hamburg-Eppendorf, Hamburg, Germany
nierhaus@uke.de

Marlies Ostermann   Department of Critical Care, King's College London, Guy's & St Thomas' NHS Foundation Trust, London, UK
marlies.ostermann@gstt.nhs.uk

D. Payen   Université Paris 7, Denis Diderot, UFR de Médecine, Sorbonne Cité, Paris, France

Annemieke M. Peters van Ton   Department of Intensive Care Medicine, Radboud University Medical Center, Radboud Institute for Molecular Life Sciences, Nijmegen, The Netherlands
nienke.petersvanton@radboudumc.nl

Peter Pickkers   Department of Intensive Care Medicine, Radboud University Medical Center, Radboud Institute for Molecular Life Sciences, Nijmegen, The Netherlands
peter.pickkers@radboudumc.nl

Adrian T. Press   Department of Anesthesiology and Intensive Care Medicine, Jena University Hospital, Jena, Germany
Medical Faculty, Friedrich Schiller University, Jena, Germany
adrian.press@med.uni-jena.de

Zudin Puthucheary   William Harvey Research Institute, Queen Mary University of London, London, UK
Adult Critical Care Unit, The Royal London Hospital, Barts Health NHS Trust, London, UK
z.puthucheary@qmul.ac.uk

Christopher Rugg   Department of Anaesthesiology and Critical Care Medicine, Medical University of Innsbruck, Innsbruck, Austria

christopher.rugg@tirol-kliniken.at

Philipp Schuetz   Department of Internal Medicine, Kantonsspital Aarau, Aarau, Switzerland

University of Basel, Basel, Switzerland

Philipp.Schuetz@unibas.ch

B. Seitz-Polski   Université de Nice, Laboratoire d'Immunologieet Service de Néphrologie-Dialyse-Transplantation CHU de Nice, Université Côte d'Azur, Nice, France

seitz-polski.b@chu-nice.fr

Charlotte Summers   Department of Medicine, University of Cambridge, Cambridge, UK

cs493@medschl.cam.ac.uk

Fabio Silvio Taccone   Department of Intensive Care Medicine, Université libre de Bruxelles (ULB), Erasme Hospital, Brussels, Belgium

fabio.taccone@ulb.be

Jean-Louis Vincent   Department of Intensive Care, Erasme Hospital, Université libre de Bruxelles, Brussels, Belgium

jlvincent@intensive.org

The Host Immune Response

Contents

Phenotypes

Nanon F. L. Heijnen, Carolyn S. Calfee, and Lieuwe D. J. Bos

Contents

1

⊛ **Learning Objectives**

In this chapter, we elaborate on the heterogeneity of the critically ill and how subgroups are defined within syndromes, introduce the concept of precision medicine, discuss previously identified data-driven subphenotypes within the critically ill phenotypes, provide insight into the role of the immune response in subphenotypes, and enumerate future challenges. After reading this chapter, you will understand more about the purpose and application of phenotyping patient populations, specifically the critically ill, and the overarching role of the immune response in that phenotyping process.

1.1 Introduction: The Critically Ill, a Heterogeneous Population

Critically ill patients require intensive care unit admission for organ support. Key features of the critically ill patient are severe respiratory, cardiovascular, and/or neurological derangement, often in combination, reflected in abnormal physiological observations. These symptoms are aggregated into clinical syndromes like acute kidney injury (AKI), sepsis, acute respiratory distress syndrome (ARDS), and delirium and are used to classify the ICU population. So far, targeted pharmacologic intervention for these syndromes has proven largely unsuccessful [1–3].

A complex of recognizable symptoms characterizing a condition for which the pathophysiology is not completely understood and/or uniform constitutes the definition of a syndrome. As a result, patients with a variety of underlying pathophysiological mechanisms may fall under the umbrella of the same syndrome. This heterogeneity in biology may contribute to the failure to discover beneficial treatment effects in randomized controlled trials (RCTs) [1–3]. The identification of subgroups within syndromic diagnoses, grouping for example more biologically alike patients, may lead to new insight in pathophysiological mechanisms and treatments.

Definitions have been proposed to standardize the terminology used for subgroups in the critically ill and associated broadly defined syndromes, like sepsis. Although terminology is still somewhat in flux in the field, the proposed definitions to be utilized in this chapter are as follows: (1) Phenotype: "*A set of clinical features in a group of patients who share a common syndrome or condition.*" (2) Subphenotype: "*A set of features in a group of patients who share a phenotype, such as shared risk factor, trait, diagnostic feature, expression marker, mortality risk, or outcome in response to treatment, which distinguishes the group from other groups of patients with the same phenotype.*" (3) Endotype: "*A distinct biological mechanism of disease, often associated with an anticipated response to treatment, that is shared by a subgroup of patients and might be indicated by shared mortality risk, clinical course, or treatment responsiveness.*" (4) Treatable trait: "*A subgroup characteristic that can be successfully targeted by an intervention*" [4].

In the critically ill, various subphenotypes have been identified in a range of syndromes. Secondary analyses of RCTs and prospective observational cohort studies in the critically ill have identified associations between specific subphenotypes and worse outcome [5–11], and some subphenotypes have been associated with difference in treatment response [12–16]. This constellation of findings implies that subphenotype identification may enable both prognostic enrichment (e.g., selecting for patients at higher risk for poor outcomes [17]) and predictive enrichment (e.g., selecting for patients more likely to respond to a given therapy [17]).

It is important to realize that the identification of a subphenotype does not necessarily imply identification of an endotype. A mechanistic difference between the subphenotypes needs to be discovered in order to speak of an endotype. The same goes for a treatable trait: not every endotype harbors a treatable trait. Only when a mechanistic difference can be successfully targeted can a treatable trait be identified [4]. Based on the successful identification of subphenotypes with prognostic and predictive value, it has been suggested that phenotyping the critically ill may reveal subsets of patients with a possible targetable treatable trait. This concept forms the foundation of precision medicine: *"treatments targeted to the need of individual patients on the basis of genetic, biomarker, phenotypic, or psychosocial characteristics that distinguish a given patient from other patients with similar clinical presentations"* [18].

Precision medicine has already successfully led to novel therapeutic strategies in other medical fields like asthma and cancer. For example, the diagnosis of asthma, a heterogeneous disease, evolved over time into an umbrella term, encompassing multiple endotypes with different treatment strategies [19]. Eosinophilic and allergic asthma are examples of identified endotypes. The discovery of the important role of eosinophils in the pathogenesis in severe asthma led to the identification of interleukin-5 (IL-5, an important regulator of growth, differentiation, recruitment, activation, and survival of eosinophils) as a possible treatable trait, which turned out to be successfully targetable with mepolizumab and reslizumab (biologicals, antibodies against IL-5), benralizumab (against IL-5R), and dupilumab (against IL-4R) in patients with the eosinophilic phenotype [20, 21]. Similarly, immunoglobulin E (IgE) was found to be a treatable trait targetable with omalizumab (recombinant DNA-derived humanized IgG1k monoclonal antibody) in allergic asthma [22, 23]. Unfortunately, true treatable traits have not been identified yet in the critically ill. However, increasing evidence points to underlying biological heterogeneity within critical illness syndromes, and deeper phenotyping may reveal mechanistic differences paving the way for precision medicine in the critically ill.

1.2 Subphenotypes Identified in Critically Ill Patients

Subphenotypes can be identified based on a variety of statistical methods and a wide range of variables, covering the aspects of etiology, clinical presentation, physiology, and biology. In this subsection, we focus on data-driven subphenotypes that include variables reflecting the immune response in the clustering model or describe differences in immune response between the identified subphenotypes. Importantly, we are not including in this review phenotyping strategies based solely on clinical data, including physiologic data, given the stated focus on the immune response.

1.2.1 Sepsis

The foundation for biologic phenotyping of critically ill patients was laid in critically ill children presenting with sepsis or septic shock. Using genome-wide expression profiling, Wong and colleagues identified three subphenotypes of distinct expression profiles related to the innate and adaptive immune response, with different clinical characteristics identified [24–26]. One of the genes repeatedly found to distinguish the subphenotypes was matrix metalloproteinase 8 (MMP8). Interestingly, increased survival was seen in a murine model of sepsis when MMP8 was suppressed, which implies that MMP8 could be a targetable treatable trait to be investigated in future studies [27]. Perhaps inspired by this approach in pediatric sepsis and septic shock, peripheral blood leukocyte gene expression profiles were subsequently used in adult critically ill septic patients to directly focus on identifying subphenotypes. Analyzing 5000 genes using unsupervised consensus clustering and machine learning resulted in the discovery of four molecular subphenotypes, MARS1–4 (◘ Table 1.1). The MARS1 subphenotype was associated with the highest risk of mortality (hazard ratio [HR] versus all other subphenotypes: MARS1 1.86 (95% CI 1.21–2.86, $p = 0.0045$) versus MARS2 0.64 (95% CI 0.40–1.04, $p = 0.061$) versus MARS3 0.71 (95% CI 0.41–1.22, $p = 0.19$) versus MARS4 1.13 (95% CI 0.63–2.04, $p = 0.69$)). This high-risk MARS1 subphenotype was associated with downregulated expression of genes involved in innate and adaptive immune functions [28].

Along the same lines, unsupervised hierarchical clustering analysis of septic patients with community-acquired pneumonia (CAP) and evidence of organ dysfunction revealed two distinct subphenotypes, namely sepsis response signature groups 1 and 2 (SRS1 and SRS2) (◘ Table 1.1). Of the 3080 differently expressed genes between SRS1 and SRS2, 2260 (73.4%) were downregulated in SRS1. SRS1 was characterized as relatively immunosuppressed with features of endotoxin tolerance, T-cell exhaustion, and metabolic derangement and was associated with a higher early (14-day) mortality risk (HR 2.4, 95% CI 1.3–4.5, $p = 0.005$) [9]. Similar subgroups based on transcriptomics have been identified in patients with sepsis due to fecal peritonitis. The source of infection was only responsible for a small number of differently expressed genes (263 out of 27,159 genes). The association of SRS1 membership with worse clinical outcome remained consistent in these patients (HR 4.78, 95% CI 1.29–17.65, $p = 0.0096$) [8]. A secondary analysis of the Vasopressin versus Norepinephrine as Initial Therapy in Septic Shock (VANISH) trial showed no difference in vasopressor treatment effect between the SRS1 and SRS2 subphenotypes. However, SRS subphenotype was associated with a different response to corticosteroids (interaction between treatment and SRS subphenotype $p = 0.03$). Patients classified as SRS2 had significantly higher mortality when receiving corticosteroids compared with placebo (odds ratio [OR] 8.3, 95% CI 1.4–47.8) [15]. Notably, when receiving a placebo, patients classified as SRS2 had also a significantly lower mortality risk compared to the SRS1 subphenotype (OR 0.13, 95% CI 0.02–0.74, $p = 0.02$).

1.2.2 Acute Respiratory Distress Syndrome

In ARDS, as defined by the Berlin definition [29], two subphenotypes have been consistently identified, the "hyperinflammatory" and "hypoinflammatory" subphenotypes (◘ Table 1.1) [12–14, 30]. Using a latent class analysis (LCA) model based on clinical and biological data, patients classified as "hyperinflammatory" had higher plasma levels of inflammatory biomarkers (IL-6, IL-8, sTNFR1), lower plasma protein C levels, higher prevalence of vasopressor use, lower bicarbonate concentrations, and higher prevalence of sepsis. The "hyperinflammatory" subphenotype seemed to represent a population with more severe inflammation, shock, and metabolic acido-

■ **Table 1.1** Overview of prevalence and prognostic and predictive enrichment per subphenotype

Syndrome	Author	Subphenotypes	Prevalence	Biological biomarkers	Prognostic enrichment	Predictive enrichment
Sepsis	Scicluna et al. (2017) [28]	MARS1	90 (29.4%)	5000 blood leukocyte genes	MARS1: higher 28-day mortality (39% vs. 22%, 23%, 33%, p = 0.0045)	–
		MARS2	105 (34.3%)			
		MARS3	71 (23.3%)			
		MARS4	40 (13.1%)			
	Davenport et al. (2016) [9]	SRS1	108 (41%)	26,185 blood leukocyte genes	SRS1: higher 28-day mortality (17% vs. 27%, p = 0.037)	Steroids: SRS2: increased mortality with hydrocortisone (interaction p = 0.02)
		SRS2	157 (59%)			
ARDS	Bos et al. (2017) [34]	Uninflamed	218 (48%)	IL-13, TNFa, GMCSF, IL-1b, ANG2/1, IFNγ, IL-10, fractalkine, IL-8, IL-9, MMP8, e-selectin, p-selectin, D-dimer, TIMP1, antithrombin, PAI-1, tPA, ICAM	Reactive: higher 30-day mortality (21.6% vs. 37.7%, p < 0.001)	–
		Reactive	236 (52%)			
	Calfee et al. (2014) [13]	Hypoinflamma-tory	318 (67%)	SPD, vWF, ICAM-1, IL-6, IL-8, sTNFR-1, PAI-1, protein C	Hyperinflammatory: higher 90-day mortality (23% vs. 44%, p = 0.006)	Fluid: Hyperinflammatory: increased survival with liberal fluid strategy (interaction p = 0.0039)
		Hyperinflam-matory	155 (33%)			PEEP: Hyperinflammatory: increased survival with higher PEEP strategy (interaction p = 0.049)

(continued)

□ Table 1.1 (continued)

Syndrome	Author	Subphenotypes	Prevalence	Biological biomarkers	Prognostic enrichment	Predictive enrichment
	Kitsios et al. (2019) [42]	Hypoinflammatory	65 (62%)	IL-6, IL-8, IL-10, sTNFR-1, ANG-2, pentraxin-3, fractalkine, ST-2, procalcitonin, RAGE	not significant	Simvastatin: Hyperinflammatory: increased survival with simvastatin (interaction $p = 0.14$)
		Hyperinflammatory	39 (38%)			–
AKI	Wiersema et al. (2020) [35]	Subphenotype 1	133 (44%)	Syndecan-1, ANG-2, IL-6, VAP-1, HBP, CD73, FGF13, OLFM4, MMP8, PRTN3, ELA	Subphenotype 2: higher 90-day mortality (29.3% vs. 40.5%, $p = 0.045$)	–
		Subphenotype 2	168 (56%)			
	Bhatraju et al. (2019) [16]	AKI-SP1	462 (58.2%)	ANG2/1, sTNFR-1, sFAS, VCAM, IL-6, IL-8, GCSF, ANG-1, ANG-2	AKI-SP2: higher 28-day mortality (6% vs. 25%, $p < 0.001$)	Vasopressin: AKI-SP1: increased survival with vasopressin ($p = 0.05$)
		AKI-SP2	332 (41.8%)			

ARDS acute respiratory distress syndrome, *AKI* Acute kidney injury, *SRS* sepsis response signature, *AKI-SP* acute kidney injury-subphenotype. Biomarker abbreviations: *IL* interleukin, *TNFa* tumor necrosis factor-alpha, *GMCSF* granulocyte-macrophage colony-stimulating factor, *ANG* angiopoietin, *IFNy* interferon gamma, *MMP8* matrix metalloproteinase-8, *TIMP1* metallopeptidase inhibitor 1, *PAI-1* plasminogen activator inhibitor-1, *tPA* tissue plasminogen activator, *ICAM* intercellular adhesion molecule, *SPD* surfactant protein D, *vWF* von Willebrand factor, *sTNFR-1* soluble tumor necrosis factor receptor-1, *ST-2* suppression of tumorigenicity 2, *RAGE* receptor of advanced glycation end products, *VAP-1* vascular adhesion protein 1, *HBP* heparin-binding protein, *FGF13* fibroblast growth factor 13, *OLFM4* olfactomedin 4, *PRTN3* proteinase 3, *ELA* neutrophil elastase 2, *VCAM* vascular cell adhesion molecule, *GCSF* granulocyte colony-stimulating factor

sis, which was also reflected by its higher 90-day mortality rate (44% versus 23%, $p = 0.006$), fewer ventilator-free days (7.7 versus 17.8, $p < 0.001$), and less organ failure-free days (8.0 versus 14.5, $p < 0.001$) compared to the "hypoinflammatory" subphenotype.

In addition to the prognostic value of these subphenotypes, they also have repeatedly been validated in secondary analyses of RCTs in ARDS patients, some of which revealed subphenotype-dependent treatment effects. The multicenter trials (1) Assessment of Low Vt and Elevated End-Expiratory Pressure to Obviate Lung Injury (ALVEOLI) [13, 31], (2) Fluid and Catheter Treatment Trial (FACTT) [12, 32], and (3) Hydroxymethylglutaryl-CoA reductase inhibition with simvastatin in Acute lung injury to Reduce Pulmonary dysfunction (HARP-2) [30, 33] identified no mortality benefit with the tested therapies in ARDS patients, although conservative fluid management decreased ventilator-free days compared to liberal fluid management. However, when stratified by the identified subphenotypes, "hyperinflammatory" patients responded differently to positive end-expiratory pressure (PEEP) [13] and to fluid strategy [12] and had a significant survival benefit with simvastatin compared to placebo [14], whereas the "hypoinflammatory" subphenotype showed either inverse effects or no effect of the tested interventions.

In addition to using combined clinical and biological data, subphenotypes have also been identified based solely on biological data. A cluster analysis of 20 plasma biomarkers reflecting inflammation, coagulation, and endothelial activation revealed two subphenotypes in a cohort of ARDS patients: "reactive" and "uninflamed" (◻ Table 1.1). Patients classified as "reactive" had higher levels of inflammation, coagulation, and endothelial activation and had worse clinical outcomes (higher ICU and 30-day mortality and less ventilator-free days) [34]. Importantly, although inflammatory biomarkers were used to identify these subphenotypes, it is unclear whether the inflammatory or immune response is the fundamental mechanistic difference between either the "reactive" and "uninflamed" subphenotype or between the "hyper-" and "hypoinflammatory" subphenotype. Indeed, further biological characterization of these subphenotypes will be needed in order to identify the key pathways driving outcomes in each group.

1.2.3 Acute Kidney Injury

In a cohort of critically ill patients with AKI based on the Kidney Disease: Improving Global Outcomes (KDIGO) score, two subphenotypes named "AKI subphenotype 1" (AKI-SP1) and "AKI subphenotype 2" (AKI-SP2) were identified using latent class analysis (LCA) (◻ Table 1.1). The model consisted of 29 variables including clinical parameters and plasma biomarkers, reflecting endothelial activation/dysfunction and inflammation/apoptosis [16]. AKI-SP2 was characterized by worse renal function, higher sepsis rates, more vasopressor use, and a higher proportion of patients also diagnosed with ARDS. In addition, patients had higher values of angiopoietin 2/1 ratio (ANG 2/1), soluble tumor necrosis factor receptor-1 (sTNFR1), soluble Fas (sFAS), soluble vascular cell adhesion molecule (sVCAM), interleukin-6 (IL-6), and IL-8. Patients classified as AKI-SP2 had almost double the risk of (1) no renal recovery at 7 days (RR: 1.6; 95% CI 1.1–2.2; $p = 0.006$) and (2) 28-day mortality (RR: 2.2; 95% CI 1.3–3.5; $p = 0.002$). A secondary analysis of the Vasopressin and

Septic Shock Trial (VASST), comparing the use of vasopressin versus norepineph-rine infusion in patients with septic shock, revealed that septic patients classified as AKI-SP1 might benefit from vasopressin therapy with reduced risk at 90-day mortal-ity (RR: 0.54, 95% CI 0.32–0.92; $p = 0.02$; interaction between AKI subphenotypes and treatment $p = 0.05$), contrary to AKI-SP2 which showed no significant risk reduction [16].

A similar approach was applied to a more specific cohort including only patients with sepsis and AKI. An LCA model including 30 variables (clinical and plasma biomarkers reflecting endothelial injury and inflammation) revealed two subpheno-types, namely "subphenotype 1" and "subphenotype 2" (▢ Table 1.1) [35]. Compared to "subphenotype 1," "subphenotype 2" was characterized by higher vasopressor use, higher levels of inflammatory and endothelial injury markers (heparin-binding protein (HBP), neutrophil elastase 2 (ELA), proteinase 3 (PRTN3), olfactomedin 4 (OLFM4), matrix metalloproteinase 8 (MMP8)), lower percentage of patients with renal recovery at day 5 (46.4% versus 63.9%, $p = 0.003$), and a higher percentage of in-hospital mortality (18.8% versus 35.7%, $p = 0.001$) and 90-day mortality (29.3% and 40.5%, $p = 0.045$). Despite the difference in included study population and plasma biomarkers, "subphenotype 2" and AKI-SP2 both seem to represent a more severe form of AKI.

1.2.4 Implications of Identified Subphenotypes

The aforementioned examples indicate that the heterogeneous critically ill popula-tion, as clinically classified by syndromes, likely encompasses discrete underlying subtypes with differences in risk profiles and treatment effects. If the subphenotypes and endotypes are properly identified, this approach could ultimately lead to the discovery of treatable traits, which in turn could revolutionize treatment strategies for the critically ill. A possible treatable trait could be found in the subphenotype-dependent difference in immune response.

1.3 The Immune Response in Subphenotypes

Additional in-depth analyses have provided a richer understanding of the immune response in several of the aforementioned subphenotypes. To provide some structure, we divided this subsection into topics covering (1) the innate immune response and (2) the adaptive immune response. We acknowledge that such classification is reduc-tive and does not fully capture the complexity of the immune response.

1.3.1 Innate Immune Response

Plasma protein and transcriptomic biomarkers indicative of pro-inflammatory innate host response (e.g., IL-1beta, IL-6, and interferon gamma) are part of the set of variables used to distinguish subphenotypes in patients with ARDS and AKI. Examining these subphenotypes in more detail, the most important class-defining variables (among the highest standardized mean differences) and differences in transcriptional signatures are related to the innate immune response.

In ARDS, whole-blood leukocyte gene expression profiles have been analyzed to improve the understanding of the biological heterogeneity in the biological subphenotypes of ARDS [36]. Gene expression profiling provides a global picture of cellular function by mapping patterns in genes expressed at the transcript level (e.g., RNA microarrays) [37]. Comparing the "reactive" and "uninflamed" subphenotypes in ARDS, approximately a third of the transcripts (3.332/11.443 (29%) genes) were differently expressed in whole blood. The top differently expressed upregulated genes in the reactive subphenotype (which had worse clinical outcomes) included matrix metallopeptidase 8 (MMP8), olfactomedin 4 (OLFM4), lipocalin-2 (LCN2), haptoglobin (HP), bactericidal/permeability-increasing protein (BPI), resistin (RETN), and transcobalamin 1 (TCN1). These genes have also been found to be positively associated with ARDS before and are related to neutrophil activation, the first line of the innate immune defense.

In AKI, the most class-defining variables also included biomarkers such as proteinase 3 (PRTN3), neutrophil elastase 2 (ELA), heparin-binding protein (HBP), MMP8, and OLFM4 [38]. MMP8, PRTN3, and ELA are all neutrophil-derived proteases with proteolytic and/or catalytic properties targeting specific proteins of the extracellular matrix, including collagens, elastin, gelatin, matrix glycoprotein, and proteoglycans. HBP is a neutrophil-derived mediator with antimicrobial and potent chemoattractant properties. HBP can also induce vascular leakage and edema. OLFM4 marks a neutrophil subset which is related to a greater risk at organ failure and mortality when highly expressed in septic shock patients [39]. All these biomarkers had higher levels in "subphenotype 2" (the subphenotype associated with worse outcomes).

These data suggest that the ARDS and AKI subphenotypes that provide prognostic and predictive enrichment may be characterized by differences in the innate immune response. In-depth analysis with leukocyte gene expression profiles has suggested that the high-risk subphenotypes may have more pronounced neutrophil activation, although the exact role and relation to the subphenotypes still have to be discovered.

1.3.2 Adaptive Immune Response

The variation and dynamic nature of the host response have been recognized in sepsis for a long time, which led to the use of transcriptional signatures of leukocyte genes as an input for classification models because these provide more insights into adaptive immune responses than readily available protein biomarker concentration in plasma [40]. In a study of consecutive patients with sepsis, four subphenotypes referred to as MARS1–4 were identified and subsequently validated in other cohorts of critically ill patients with sepsis. Although all MARS1–4 subphenotypes had distinct molecular signatures, the high-risk MARS1 subphenotype showed an inverse gene expression profile compared to MARS2–4 subphenotypes, to an extent. The MARS1 subphenotype was characterized predominantly by underexpression of genes related to (1) pattern recognition receptor and cytokine signaling (e.g., interferon signaling, TREM1 signaling, NF-KB signaling); (2) cell growth, proliferation, and mobility (e.g., integrin signaling, fMLP signaling in neutrophils, Cd42 signaling); (3) lymphocyte pathways (CD28 signaling in T-helper cells, IL-4 signaling, natural killer cell signaling, T-cell receptor signaling, B-cell receptor signaling); and (4) cell death (e.g., retinoic acid-mediated apoptosis signaling, death receptor signaling). In other words, the MARS1 expression signature was largely characterized by a decrease in expressed genes related to the innate and adaptive immune response. This pattern contrasted with the patterns observed in MARS2–4 subphenotypes; for example, MARS3 expression signature was primarily characterized by increased expression of genes related to lymphocyte pathways (e.g., CD28 signaling in T-helper cells, antigen presentation pathway, natural killer cell signaling, and IL-4 signaling).

Similarly, SRS1 and SRS2 subphenotypes have also been identified to have distinct expression signatures with differences in genes related to the immune response [41]. The SRS1 subphenotype was characterized by downregulated PTPRC, PTPN22, CBL, and PAG1 (negative regulators of TCR signal initiation) and increased expression of IRAK3 and TOLLIP, key mediators of endotoxin tolerance and negative regulators of TLR signaling. Endotoxin tolerance is a transient hyporesponsive state occurring after initial endotoxin exposure. Dysregulation of this mechanism adds to the immunosuppressive state. In addition, CD274, a main signal transduction element in the T-cell antigen receptor complex, IL7R, and CD247 genes were downregulated, indicative of T-cell exhaustion. Furthermore, human leukocyte antigen (HLA) class II regulator genes, CIITA and RFX5, were downregulated. Taken together, the SRS1 subphenotype appears to be a relative immunosuppressed subphenotype with endotoxin tolerance and T-cell exhaustion.

1.3.3 Implications of the Immune Response in Subphenotypes

Current data suggests that in the ARDS and AKI subphenotypes, respectively, the differences in immune response between their individual subphenotypes seem to be driven by differences in neutrophil activation. In sepsis, the subphenotypes comprised upregulated and downregulated transcriptional signatures covering a broader area of the immune response, sketching a more immunosuppressed or immunocompetent profile. To some extent, these differences may reflect the differences in biologic assays used to characterize the subphenotypes: ARDS and AKI subphenotypes have largely been identified using protein biomarker analyses, in contrast to sepsis subphenotypes which have been driven by whole-blood gene expression profiling. Future studies comparing subphenotypes across syndromes are needed in order to determine how these groups overlap with each other. Likewise, in-depth analyses focusing on immunology pathways (e.g., RNA sequencing and CyTOF) need to be performed to elucidate the exact role of the immune response and the link to the subphenotypes identified in the critically ill.

1.3.4 Unique or Generalizable?

All the discussed subphenotypes have been identified in critical illness syndromes that often overlap and encompass patient heterogeneity. The potential links to pathophysiological mechanisms still need to be unraveled. The variables reflecting the immune response appear to be important contributors to the phenotyping models, although this response is not yet targetable with therapeutics. Furthermore, the captured underlying inflammatory reaction might reflect a more generic mechanism, possibly generalizable to other critically ill patients.

Some indication that these subtypes may be generalizable across syndromic diagnoses has been observed using the ARDS subphenotypes, which were initially proven to be robust in highly selected ARDS patient populations. Similar subphenotypes to the "reactive"/"uninflamed" and "hyperinflammatory"/"hypoinflammatory" subphenotypes with similar characteristics and clinical outcomes have since been identified and validated in (1) observational cohorts with ARDS patients included (less highly selected), (2) patients at risk for ARDS, and (3) mechanically ventilated patients without ARDS [7, 42, 43]. In a population of mechanically ventilated consecutive adult ICU patients, the top differentially expressed blood leukocyte genes of individual subphenotypes (including reactive/uninflamed and hyperinflammatory/hypoinflammatory) were similar, irrespective of ARDS status [7]. This finding supports the hypothesis that subphenotypes identified in ARDS may be generalizable to other critically ill patients.

Another indication that these approaches to subphenotyping may be agnostic to syndromic diagnosis is the overlap of characteristics in different subphenotypes. For example, MMP8 and OLFM4 (both associated with neutrophil activation) were part of the top differently expressed genes and were upregulated in both the ARDS "reactive" subphenotype and AKI "subphenotype 2" [36, 38, 44]. It could be postulated that these genes play a significant role in both subphenotypes, as they are not related to an organ-specific mechanism. It is important to realize that fulfilling the criteria of, for example, AKI does not rule out the possibility of also fulfilling the criteria of ARDS, or sepsis, or vice versa. These syndromes often occur simultaneously in the same patients, as is also reflected by for example the upregulated lipocalin-2 (LCN2, also known as NGAL, a biomarker for acute kidney injury) in the "reactive" ARDS subphenotype [36]. Overlap between subphenotypes should always be taken into account, given the "generic" biological and clinical data often used as input variables in the phenotyping models.

This overlap does not necessarily prevent the search for new treatment strategies based on phenotype characteristics, as we have learned from other fields in medicine. For example, the antibody IgE plays an essential role in the development of IgE-mediated allergic diseases, like allergic asthma. The discovery of omalizumab (anti-IgE) as a treatment for allergic asthma led to the identification of its beneficial effects in allergic dermatitis (another IgE-mediated allergic disease) later on [22, 23, 45]. Similarly, targeting IL-5 in eosinophilic asthma with mepolizumab (antibody against IL-5) revealed beneficial effects, and mepolizumab is now also registered as a treatment for eosinophilic granulomatosis with polyangiitis (EGPA) [46, 47]. As some biological signatures in asthma translate well to other diseases, it is certainly plausible that biological signatures of ARDS and AKI can be translated to other critically ill populations.

1.4 Future Challenges

Data-driven subphenotypes with the potential for prognostic and predictive enrichment, *and* evidence for differences in immune response, have been identified in the critically ill. As of yet, however, the ultimate goal of identifying treatable traits as part of precision medicine has not yet been reached. Before this can be accomplished, some key challenges need to be addressed including (1) elucidating the pathophysiological mechanisms reflected by subphenotypes and (2) clinical application of the subphenotypes.

First, it will be pivotal to increase our knowledge about the pathophysiological mechanisms reflected by the subphenotypes. The current models are mainly based on "generic" plasma biomarker and clinical data, omitting, for example, the pulmonary biology in ARDS and renal biology in AKI. Put more directly, although differences in inflammation and potentially the immune response appear to be important in characterizing the biologic differences between ARDS and AKI phenotypes, they may be entirely irrelevant to the differences in clinical outcomes and/or treatment responses in these patients. The observed differences may be a classic example of "looking only under the light" (i.e., we only observe differences in pathways we have studied) and reflect our current superficial understanding of differences in subphenotype pathogenesis. Deeper phenotyping—specifically, a comprehensive assessment of distinct phenotype-related manifestations, components, and mechanisms—could allow us to elucidate the link between subphenotype-related biological differences and pathophysiological mechanisms. Firstly, deeper phenotyping could aid in differentiating organ-specific pathways from more generic pathways. This distinction is important for the development of new therapeutics, which rely on the identification of possible treatable traits. Secondly, deeper phenotyping could help clarify the meaning and potential use of overlapping underlying mechanisms between subphenotypes. Ultimately, it could aid in determining whether a marker also behaves as a mediator. Basic characteristics of the subphenotypes, like the evolution over time and relation to the course of the underlying disease, should not be disregarded. Deeper phenotyping could improve our research strategies from preclinical models to clinical trials in search for treatable traits and new treatments.

A second challenge will be clinical implementation of phenotyping, as the models for subphenotype identification used currently are not yet suitable for bedside implementation. A predictive model of six genes (CD163, ZDHHC19, MME, FAM89A, ZBP1, B3GNT2) was able to properly classify patients into SRS1 and SRS2 subphenotypes (4.1% misclassification) [8]. However, the analyses required to perform this in a clinical setting are error-prone and time consuming, making this unsuitable as a bedside test. Fortunately, the majority of the subphenotypes found less complex predictive models to classify patients. In ARDS, these models are consistent of only 3–4 plasma biomarkers [12, 13, 28, 32, 46], which is likely more practical in a clinical setting. Point-of-care tests are currently under evaluation in a clinical setting for ARDS subphenotypes (▶ ClinicalTrials.gov Identifier: NCT04009330). While awaiting these results, a predictive model using readily available clinical data has been developed, classifying ARDS subphenotypes with high accuracy (AUC: 0.95; 95% CI 0.94–0.96) [48]. These findings are promising and open the door for phenotyping at the bedside in prospective studies.

Summary

In the heterogeneous critically ill population, subphenotypes have been identified with prognostic and potentially predictive enrichment. These subphenotypes have also shown differences in immune response. In-depth analysis showed that the subphenotypes identified in AKI and ARDS mainly differed in neutrophil activation. The subphenotypes identified in sepsis showed different transcriptional signatures with evidence for T-cell exhaustion and endotoxin tolerance, which suggests a more immunosuppressed and immunocompetent profile, respectively. Although phenotyping seems promising in the critically ill, real treatable traits have not yet been identified, and it is still unclear whether the observed differences in inflammatory markers and pathways related to the immune response represent targetable nodes in subphenotype pathogenesis. Increasing our understanding about the identified subphenotypes by deeper phenotyping will hopefully pave the way for precision medicine in the critically ill.

Take-Home Messages

- Data-driven subphenotypes in the critically ill based on models which included inflammatory biomarkers provide prognostic and predictive enrichment.
- Transcriptomic analyses indicate that neutrophil activation might distinguish subphenotypes in ARDS.
- Leukocyte gene expression signatures (MARS1–4 and SRS1–2) in sepsis distinguish subphenotypes resembling an immunosuppressed and immunocompetent profile.
- Deeper phenotyping can reveal the link between differences found in subphenotypes and pathophysiological mechanisms, a pivotal step in identifying treatable traits.
- Predictive models that can be used at the bedside need to be developed.

References

1. Matthay MA, McAuley DF, Ware LB. Clinical trials in acute respiratory distress syndrome: challenges and opportunities. Lancet Respir Med. 2017;5(6):524–34.
2. Marshall JC. Why have clinical trials in sepsis failed? Trends Mol Med. 2014;20(4):195–203.
3. Cavaillon J, Singer M, Skirecki T. Sepsis therapies: learning from 30 years of failure of translational research to propose new leads. EMBO Mol Med. 2020;12(4):e10128.
4. Reddy K, Sinha P, O'Kane CM, Gordon AC, Calfee CS, McAuley DF. Subphenotypes in critical care: translation into clinical practice. Lancet Respir Med. 2020;8(6):631–43.
5. Girard TD, Thompson JL, Pandharipande PP, Brummel NE, Jackson JC, Patel MB, et al. Clinical phenotypes of delirium during critical illness and severity of subsequent long-term cognitive impairment: a prospective cohort study. Lancet Respir Med. 2018;6(3):213–22.
6. Geri G, Vignon P, Aubry A, Fedou AL, Charron C, Silva S, et al. Cardiovascular clusters in septic shock combining clinical and echocardiographic parameters: a post hoc analysis. Intensive Care Med. 2019;45(5):657–67.
7. Heijnen NFL, Hagens LA, Smit MR, Cremer OL, Ong DSY, van der Poll T, et al. Biological subphenotypes of acute respiratory distress syndrome show prognostic enrichment in mechanically

ventilated patients without acute respiratory distress syndrome. Am J Respir Crit Care Med. 2021;203(12):1503–11.

8.   Burnham KL, Davenport EE, Radhakrishnan J, Humburg P, Gordon AC, Hutton P, et al. Shared and distinct aspects of the sepsis transcriptomic response to fecal peritonitis and pneumonia. Am J Respir Crit Care Med. 2017;196(3):328–39.

9.   Davenport EE, Burnham KL, Radhakrishnan J, Humburg P, Hutton P, Mills TC, et al. Genomic landscape of the individual host response and outcomes in sepsis: a prospective cohort study. Lancet Respir Med. 2016;4(4):259–71.

10. Gårdlund B, Dmitrieva NO, Pieper CF, Finfer S, Marshall JC, Thompson BT. Six subphenotypes in septic shock: latent class analysis of the PROWESS shock study. J Crit Care. 2018;2018(47):70–9.

11. Lindroth H, Khan BA, Carpenter JS, Gao S, Perkins AJ, Khan SH, et al. Delirium severity trajectories and outcomes in ICU patients. Defining a dynamic symptom phenotype. Ann Am Thorac Soc. 2020;17(9):1094–103.

12. Famous KR, Delucchi K, Ware LB, Kangelaris KN, Liu KD, Thompson BT, et al. Acute respiratory distress syndrome subphenotypes respond differently to randomized fluid management strategy. Am J Respir Crit Care Med. 2017;195(3):331–8.

13. Calfee CS, Delucchi K, Parsons PE, Thompson BT, Ware LB, Matthay MA, et al. Subphenotypes in acute respiratory distress syndrome: latent class analysis of data from two randomised controlled trials. Lancet Respir Med. 2014;2(8):611–20.

14. Calfee CS, Delucchi KL, Sinha P, Matthay MA, Hackett J, Shankar-Hari M, et al. Acute respiratory distress syndrome subphenotypes and differential response to simvastatin: secondary analysis of a randomised controlled trial. Lancet Respir Med. 2018;6(9):691–8.

15. Antcliffe DB, Burnham KL, Al-Beidh F, Santhakumaran S, Brett SJ, Hinds CJ, et al. Transcriptomic signatures in sepsis and a differential response to steroids from the VaNISH randomized trial. Am J Respir Crit Care Med. 2019;199(8):980–6.

16. Bhatraju PK, Zelnick LR, Herting J, Katz R, Mikacenic C, Kosamo S, et al. Identification of acute kidney injury subphenotypes with differing molecular signatures and responses to vasopressin therapy. Am J Respir Crit Care Med. 2019;199(7):863–72.

17. Food and Drug Administration. Enrichment strategies for clinical trials to support determination of effectiveness of human drugs and biological products. Guidance for industry 2019;(March):1–41.

18. Jameson JL, Longo DL. Precision medicine—personalized, problematic, and promising. N Engl J Med. 2015;372(23):2229–34.

19. Anderson GP. Endotyping asthma: new insights into key pathogenic mechanisms in a complex, heterogeneous disease. Lancet. 2008;372(9643):1107–19.

20. Wenzel SE. Eosinophils in asthma—closing the loop or opening the door? N Engl J Med. 2009;360(10):1026–8.

21. Pavord ID, Korn S, Howarth P, Bleecker ER, Buhl R, Keene ON, et al. Mepolizumab for severe eosinophilic asthma (DREAM): a multicentre, double-blind, placebo-controlled trial. Lancet. 2012;380(9842):651–9.

22. Solèr M, Matz J, Townley R, Buhl R, O'Brien J, Fox H, et al. The anti-IgE antibody omalizumab reduces exacerbations and steroid requirement in allergic asthmatics. Eur Respir J. 2001;18(2):254–61.

23. Niven R, Chung KF, Panahloo Z, Blogg M, Ayre G. Effectiveness of omalizumab in patients with inadequately controlled severe persistent allergic asthma: an open-label study. Respir Med. 2008;102(10):1371–8.

24. Wong HR, Cvijanovich N, Allen GL, Lin R, Anas N, Meyer K, et al. Genomic expression profiling across the pediatric systemic inflammatory response syndrome, sepsis, and septic shock spectrum. Crit Care Med. 2009;37(5):1558–66.

25. Wong HR, Cvijanovich N, Lin R, Allen GL, Thomas NJ, Willson DF, et al. Identification of pediatric septic shock subclasses based on genome-wide expression profiling. BMC Med. 2009;7:34.

26. Wong HR, Shanley TP, Sakthivel B, Cvijanovich N, Lin R, Allen GL, et al. Genome-level expression profiles in pediatric septic shock indicate a role for altered zinc homeostasis in poor outcome. Physiol Genomics. 2007;30(2):146–55.

27. Wong HR. Genetics and genomics in pediatric septic shock. Crit Care Med. 2012;40(5):1618–26.

28. Scicluna BP, van Vught LA, Zwinderman AH, Wiewel MA, Davenport EE, Burnham KL, et al. Classification of patients with sepsis according to blood genomic endotype: a prospective cohort study. Lancet Respir Med. 2017;5(10):816–26.

29. ARDS Definition Task Force, Ranieri VM, Rubenfeld GD, Thompson BT, Ferguson ND, Caldwell E, et al. Acute respiratory distress syndrome: the Berlin definition. JAMA [Internet]. 2012;307(23):2526–33. http://www.ncbi.nlm.nih.gov/pubmed/22797452.

30. Sinha P, Delucchi KL, Thompson BT, McAuley DF, Matthay MA, Calfee CS, et al. Latent class analysis of ARDS subphenotypes: a secondary analysis of the statins for acutely injured lungs from sepsis (SAILS) study. Intensive Care Med. 2018;44(11):1859–69.

31. Brower RG, Lanken PN, MacIntyre N, Matthay MA, Morris A, Ancukiewicz M, et al. Higher versus lower positive end-expiratory pressures in patients with the acute respiratory distress syndrome. N Engl J Med. 2004;351(4):327–36.

32. National Heart, Lung and BIARDS (ARDS) CTN, Wiedemann HP, Wheeler AP, Bernard GR, Thompson BT, Hayden D, et al. Comparison of two fluid-management strategies in acute lung injury. N Engl J Med. 2006;354(24):2564–75.

33. McAuley DF, Laffey JG, O'Kane CM, Perkins GD, Mullan B, Trinder TJ, et al. Simvastatin in the acute respiratory distress syndrome. N Engl J Med. 2014;371(18):1695–703.

34. Bos LD, Schouten LR, van Vught LA, Wiewel MA, Ong DSY, Cremer O, et al. Identification and validation of distinct biological phenotypes in patients with acute respiratory distress syndrome by cluster analysis. Thorax. 2017;72(10):876–83.

35. Wiersema R, Jukarainen S, Vaara ST, Poukkanen M, Lakkisto P, Wong H, et al. Two subphenotypes of septic acute kidney injury are associated with different 90-day mortality and renal recovery. Crit Care. 2020;24(1):150.

36. Bos LDJ, Scicluna BP, Ong DSY, Cremer O, van der Poll T, Schultz MJ. Understanding heterogeneity in biologic phenotypes of acute respiratory distress syndrome by leukocyte expression profiles. Am J Respir Crit Care Med [Internet]. 2019;200(1):42–50. http://www.ncbi.nlm.nih.gov/pubmed/30645145.

37. Verbist B, Klambauer G, Vervoort L, Talloen W, QSTAR Consortium, Shkedy Z, et al. Using transcriptomics to guide lead optimization in drug discovery projects: lessons learned from the QSTAR project. Drug Discov Today [Internet]. 2015;20(5):505–13. http://www.ncbi.nlm.nih.gov/pubmed/25582842.

38. Wiersema R, Jukarainen S, Vaara ST, Poukkanen M, Lakkisto P, Wong H, et al. Two subphenotypes of septic acute kidney injury are associated with different 90-day mortality and renal recovery. Crit Care [Internet]. 2020;24(1):150. http://www.ncbi.nlm.nih.gov/pubmed/32295614.

39. Kangelaris KN, Clemens R, Fang X, Jauregui A, Liu T, Vessel K, et al. A neutrophil subset defined by intracellular olfactomedin 4 is associated with mortality in sepsis. Am J Physiol Lung Cell Mol Physiol. 2021;320(5):L892–902.

40. Scicluna BP, van Vught LA, Zwinderman AH, Wiewel MA, Davenport EE, Burnham KL, et al. Classification of patients with sepsis according to blood genomic endotype: a prospective cohort study. Lancet Respir Med [Internet]. 2017;5(10):816–26. http://www.ncbi.nlm.nih.gov/pubmed/28864056.

41. Davenport EE, Burnham KL, Radhakrishnan J, Humburg P, Hutton P, Mills TC, et al. Genomic landscape of the individual host response and outcomes in sepsis: a prospective cohort study. Lancet Respir Med [Internet]. 2016;4(4):259–71. https://doi.org/10.1016/S2213-2600(16)00046-1.

42. Kitsios GD, Yang L, Manatakis DV, Nouraie M, Evankovich J, Bain W, et al. Host-response subphenotypes offer prognostic enrichment in patients with or at risk for acute respiratory distress syndrome. Crit Care Med [Internet]. 2019;47(12):1724–34. http://www.ncbi.nlm.nih.gov/pubmed/31634231.

43. Sinha P, Delucchi KL, Chen Y, Zhuo H, Abbott J, Wang C, et al. Latent class analysis-derived subphenotypes are generalisable to observational cohorts of acute respiratory distress syndrome: a prospective study. Thorax [Internet]. 2022;77:13–21. http://www.ncbi.nlm.nih.gov/pubmed/34253679.

44. Bos LD, Schouten LR, van Vught LA, Wiewel MA, Ong DSY, Cremer O, et al. Identification and validation of distinct biological phenotypes in patients with acute respiratory distress syndrome by cluster analysis. Thorax [Internet]. 2017;72(10):876–83. http://www.ncbi.nlm.nih.gov/pubmed/28450529

1

45. Chan S, Cornelius V, Cro S, Harper JI, Lack G. Treatment effect of omalizumab on severe pediatric atopic dermatitis: the ADAPT randomized clinical trial. JAMA Pediatr. 2020;174(1):29–37.

46. Wechsler ME, Akuthota P, Jayne D, Khoury P, Klion A, Langford CA, et al. Mepolizumab or placebo for eosinophilic granulomatosis with polyangiitis. N Engl J Med [Internet]. 2017;376(20):1921–32. http://www.ncbi.nlm.nih.gov/pubmed/28514601

47. Pavord ID, Korn S, Howarth P, Bleecker ER, Buhl R, Keene ON, et al. Mepolizumab for severe eosinophilic asthma (DREAM): a multicentre, double-blind, placebo-controlled trial. Lancet [Internet]. 2012;380(9842):651–9. https://doi.org/10.1016/S0140-6736(12)60988-X.

48. Sinha P, Churpek MM, Calfee CS. Machine learning classifier models can identify acute respiratory distress syndrome phenotypes using readily available clinical data. Am J Respir Crit Care Med. 2020;202(7):996–1004.

The Dysregulated Host Response

D. Payen, M. Carles, and B. Seitz-Polski

Contents

© The Author(s), under exclusive license to Springer Nature Switzerland AG 2023
Z. Molnar et al. (eds.), *Management of Dysregulated Immune Response in the Critically Ill*,
Lessons from the ICU, https://doi.org/10.1007/978-3-031-17572-5_2

2

🎯 **Learning Objectives**

The learning objectives are to (1) give an integrated picture of systemic immune host response during severe infection, with consequences on tissue fitness and potential organ failure; (2) describe the main metabolic pathway supplying energy for resting and stimulated immune cells; (3) describe the shift in metabolic pathways after stimulation related to infection, particularly the activation of "aerobic metabolism"; and (4) describe the relation within metabolic shift and changes in immune cell functions towards immunodepressed phenotype.

2.1 Introduction

As recently stated in Frontiers in Medicine about the scenario of COVID-19 breakthrough, "the field of Translational Medicine is of vital importance for the research breakthroughs stemming from the bench into clinical practices with the ultimate goal of improving patient outcomes. Cross-disciplinary interactions between basic life science researchers, and clinical practitioners have never been more important" [1]. The wording to characterize the systemic inflammatory response (host response) induced by an infection called "sepsis" is important to consider. The term "dysregulated" host response implies a condition in which the host response is not controlled in the way that it normally should be, according to the Cambridge Dictionary. This way may then alter the homeostasis, a process by which biological systems maintain equilibrium adjusting cellular functions to inflammation, which promotes survival. The rupture of this equilibrium leads to the following questions: (1) Is the dysregulation describing a real abnormal systemic response, or an adapted response but tolerable or not by the tissue cells, previously altered by chronic diseases and/or treatments? (2) Are the factors of the dysregulation reversible or not?

The host response domain gained credence in the medical practice because of the revolution for treating solid tumors [2] and the COVID-19 outbreak [3]. The care of COVID-19 illustrates well the concept of host response that is a major factor for sickness in the absence of a demonstrated efficient antiviral drug. The clinical patterns facing a similar SARS-CoV-2 virus vary from no symptoms to the most severe as ARDS in parallel with the intensity of host response [4]. More than the initial measurement, it is the longitudinal analysis of the host response that demonstrates the time evolution of the inflammatory response. An early (several days) and a late phase (several weeks) were observed in sepsis, which correspond to changes in gene expression, protein synthesis, metabolic shift, and finally cellular functions [5]. The early phase results from an activation of inflammation, particularly the immune cells releasing a large amount of cytokines (cytokine storm) [6]. The next phase is characterized by an "immunosuppressed" profile, which has been shown to facilitate the occurrence of secondary infections [7, 8]. This immunodepressed phenotype seems also to be associated with a higher rate of cancer occurrence [9]. After listing the major metabolic factors implicated in immune energy supply, the chapter will focus on the metabolic shift of the immune cells and its potential consequences on the functional changes in immune cells.

2.2 The Inflammatory Response in Severe Infection

For many years, a disproportionate inflammatory response to invasive infection was considered the main mechanism for sepsis pathophysiology. Now it is clear that the host response is disturbed in a much more complex way, with concomitant sustained inflammation and immune depression, with some patients having a non-repairing ability to maintain homeostasis. The recent years' publications suggest a "reprogramming" of immune cell processes in relation to metabolic shifts [10].

The cellular homeostasis is disturbed during sepsis (◘ Fig. 2.1). During infection, the invading pathogen encounters the host innate immune system reacting via the pattern recognition receptors (PRRs) recognizing the pathogen-associated molecular patterns (PAMPs). When a local host response is overwhelmed, the process is extended to the circulation compartment, with potential harmful effects on organ functions not directly concerned by the initial infection. In this severe clinical

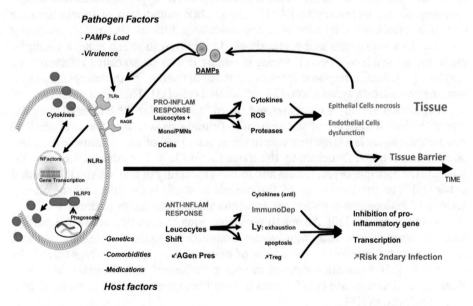

◘ **Fig. 2.1** Schematic representation of the host response to pathogen factors and/or tissue lesion. Bacterial, viral or parasite are activating the innate immunity through the pattern recognition receptors (PRRs), classified in two major types: the pathogen-associated molecular patterns (PAMPs) and the damage-associated molecular patterns (DAMPs). The recognition leads to a cascade of activation/phosphorylation that induces the stereotypic inflammatory response. Four types of receptors have been identified: Toll-like receptors (TLRs), the Nod-like receptors (NLRs), the RIG-like receptors (RLRs), and C-type lectin receptors (CLRs). Among these, TLRs (10 types in human being) have received the most attention, mainly the TLR4 the receptor for lipopolysaccharide. The TLRs induce a cascade of activation that via in nuclear transcription factors as NFκB leads to generate inflammatory cytokines. NLRs are soluble cytosolic PRRs that shares common nucleotide-binding oligomerization domain (NOD), with particular attention for NOD1 and NOD2 binding bacterial peptidoglycan. The activation of the inflammasome, especially NLRP3, the IL-1, a member of IL-1 family, promotes the amplification cascade and induces the synthesis of several inflammatory cytokine genes as IL-6. *Ly* lymphocyte, *ROS* reactive oxygen species, *Agene* antigen, *Treg* T regulatory cell, *DCells* dendritic cells, *Immunodep* immunodepression situation, recent investigations have shown a combination of excessive inflammation with immune suppression [11]. Although relatively few clinical studies on sepsis have reported longitudinal measurements after intensive care admission, these studies have shown a persistent inflammation despite appropriate treatment of the primary infection [12] with lasting organ dysfunction. This phasic change fits well with the model proposed by P Matzinger [13], suggesting a maintenance of inflammation in relation with tissue damage-associated molecular patterns (DAMPs), stimulating also the immune cells via the PRRs [6].

The most important features of the host response in sepsis are well described in other chapters and will only be summarized here to illustrate the "dysregulation" of host response.

The time evolution of acute inflammation was shown to be a fast-track process for cells to move from quiescent to activated status observed in many diseases. After activation, the immune response oscillates between pro- and anti-inflammation profile corresponding to different immune phenotypes. The hyper-inflammation in sepsis (early phase) secondary to PAMP and DAMP stimulation of innate immune system is associated clinically with approximately 50% of the overall mortality observed in severe sepsis and septic shock. In addition to shock state, a multiple-organ failure syndrome occurs, which is mainly driven by excessive inflammatory response [14]. Such a response interconnects the activation of the complement system, the coagulation system, and the endothelial cells [15]. The strong activation of the coagulation system is characterized by an intravascular disseminated coagulation with clinical evidence of microvascular thrombosis and local hemorrhage. The rapid consequence is a large decrease in the plasma level of coagulation factors and platelet number, mainly driven by the tissue factor (TF). The inhibition of this TF prevents the multiple-organ failure and reduces mortality in baboon model of lethal sepsis [15]. The predominance of thrombosis in sepsis is amplified by the altered activity of anticoagulant pathways: anti-thrombin, tissue factor pathway inhibitor, and protein C system [15]. Although reversible, such coagulation activation participates in organ failure and endothelium dysfunction. Vascular inflammation and coagulation are amplified by the release of neutrophil extracellular traps (NETs) by neutrophils [16]. Nets are supposed to entrap pathogens that facilitates pathogen elimination. The increase in NET level in blood in septic patients is associated with organ dysfunction [16].

The alteration of endothelial barrier is also a hallmark of severe sepsis, which creates a leakage of intravascular proteins and plasma to the extravascular compartment with a reduced microvascular perfusion.

2.3 The Immune Depression in Sepsis (Early and Late Phase)

The well-admitted phases of inflammation along time seem to drive mortality by different mechanisms. The early death rate (before day 7) (close to 50% of the total death) occurs in a context of hyper-inflammation. The later death (after day 7) occur in a context of immnodepressive phase [12]. The demonstrated immune depression in sepsis associates both innate and adaptive immunity elements and sounds to be most often reversible in clinic [17–20].

2.3.1 The Immune Phases

This concept of wave in inflammatory process has been confirmed in GWAs in septic shock [12] and in transcriptomic studies on blood monocytes [21, 22], on proteomic reports [23–25], and finally on cell functions [26]. Differential gene SNPs were found to be related to early versus late phases in human septic shock [12, 21, 25]. Recently, a GWA analysis on 832 multicentric septic shock patients has identified 139 SNPs associated with mortality. Among these, the leading one was the cytokine regulation gene *CISH* gene [12]. *CISH* is the first gene member of the suppressor of cytokine signaling (SOCS) family. When its level of expression is low, this enhances activation of lymphocyte Treg, an important factor of immune depression [27]. Conversely, LPS and INFγ induce a high expression of *CISH* in human monocytes in transcriptomic study [28] and high level of cytokines. When the global mortality was separated in early (<7 days) and late phases (between days 8 and 28), SNPs associated with early death (12 SNPs) differed from those associated with late mortality (16 SNPs), supporting the difference in molecular mechanisms along time. After completion of protein mapping corresponding to the gene SNPs related to mortality, 79 biological pathways have been identified including the renin-angiotensin-aldosterone system and immune systems, which can be then disrupted by genetic differences [12].

2.3.2 The "Downregulation" of Monocyte/Macrophages

The blood monocytes in septic patients are major players in the "dysregulated host response" [21, 29]. The longitudinal transcriptome analysis of human blood monocytes at the initial phase (early phase) followed by the recovery phase (late phase) has been compared with cells from healthy donors [21]. The hierarchical clustering of the monocyte transcriptomes showed clearly two different populations corresponding to acute-phase monocytes and to "recovery monocytes" having different gene expressions. In the acute phase, the statistically categorized top ten showed an overexpression of genes dealing with immune response (cytokines, chemokines, surface molecules), with a hyper-expression of IL-10. The downregulated expressed genes mainly related to the metabolic processes [21]. In the late phase, a decreased expression of key costimulatory factors and MHC class II molecules was shown ex vivo, which explains the observed alteration of monocyte surface HLA-DR [7, 30]. The downregulation of HLA-DR expression was profound in "classic" monocytes (CD14+ CD16−), but relatively modest in "nonclassical" recovery monocyte (CD14+ CD16+) [31]. Such differences in blood monocytes have recently been observed in severe ARDS COVID-19, confirming the relative independence of the original stimulus of inflammation [32, 33].

2.3.3 The Immunodepression and Adaptive Immunity

Adaptive immunity is also implicated in immunodepression status. First, a low absolute number of lymphocytes is frequently observed in severe sepsis, septic shock, and severe COVID-19 patients [17, 33, 34]. More importantly, the repertoire of T cells is altered [35] and classically called "lymphocyte exhaustion" [36–38]. The cell depletion can be profound for CD4 and CD8 T cells mainly due to apoptosis [37]. The observed improved outcome in sepsis model using pharmacologic inhibitor of apoptosis strongly suggests a causal role in sepsis mortality, which was confirmed in human clinic [39]. CD4 Th1, Th2, and Th17 functions are also depressed in septic patients [37]. CD4 T cells from patients who died from sepsis overexpressed the programmed cell death (PD1) [40]. The recent clinical testing of monoclonal antibodies blocking PD1 or PDL1 ligand showed promising immune results in human severe sepsis [41, 42]. The proportion of regulatory T cell was found elevated in severe septic patients [36, 43], a factor participating in immune-depression syndrome, as suggested by the improved immune function after experimentally blocking Treg cell function [44].

2.3.4 The Proteomic Consequences

Proteomic evaluation of immune "dysregulation" in sepsis has been focused mainly on cytokine and lymphokine release as key mediators. They may amplify the cytokine production amplifying the cytokine response, which may induce cell and tissue damage [6] participating in organ failures. Such release had been called "cytokine storm," a particularly famous wording during the COVID-19 breakthrough. Although initially introduced to describe the graft-versus-host syndrome [45], it was observed in severe sepsis and septic shock, corresponding to systemic inflammation related to a proven or a highly suspected infection. Cytokines are relatively small-size proteins with autocrine, paracrine, and endocrine activities modulating immunity, which can be separated in interleukins, chemokines, interferons, or growth factors. Binding to their specific receptors, cytokines induce activation/inhibition, proliferation/destruction, and migration of target cells. Although artificially divided into pro- and anti-inflammatory mediators, it is useful to consider the cytokines responsible for cell activation and apoptosis/necrosis as pro- and those damping or reversing the inflammation as anti-inflammatory cytokines. Because of the complexity of cytokine network and their interrelations, only the leading molecules assessed in sepsis are currently presented as players of the "dysregulated host response."

In studies looking at the pro-inflammatory cytokine group during sepsis, IL-1β, IL-6, IL-12, and IL-17 have a key role. IL-1β, produced after activation of inflammasome, induces the synthesis of various inflammatory molecules in parallel to IL-18 and IL-33 [46]. IL-6 seems actually the "star" of pro-inflammatory marker, including in COVID-19 [47], despite complex interactions with other released cytokines. IL-6, a family of proteins, is in fact mainly produced by monocyte/macrophages binding to IL-6 receptors (two subunits). Interestingly, the receptor expression itself regulates partially the effect of IL-6: low level of receptors with high level of IL-6 will induce relatively modest effect. A large number of clinical studies on sepsis have shown the association between high level of IL-6 and severity and poor outcome of patients [20], which was also observed in COVID-19 [47]. The therapeutic development of IL-6 monoclonal antibodies emphasized the admitted importance of this cytokine, especially for COVID-19, but with controversial results [48–50]. Similarly, the elevated level of IL-12 in severe sepsis differentiates the naïve T cells into helper T cells (TH1) and activates NK cells that produce high levels of INFγ. IL-17, produced by

TH17 T cells, is finely tuned among different cytokines. Interferons are classified into three types according to their receptor specificity: type 1 interferon, type 2 interferon (INFγ), and interferon λ. INFγ produced by CD4 and CD8 T cells and to a lesser extent by NK cells defines the TH1-type cells' response. Consequently, INFγ is a key player of inflammatory response in sepsis, which had been shown to be damped in longitudinal studies. This damping may result from the altered lymphocyte responsiveness [19]. This impaired lymphocyte function can be replaced by exogenous INFγ administration, with a spectacular correction of monocyte/macrophage immune depression [19, 20].

Among the anti-inflammatory cytokines, the most studied in human context are IL-10, IL-4, and IL-l-RA. IL-10 is the major anti-inflammatory cytokine that is blocking the production of pro-inflammatory cytokines produced by myeloid cells, NK cells, and T cells [51]. Although anti-inflammatory, the level of IL-10 varies in parallel with the pro-inflammatory cytokines (IL-6), suggesting to consider the inflammatory response as a global phenomenon, with a balance regulating the final phenotype as immune depression.

The cytokine release induced by acute infection is a redundant process that auto-amplifies the inflammatory response that helps to eliminate the pathogens, but also to preserve the best fitness of the tissues by regulating the host response. In this longitudinal view, cytokines play a key role as a microenvironment of the cells able to change the cells' functions. When such regulation is insufficient or non-adapted to the tissue cells' capability, it may induce pathways leading to cell destructions or irreversible functional alterations, including for the immune system. Although important in such intimal mechanism, the roles of epigenetic [52] and neuro-inflammatory reflex [53, 54] are not discussed in this chapter.

2.4 The Role of Cellular Metabolism

The need for rapid adaptation of immune cells to an acute circumstance as sepsis implies that these cells are extremely dynamic, depending on the environmental signals. Several aspects are quickly changing when the cells move from resting state to activation, with the latter being strongly modulated to maintain the capacity of the cell tissues to recover. Moving from resting state to hyper-inflammation and further to immune tolerance (immune depression) correlates well with their specific metabolic profile. More importantly than the correlation, it appears clear that cellular metabolism has direct roles in regulating immune function [55, 56] in relation with anabolic and catabolic processes. The chapter then summarizes the intracellular metabolic changes having an integral role in controlling immune responses [10, 26, 55, 57–60].

The microenvironment in healthy conditions contains mediators and nutrients that are changing rapidly during acute host response, with competition for nutrients. For example, bacterial infections can compete with immune cells to use oxygen and glucose. Consequently, the level of glucose available for immune cells could be reduced [61]. In viral infection, the virus can upregulate glucose uptake and global cell metabolism to facilitate the viral replication [62]. The site of inflammation can also become hypoxic because of microvessel thrombi and also because of influx of activated inflammatory cells. To achieve such functional changes, energetic requirements and nature of useful substrates have to be adapted to provide sufficient ATP to meet cellular demands.

Knowledge on macrophage/monocyte metabolism has made significant advances with clear differences in subsets of monocyte subpopulations. The pro-inflammatory M1 macrophages increase their glucose metabolism and lactate production via aerobic glycolysis, whereas more anti-inflammatory M2 macrophages rely more on oxidative phosphorylation (OxPhos) and β-oxidation of free fatty acid [62].

2.4.1   The Aerobic Glycolysis or "Warburg Effect" (◻ Fig. 2.2 [57])

ATP production is essential to provide energy for cellular functions, and proinflammatory human immune cells adopt a distinct metabolic program called "aerobic glycolysis" metabolizing glucose to lactate in the presence of abundant oxygen (◻ Fig. 2.2). This process provides immune cells with components essential for cell proliferation and cytokine synthesis [57]. In restrictive metabolic conditions, such as hypoxia, this cell metabolic reprogramming allows the cell to survive despite an

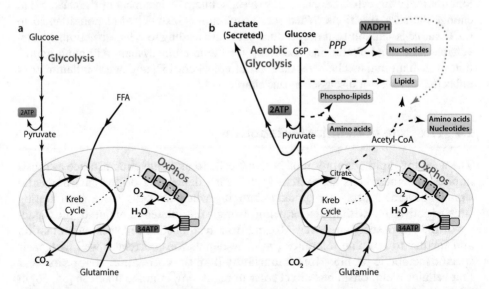

◻ **Fig. 2.2**   from{Loftus, 2016 #284}: Schematic representation of metabolism matching the immune cell function. **a** The ATP level is key for cell homeostasis and surviving. Glucose the major source of energy, is metabolized via 2 integrated pathways, glycolysis and oxidative phosphorylation (OxPhos) to generate ATP. Glycolysis converts glucose to pyruvate, generating 2 molecules of ATP. After pyruvate transport to mitochondria is metabolized in the tri-carboxylic acid (TCA) cycle, which drives OxPhos, generating 34 ATP per molecule of glucose. Alternative substrates are also metabolized, such as lipids and glutamine, reaching the TCA at acetyl-CoA. Faty acid oxidation (FFA) and glutaminolysis produce acetyl-CoA for the TCA. **b** The aerobic glycolysis ("Warburg effect") takes large amount of glucose associated with a high glycolytic flux. Various intermediate pathways are diverting glycolytic molecules such as the pentose phosphate pathways (PPP) to support nucleotide synthesis and NADPH synthesis for NADPH oxidase. A significant proportion of pyruvate is converted in acetyl-CoA for lipid synthesis. Pyruvate is also converted in lactate and secreted from the cell

altered mitochondrial OxPhos [5, 57]. The high rate of glycolysis generates enough ATP to maintain energy homeostasis. After importation into the cell by GLUT1 (not controlled by insulin), glucose is phosphorylated and enters the glycolytic pathways. It is converted into pyruvate after successive enzymatic reactions, from which some are limiting steps as hexokinase or phosphofructokinase. This pathway produces two molecules of ATP. After pyruvate transportation into the mitochondria, pyruvate enters the tricarboxylic acid (TCA) circle (or Krebs cycle) and drives the oxidative phosphorylation (OxPhos) and proton translocation across the inner membrane of mitochondria (◘ Figs. 2.2 and 2.3). This pathway produces 34 ATP molecules per molecule of glucose. Alternative substrates such as lipids and glutamine may feed the TCA and also drive OxPhos. Fatty acid-β-oxidation and glutaminolysis are fueling also the TCA via the intermediate molecule acetyl-CoA to produce ATP. During the acute inflammatory process, the activation of aerobic glycolysis allows to take up larger amount of glucose, which maintains sufficient cellular ATP level for cellular metabolic homeostasis, even in the presence of altered mitochondrial ATP synthesis [57]. Moreover, the elevated glucose flux also fuels glycolytic intermediates that are diverted into other pathways as the pentose phosphate pathways (PPPs). The PPP pathway is essential to support the nucleotide synthesis and to generate NADPH, an essential cofactor for lipid synthesis and for NADPH oxidase function to produce reactive oxygen species (ROS) [5, 57, 63]. The conversion of glucose into cytoplasmic acetyl-CoA can in turn be used to produce cholesterol and FFA. In addition, a consistent part of pyruvate produced by aerobic glycolysis is converted into lactate and secreted. Interestingly, hyperlactatemia is a hallmark biomarker in severe sepsis or septic shock, which is classically interpreted as a result of tissue hypoperfusion with tissue hypoxia. Being also present in the absence of shock in several life-threatening conditions or stress conditions as major surgery [64, 65], it can be suggested that a significant part of elevated serum lactate in severe sepsis originates from activated aerobic glycolysis in immune cells [64].

◘ **Fig. 2.3** The tricaboxylic acid (TCA) cycle

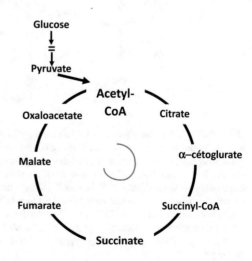

2.4.2 The Hypoxia-Inducible Factor (HIF)

The human monocyte is reprogrammed in the human sepsis, passing from an inflammatory state to an immune-depressive state. This reprogramming is under the dependence of the key transcription factor "hypoxia-inducible factor (HIF)," which is a heterodimer with two protein subunits, HIF-1α and β. HIF-1β is constitutively expressed in cell, and HIF-1α is constitutively transcribed with a rapid degradation. HIF-1α was initially identified as a major regulator of cellular response to hypoxia [66] (◘ Fig. 2.4). Recently, it was also demonstrated that HIF-1α is a crucial regulator of immune cell functions coupling the shift of cellular metabolism to the immune cell-specific transcriptional outputs. The induction of aerobic glycolysis and the HIF-1α stabilization in the macrophages drive the macrophage activation to produce cytokines as IL1-β and to control intracellular infection. Increased glycolytic flux leads to HIF-1α stabilization. Subsequently, HIF-1α stabilization increases the expression of numerous glycolytic genes setting up a positive feedback loop for macrophage activation [67]. To summarize, the emerging principle is that HIF-1α couples metabolic cues with immune responses essential for control of infection. If the testing of pharmacologic agents that activate HIF-1α is missing, this represents an important target for therapies fighting against drug-resistant infections.

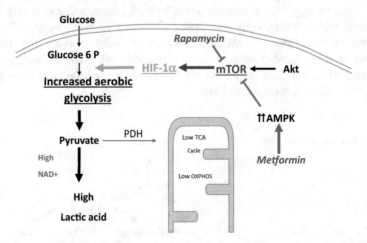

◘ **Fig. 2.4** Under stimulation by b-glucan recognition, the Akt-mTOT-HIF-1α pathway is activated and shifts the glucose metabolism from oxidative phosphorylation (OXPHOS) to aerobic glycolysis ("Warburg effect"). This metabolic switch was reported earlier as a feature of cell activation and proliferation. It was demonstrated a play a role both in trained monocytes but also in effector T cell and NK cells. (adapted from Cheng et al Science2014) mTOR and aerobic glycolysis are activated in trained monocytes, which was blocked by rapamycin and AMPK activator. The mTOR induction of glycolysis is mediated the activation of HIF-1α and activation of expression of glycolytic enzymes. *AMPK* adenosine monophosphate-activated protein kinase, *HIF-1α* hypoxia inducible factor–1α, *Akt* family of protein kinase, *PDH* pyruvate dehydrogenase, *mTOR* mammalian target of rapamycin, *OXPHOS* oxidative phosphorylation

2.4.3 The Regulation of the Immune Response by mTOR [68]

Discovered during experimental research for antibiotic molecules, it has been found that rapamycin, a macrolide antibiotic, was capable of inhibiting fungal growth with immunosuppressive and antitumor properties. Target of rapamycin ("mammalian target of rapamycin (MOR)") is recognized as the central regulator of immune responses, in particular the signaling cascade that integrates microenvironmental information. The activation of kinase mTOR regulates cellular metabolism and makes the link between metabolic demand and cellular innate and adaptive responses. The activation of mTOR via HIF-α increases the expression of the proteins involved in glycolysis and glucose capture. mTOR exists in two structurally distinct complexes (mTORC1 and mTORC2) that mediate separate and overlapping cellular function (◘ Fig. 2.4). Rapamycin inhibits mTORC1 activity and amplifies mTORC2 activity. mTORC1 controls directly the anabolic pathways and consequently the cellular growth and proliferation, while mTORC2 regulates downstream signal transduction and cytoskeleton. The administration of rapamycin in various inflammatory contexts showed that mTORC1 can either promote or inhibit inflammation. This suggests that the role mTOR plays in innate immune cells is complex and dependent on the cellular context. Inhibition of mTORC1 with rapamycin promotes pro-inflammatory cytokine production while inhibiting IL-10 production, whereas mTORC1 activation in monocytes results in enhanced production of IL-10 and diminished production of pro-inflammatory cytokines in response to LPS. mTOR plays a dominant role in the regulation of metabolism as observed in inflammatory phenotype induced by TLR agonists with aerobic. This pathway can be associated with an enhanced FAO when the alternative activation induced by IL-4 is present.

When these metabolic pathways are blocked, activation of T-lymphocytes is inhibited, as observed when metformin is used. The inhibition of mTOR leads to the increase in controller T4 lymphocyte and decrease in immunosuppressive cell T_{reg}. Similar data has been observed for T8 lymphocytes. The later effect was nicely demonstrated to be linked with the promotion of catabolic process of FAO and autophagy when rapamycin is used. The cellular Treg is also dependent on FAO [69] suggesting that the rapamycin promotes these cells by an induced metabolic bias. Depending on the microenvironment of cells, particularly the cytokines generated by the antigen-presenting cells, CD4 T cells become activated and differentiate in distinct T helper (Th1, Th2, Th17, Treg). Rapamycin was shown to inhibit Th1, Th2, and Th17 and to promote Treg cell differentiation. All of this confirms the role of mTOR in promoting glycolysis and repressing FAO, crucial metabolic pathways for the development of Teff and Treg. Ultimately, the roles of mTOR in B cells are less known.

2.4.4 The Combination of Mediated mTOR and HIF-1α Aerobic Glycolysis: A Basis for Trained Immunity [3, 5] (◘ Fig. 2.4)

Trained immunity (TI) is an innate immune memory program induced in monocytes or macrophages by exposure to pathogens, microbial component, or vaccines as a mechanism to prevent repeated infections [70, 71]. Trained immunity is characterized by immunometabolic changes and histone posttranslational modifications, leading to stronger gene transcription upon stimulation, in particular enhancing the production of pro-inflammatory cytokines. The interaction between aerobic glycolysis, mTOR, and HF-1α had been well reported in 2014 by Cheng et al. [5] Among the cytokines involved, the LI-1 family cytokines were shown to induce monocyte-trained immunity in vitro. These reported factors modulating glycolysis highlight the crucial regulatory role of cellular metabolism in host defense, which is a credible therapeutic target. The incidental observation of the role of metformin (AMPK inhibitor) [72] and then mTOR inhibitor was demonstrated in vitro to suppress the trained immunity. Since accurate control of TI is essential in inflammation, interest has been growing for IL-37 [73]. IL-37 is the unique IL-1 member family that inhibits innate inflammation by suppressing cytokine production and modulates metabolic pathways. It abrogates the protective effect of TI in vivo and suppresses cytokine production in response to infection. According to the inflammatory status, use of IL-37 system is a potential therapeutic target in immune pathologies.

2.4.5 The Liaison Between Metabolic Shift Modifications and Functions of Immune Cells

In their landmark paper, Cheng et al. [74] have identified the cellular metabolic processes being the potential target for therapies in sepsis. The study demonstrated the metabolic defects in PBMC from septic patients. PBMCs from immunodepressed septic patients were unable to produce lactate after ex vivo stimulation with LPS. Such alteration was shown to be associated with an altered maximal oxygen consumption of PBMC compared to control subjects [26, 74] corrected in patients who recovered from sepsis. To restore these metabolic abnormalities, IFN-γ was tested after positive results were obtained in clinic [19, 20], a molecule known to upregulate cytokine production in innate tolerance [30]. By autocrine action, IFN-γ production is involved in the mTOR-HIF-1α-dependent metabolic switch. Other mechanisms of actions of IFN-γ have been reported: involvement in epigenetic inducing histone acetylation at promoter and enhancer sites of genes encoding pro-inflammatory cytokines [75] with a metabolic restoration to produce succinate, an important positive regulator of IL-1β.

Summary

Host response to infection includes coagulation, immunity, and cell metabolic factors, which all can participate in the possible overwhelming of individuals. If the immune cells' microenvironment containing mediators drives the cell response, this requires energy to produce adequate ATP and to fuel intermediate metabolic pathways. The metabolic shift in glucose metabolism to "aerobic glycolysis" provides sufficient ATP production and stimulates the pentose phosphate pathways and production of pyruvate. All are essential to tune the functional capabilities of immune cells as monocytes/macrophages and lymphocytes. Such metabolic shift depends on genetic predisposition, functional transcription, and translation for activation of key enzymes. These metabolic modifications have been linked to trained immunity, evolution towards immunodepression phenotype, and cell death. The recent knowledge motivates the development of therapies targeting cell metabolism to control the "dysregulated host response."

Take-Home Message

- Host response has a kinetic moving from hyper-inflammation to immunodepression.
- The shift in immune cell phenotype is related to metabolic reprogramming of the cells, mainly shifting towards "aerobic glycolysis."
- Such a shift is controlled by the HF1-α and mTOR that increase glucose consumption and activate intermediate pathways.
- The metabolic changes are responsible for immune cell function changes.

Conclusion and Road Map for the Future

In the recent years, after failure of randomized trials testing anti-inflammatory drugs or methods, important progresses, new approaches, and understanding have changed the pathophysiological picture of the host response related to severe infection. Among the main novelties, the evidence of time-related phases in sepsis highlights the rapid shift in immune cell phenotypes for both innate and adaptive immunity. The rapid shift from hyper-inflammation to immunodepression phenotype implies first the innate immune cells, mainly the monocyte/macrophage with an altered antigen presentation to lymphocyte. The association of exhausted and/or apoptotic lymphocytes amplifies the immunodepression syndrome, which seems an adapted modification to preserve the tissue fitness. The persistence of this immunodepression exposes the occurrence of secondary infections and delays tissue recovery. The second major input came from the evidence of the role of cell metabolic shift, especially the shift to aerobic glycolysis or "Warburg effect." This metabolic shift leads to increase in glucose flux with increase in the activity of intermediate pathways as pentose phosphate pathway, essential for nucleotide synthesis and NADPH synthesis, the substrate of NADPH oxidase. The underlying mechanisms for such metabolic shift show the key role of both HIF-1α and mTOR. The metabolic shift is now well documented as a major mechanism to change the immune cell function. These new aspects may rapidly lead to develop therapies interfering with these metabolic changes to modulate the host response related to sepsis.

References

1. Bunik V. Experts' opinion in translational medicine. Fr Med. 2021; Research Topic.
2. Abrams DI, Velasco G, Twelves C, Ganju RK, Bar-Sela G. Cancer treatment: preclinical & clinical. J Natl Cancer Inst Monogr. 2021;2021(58):107–13.
3. Knoll R, Schultze JL, Schulte-Schrepping J. Monocytes and macrophages in COVID-19. Front Immunol. 2021;12:720109.
4. Chen ATC, Coura-Filho GB, Rehder MHH. Clinical characteristics of Covid-19 in China. N Engl J Med. 2020;382:1708–20.
5. Cheng SC, Quintin J, Cramer RA, et al. mTOR- and HIF-1alpha-mediated aerobic glycolysis as metabolic basis for trained immunity. Science. 2014;345(6204):1250684.
6. Chousterman BG, Swirski FK, Weber GF. Cytokine storm and sepsis disease pathogenesis. Semin Immunopathol. 2017;39(5):517–28.
7. Lukaszewicz AC, Grienay M, Resche-Rigon M, et al. Monocytic HLA-DR expression in intensive care patients: interest for prognosis and secondary infection prediction. Crit Care Med. 2009;37(10):2746–52.

2

8. Monneret G, Venet F, Meisel C, Schefold JC. Assessment of monocytic HLA-DR expression in ICU patients: analytical issues for multicentric flow cytometry studies. Crit Care. 2010;14(4):432.
9. Liu Z, Mahale P, Engels EA. Sepsis and risk of cancer among elderly adults in the United States. Clin Infect Dis. 2019;68(5):717–24.
10. Arts RJ, Gresnigt MS, Joosten LA, Netea MG. Cellular metabolism of myeloid cells in sepsis. J Leukoc Biol. 2017;101(1):151–64.
11. Hotchkiss RS, Monneret G, Payen D. Immunosuppression in sepsis: a novel understanding of the disorder and a new therapeutic approach. Lancet Infect Dis. 2013;13(3):260–8.
12. Rosier F, Brisebarre A, Dupuis C, et al. Genetic predisposition to the mortality in septic shock patients: from GWAS to the identification of a regulatory variant modulating the activity of a CISH enhancer. Int J Mol Sci. 2021;22(11):5852.
13. Matzinger P. The danger model: a renewed sense of self. Science. 2002;296(5566):301–5.
14. van der Poll T, van de Veerdonk FL, Scicluna BP, Netea MG. The immunopathology of sepsis and potential therapeutic targets. Nat Rev Immunol. 2017;17(7):407–20.
15. Levi M, van der Poll T. Coagulation and sepsis. Thromb Res. 2017;149:38–44.
16. Yipp BG, Kubes P. NETosis: how vital is it? Blood. 2013;122(16):2784–94.
17. Boomer JS, To K, Chang KC, et al. Immunosuppression in patients who die of sepsis and multiple organ failure. JAMA. 2011;306(23):2594–605.
18. Nalos M, Santner-Nanan B, Parnell G, Tang B, McLean AS, Nanan R. Immune effects of interferon gamma in persistent staphylococcal sepsis. Am J Respir Crit Care Med. 2012;185(1):110–2.
19. Delsing CE, Gresnigt MS, Leentjens J, et al. Interferon-gamma as adjunctive immunotherapy for invasive fungal infections: a case series. BMC Infect Dis. 2014;14:166.
20. Payen D, Faivre V, Miatello J, et al. Multicentric experience with interferon gamma therapy in sepsis induced immunosuppression. A case series. BMC Infect Dis. 2019;19(1):931.
21. Shalova IN, Lim JY, Chittezhath M, et al. Human monocytes undergo functional re-programming during sepsis mediated by hypoxia-inducible factor-1alpha. Immunity. 2015;42(3):484–98.
22. Herwanto V, Tang B, Wang Y, et al. Blood transcriptome analysis of patients with uncomplicated bacterial infection and sepsis. BMC Res Notes. 2021;14(1):76.
23. Venet F, Demaret J, Gossez M, Monneret G. Myeloid cells in sepsis-acquired immunodeficiency. Ann N Y Acad Sci. 2021;1499(1):3–17.
24. Tawfik VL, Huck NA, Baca QJ, et al. Systematic immunophenotyping reveals sex-specific responses after painful injury in mice. Front Immunol. 2020;11:1652.
25. Payen D, Lukaszewicz AC, Belikova I, et al. Gene profiling in human blood leucocytes during recovery from septic shock. Intensive Care Med. 2008;34(8):1371–6.
26. Belikova I, Lukaszewicz AC, Faivre V, Damoisel C, Singer M, Payen D. Oxygen consumption of human peripheral blood mononuclear cells in severe human sepsis. Crit Care Med. 2007;35(12):2702–8.
27. Khor CC, Hibberd ML. Shared pathways to infectious disease susceptibility? Genome Med. 2010;2(8):52.
28. Fairfax BP, Knight JC. Genetics of gene expression in immunity to infection. Curr Opin Immunol. 2014;30:63–71.
29. Biswas SK, Lopez-Collazo E. Endotoxin tolerance: new mechanisms, molecules and clinical significance. Trends Immunol. 2009;30(10):475–87.
30. Docke WD, Randow F, Syrbe U, et al. Monocyte deactivation in septic patients: restoration by IFN-gamma treatment. Nat Med. 1997;3(6):678–81.
31. Wong HR, Wheeler DS, Tegtmeyer K, et al. Toward a clinically feasible gene expression-based subclassification strategy for septic shock: proof of concept. Crit Care Med. 2010;38(10):1955–61.
32. Roquilly A, Jacqueline C, Davieau M, et al. Alveolar macrophages are epigenetically altered after inflammation, leading to long-term lung immunoparalysis. Nat Immunol. 2020;21(6):636–48.
33. Payen D, Cravat M, Maadadi H, et al. A longitudinal study of immune cells in severe COVID-19 patients. Front Immunol. 2020;11:580250.
34. Rimmele T, Payen D, Cantaluppi V, et al. Immune cell phenotype and function in sepsis. Shock. 2016;45(3):282–91.
35. Venet F, Filipe-Santos O, Lepape A, et al. Decreased T-cell repertoire diversity in sepsis: a preliminary study. Crit Care Med. 2013;41(1):111–9.
36. Monneret G, Venet F. A rapidly progressing lymphocyte exhaustion after severe sepsis. Crit Care. 2012;16(4):140.

37. Hotchkiss RS, Monneret G, Payen D. Sepsis-induced immunosuppression: from cellular dysfunctions to immunotherapy. Nat Rev Immunol. 2013;13(12):862–74.

38. Zheng HY, Zhang M, Yang CX, et al. Elevated exhaustion levels and reduced functional diversity of T cells in peripheral blood may predict severe progression in COVID-19 patients. Cell Mol Immunol. 2020;17:541–3.

39. Venet F, Foray AP, Villars-Mechin A, et al. IL-7 restores lymphocyte functions in septic patients. J Immunol. 2012;189(10):5073–81.

40. Patera AC, Drewry AM, Chang K, Beiter ER, Osborne D, Hotchkiss RS. Frontline science: defects in immune function in patients with sepsis are associated with PD-1 or PD-L1 expression and can be restored by antibodies targeting PD-1 or PD-L1. J Leukoc Biol. 2016;100(6):1239–54.

41. Shindo Y, McDonough JS, Chang KC, Ramachandra M, Sasikumar PG, Hotchkiss RS. Anti-PD-L1 peptide improves survival in sepsis. J Surg Res. 2017;208:33–9.

42. Hotchkiss R, Olston E, Yende S, et al. Immune checkpoint inhibition in sepsis: a phase 1b randomized, placebo-controlled, single ascending dose study of antiprogrammed cell death-ligand 1 antibody (BMS-936559). Crit Care Med. 2019;47(5):632–42.

43. Venet F, Pachot A, Debard AL, et al. Human CD4+CD25+ regulatory T lymphocytes inhibit lipopolysaccharide-induced monocyte survival through a Fas/Fas ligand-dependent mechanism. J Immunol. 2006;177(9):6540–7.

44. Scumpia PO, Delano MJ, Kelly-Scumpia KM, et al. Treatment with GITR agonistic antibody corrects adaptive immune dysfunction in sepsis. Blood. 2007;110(10):3673–81.

45. Ferrara JL. Cytokine dysregulation as a mechanism of graft versus host disease. Curr Opin Immunol. 1993;5(5):794–9.

46. Bosmann M, Ward PA. The inflammatory response in sepsis. Trends Immunol. 2013;34(3):129–36.

47. Coomes EA, Haghbayan H. Interleukin-6 in Covid-19: a systematic review and meta-analysis. Rev Med Virol. 2020;30(6):1–9.

48. Maraolo AE, Crispo A, Piezzo M, et al. The use of tocilizumab in patients with COVID-19: a systematic review, meta-analysis and trial sequential analysis of randomized controlled studies. J Clin Med. 2021;10(21):4935.

49. RECOVERY Collaborative Group. Tocilizumab in patients admitted to hospital with COVID-19 (RECOVERY): a randomised, controlled, open-label, platform trial. Lancet. 2021;397(10285):1637–45.

50. Gupta S, Leaf DE. Tocilizumab in COVID-19: some clarity amid controversy. Lancet. 2021;397(10285):1599–601.

51. Opal SM, DePalo VA. Anti-inflammatory cytokines. Chest. 2000;117(4):1162–72.

52. Fanucchi S, Dominguez-Andres J, Joosten LAB, Netea MG, Mhlanga MM. The intersection of epigenetics and metabolism in trained immunity. Immunity. 2021;54(1):32–43.

53. Pavlov VA, Tracey KJ. The vagus nerve and the inflammatory reflex—linking immunity and metabolism. Nat Rev Endocrinol 2012;8(12):743–754.

54. Tracey KJ. The inflammatory reflex. Nature. 2002;420(6917):853–9.

55. O'Neill LA, Kishton RJ, Rathmell J. A guide to immunometabolism for immunologists. Nat Rev Immunol. 2016;16(9):553–65.

56. O'Neill LA, Pearce EJ. Immunometabolism governs dendritic cell and macrophage function. J Exp Med. 2016;213(1):15–23.

57. Loftus RM, Finlay DK. Immunometabolism: cellular metabolism turns immune regulator. J Biol Chem. 2016;291(1):1–10.

58. Mickiewicz B, Vogel HJ, Wong HR, Winston BW. Metabolomics as a novel approach for early diagnosis of pediatric septic shock and its mortality. Am J Respir Crit Care Med. 2013;187(9):967–76.

59. Dominguez-Andres J, Netea MG. Long-term reprogramming of the innate immune system. J Leukoc Biol. 2019;105(2):329–38.

60. Nalos M, Parnell G, Robergs R, Booth D, McLean AS, Tang BM. Transcriptional reprogramming of metabolic pathways in critically ill patients. Intensive Care Med Exp. 2016;4(1):21.

61. Vitko NP, Spahich NA, Richardson AR. Glycolytic dependency of high-level nitric oxide resistance and virulence in Staphylococcus aureus. mBio. 2015;6(2):e00045–15.

62. Ripoli M, D'Aprile A, Quarato G, et al. Hepatitis C virus-linked mitochondrial dysfunction promotes hypoxia-inducible factor 1 alpha-mediated glycolytic adaptation. J Virol. 2010;84(1):647–60.

63. Saha S, Shalova IN, Biswas SK. Metabolic regulation of macrophage phenotype and function. Immunol Rev. 2017;280(1):102–11.

64. Nolt B, Tu F, Wang X, et al. Lactate and immunosuppression in sepsis. Shock. 2018;49(2):120–5.

65. Delano MJ, Ward PA. The immune system's role in sepsis progression, resolution, and long-term outcome. Immunol Rev. 2016;274(1):330–53.

66. Knight M, Stanley S. HIF-1alpha as a central mediator of cellular resistance to intracellular pathogens. Curr Opin Immunol. 2019;60:111–6.

67. Braverman J, Sogi KM, Benjamin D, Nomura DK, Stanley SA. HIF-1alpha is an essential mediator of IFN-gamma-dependent immunity to Mycobacterium tuberculosis. J Immunol. 2016;197(4):1287–97.

68. Jones RG, Pearce EJ. MenTORing immunity: mTOR Signaling in the development and function of tissue-resident immune cells. Immunity. 2017;46(5):730–42.

69. Michalek RD, Gerriets VA, Jacobs SR, et al. Cutting edge: distinct glycolytic and lipid oxidative metabolic programs are essential for effector and regulatory CD4+ T cell subsets. J Immunol. 2011;186(6):3299–303.

70. Netea MG, Giamarellos-Bourboulis EJ, Dominguez-Andres J, et al. Trained immunity: a tool for reducing susceptibility to and the severity of SARS-CoV-2 infection. Cell. 2020;181(5):969–77.

71. Netea MG, Joosten LAB, van der Meer JWM. Hypothesis: stimulation of trained immunity as adjunctive immunotherapy in cancer. J Leukoc Biol. 2017;102(6):1323–32.

72. Gwinn DM, Shackelford DB, Egan DF, et al. AMPK phosphorylation of raptor mediates a metabolic checkpoint. Mol Cell. 2008;30(2):214–26.

73. Cavalli G, Tengesdal IW, Gresnigt M, et al. The anti-inflammatory cytokine interleukin-37 is an inhibitor of trained immunity. Cell Rep. 2021;35(1):108955.

74. Cheng SC, Scicluna BP, Arts RJ, et al. Broad defects in the energy metabolism of leukocytes underlie immunoparalysis in sepsis. Nat Immunol. 2016;17(4):406–13.

75. Qiao Y, Giannopoulou EG, Chan CH, et al. Synergistic activation of inflammatory cytokine genes by interferon-gamma-induced chromatin remodeling and toll-like receptor signaling. Immunity. 2013;39(3):454–69.

What Is Cytokine Storm?

Dominik Jarczak and Axel Nierhaus

Contents

3

⊜ **Learning Objectives**

The human immune system plays a crucial role in the defense against invasive pathogens and is essential for survival. A protective inflammatory response is based on a tightly controlled balance between pro- and anti-inflammation, including cytokines, interleukins, interferons, coagulation factors, complement, cellular interactions, and much more. Disturbances of this balance, in which the excessive and uncontrolled release of various mediators occurs, are referred to as "cytokine storm" and can lead to serious clinical conditions and deleterious course.

The underlying causes of such hyperinflammation are manifold: for example, congenital defects may cause inadequate pathogen recognition or impaired termination of the immune response and thus trigger a cytokine storm. Certain pathogens or particularly high loads of nonspecific pathogens can also trigger a hyperinflammatory response. Certain immunotherapies used in the treatment of some oncological diseases are also associated with an increased risk of hypercytokinemia.

This overview summarizes the basic functioning of the innate and acquired immune system and the possible disturbances leading to an immunological disbalance with formation of a cytokine storm.

3.1 Introduction

Various pathogens, autoimmune and malignant diseases, but also genetic disorders and certain therapeutic interventions can lead to life-threatening systemic inflammatory syndromes in the human body. Their common feature is a massive release of cytokines due to excessive activation of immune cells. This dysregulated inflammatory response leads to self-reinforcing feedback and may ultimately be life-threatening to the host.

These conditions are widely referred to as cytokine release syndrome (CRS) or, in particularly severe courses, cytokine storm (CS). The term CS was first used by James L. Ferrara in 1993 to describe acute graft-versus-host disease (GvHD) in the setting of engraftment syndrome following allogeneic stem cell transplantation [1]. The term CRS originated with L. Chatenoud, who used it in 1991 to describe a muromonab-induced anti-CD3 syndrome in the setting of immunosuppressive therapy in solid-organ transplantation [2].

CS occurs frequently in the context of certain diseases, syndromes, and therapies, for example, anaphylaxis, graft-versus-host disease, acute respiratory distress syndrome (ARDS), and systemic inflammatory response syndrome (SIRS), as well as chimeric antigen receptor-T (CAR-T) cell therapy and sepsis—the latter accounting for up to 19.7% of all deaths worldwide [3].

To date, there is no valid definition for the term CS. It is usually understood to mean an overwhelming immune response characterized by the release of cytokines, interleukins, interferons, chemokines, and other mediators (see ◘ Table 3.1). These mediators are part of an evolutionarily well-conserved innate immune response that is required for efficient elimination of infectious agents and the repair processes that immediately follow.

CS means that the dynamics and quantity of systemically released cytokines cause serious damage in the host organism. However, distinguishing between an

▣ Table 3.1 Common biomarkers affected during cytokine storm

Mediator (Abbreviation)	Main source	Major function
Cytokines		
IL-1	Macrophages, pyroptotic cells, epithelial cells	Pro-inflammatory; pyrogenic function; activation of macrophage and T_H17 cells
IL-2	T cells	Immune response; T_{eff} and T_{reg} cell growth factor; T cell differentiation
IL-4	T_H2 cells, basophils, eosinophils, mast cells, NK cells	T_H2 differentiation; adhesion; chemotaxis
IL-6	T cells, macrophages, endothelial cells	Pro-inflammatory; pleiotropic; pyrogenic function; acute phase response; lymphoid differentiation; increased antibody production,
IL-9	T_H9 cells	Pleiotropic; stimulation of B, T and NK cells; protection from helminth infections; activation of mast cells; association with type I interferon in Covid-19
IL-10	Regulatory T cells, T_H9 cells	Anti-inflammatory; inhibition of macrophage activation; inhibition of T_H1 cells and cytokine release
IL-12	Dendritic cells, macrophages	Stimulation of T and NK cells; activation of T_H1 pathway; induction of interferon-γ from T_H1 cells; cytotoxic T cells and NK cells; acting in synergy with Interleukin-18
IL-13	T_H2 cells	Differentiation of B cells; mediator of humoral immunity
IL-17	T_H17 cells, NK cells, group 3 innate lymphoid cells	Protection from bacterial and fungal infections; promotion of neutrophilic inflammation
IL-18	Monocytes, macrophages, dendritic cells	Pro-inflammatory; activation of T_H1 pathway; synergistic with Interleukin-12
IL-31	T_H2 cells, macrophages, mast cells, dendritic cells	Pro-inflammatory; cell-mediated immunity
IL-33	Macrophages, dendritic cells, mast cells, epithelial cells	Pro-inflammatory; amplification of T_H1 and T_H2 cells; activation of cytotoxic T cells, NK cells and mast cells
Interferon γ	T_H1 cells, cytotoxic T cells, group 1 innate lymphoid cells, NK cells	Pro-inflammatory; activation of monocytes and macrophages

(continued)

3

■ **Table 3.1** (continued)

Mediator (Abbreviation)		Main source	Major function
TGF-β		T_{reg} cells, monocytes, macrophages, fibroblasts, epithelial cells, cancer cells	Immunosuppressive; regulation of proliferation, differentiation, apoptosis and adhesion; inhibition of haematopoiesis
Tumor necrosis factor		T cells, NK cells, mast cells, macrophages	Pyrogenic; increasing vascular permeability
Chemokines			
MCP-1	CCL2	Macrophages, dendritic cells, cardiac myocytes	Pyrogenic; recruitment of T_H1 cells, NK cells, macrophages, eosinophils, dendritic cells
MIP-1α	CCL3	Monocytes, neutrophils, dendritic cells, NK cells, mast cells	Recruitment of T_H1 cells, NK cells, macrophages, dendritic cells
MIP-1β	CCL4	Macrophages, neutrophils, endothelium	Recruitment of B cells, $CD4^+$ T cells, dendritic cells
IL-8	CXCL8	Macrophages, epithelial cells	Recruitment of neutrophils
MIG	CXCL9	Monocytes, endothelial cells, keratinocates	Interferon-inducible chemokine; recruitment of T_H1 cells, NK cells, plasmacytoid dendritic cells
IP-10	CXCL10	Monocytes, endothelial cells, keratinocytes	Interferon-inducible chemokine; recruitment of T_H1 cells, NK cells, macrophages
BLC	CXCL13	B cells, follicular dendritic cells	Recruitment of T_H1 cells, monocytes, dendritic cells, basophils
Plasma proteins			
CRP		Hepatocytes	Interleukin-6 increases CRP expression, Interleukin-8 and MCP-1 secretion
Complement		Hepatocytes, other cells	in cytokine storm, activation of Complement contributes to tissue damage, inhibition may reduce immunopathologic effects

BLC B lymphocyte chemoattractant, *CCL* chemokine ligand, *CRP* C-reactive protein, *CXCL* C-X-C motif chemokine ligand, *IL* interleukin, *IP-10* IFN-gamma-inducible protein 10, *MCP-1* monocyte chemoattractant protein-1, *MIG monokine* induced by IFN-gamma, *MIP-1* macrophage inflammatory protein 1, *NK cell* natural killer cell T_{eff} cell, effector T cell, T_H *cell* T helper cell, T_{reg} *cell* regulatory T cell

appropriate and a pathologically dysregulated inflammatory response in critical illness is difficult or impossible. Since most of the mediators involved in the CS exhibit pleiotropic downstream effects and, in addition, are often interdependent in their biological activity, an extremely complex dynamic arises. The interaction of the mediators and the signaling pathways triggered by them are neither linear nor uniform. Moreover, their quantitative values may indicate the severity of the reactions, but not necessarily the pathogenesis. This complex interplay highlights the limitations of intervening in the acute inflammatory response based on single mediators and at undifferentiated time points.

Dysregulated hypercytokinemia with resulting systemic inflammatory response can progress from various physical symptoms to multiorgan failure if identified too late and treated inadequately. Clinically, most patients develop febrile temperatures at the onset of CS, which may progress to high fever in severe courses. Other common symptoms in the early phase may include headache, diarrhea, fatigue, rash, arthralgias, and myalgias; neuropsychiatric changes ("septic encephalopathy") are also common.

Depending on the underlying causes and therapeutic measures, CS differs from each other both in onset and duration. However, the longer the clinical course lasts, the more similar the courses become, so that with advanced progression, there is almost a uniform clinical picture—regardless of the original triggers.

From a clinical point of view, the earliest possible detection of excessive cytokine release is extremely important, as it is associated with therapeutic decisions and ultimately with prognosis and outcome.

Identifying the underlying disorder of a CS is complex and not possible by exclusion diagnostics alone, as the potential triggers can be multiple and the clinical picture highly variable. For example, patients may have hypercytokinemia due to a noninfectious cause, such as in CAR-T cell therapy, but may also have sepsis or septic shock. It is difficult to distinguish between these states based on individual clinical and laboratory parameters, especially since they can also occur together. However, early and correct diagnosis is essential, since immunosuppressive therapy, as is commonly performed for CS during CAR-T cell therapy, may harm patients with sepsis, whereas antibiotic therapy will not improve the clinical picture in CAR-T cell-induced CS.

In general, infection as the cause of a CS must be excluded early and reliably, and the function of important organ systems must be assessed based on laboratory chemistry parameters. In addition to acute-phase proteins and inflammatory parameters (e.g., IL-6, CRP, PCT, ferritin), this also includes standardized values of liver and kidney function as well as blood count and arterial blood gas analysis. These readily available parameters allow an early decision on therapy and an initial assessment of the course of the disease. If an infectious cause can be ruled out, CS can be identified based on repeatedly and profoundly elevated cytokine levels. That said, it is difficult to clearly distinguish a high-grade inflammatory response from a dysregulated host response in severe infection. Profiles of different cytokines (e.g., IL-6/IL-10 ratio) can be helpful to identify a trend for the further course based on baseline values [4]. However, they are mostly not available in a timely manner and of limited use to make prompt treatment decisions.

3.2 Pathophysiology of CS

Inflammation is the mechanism that multicellular organisms have evolved to defeat invasive pathogens and initiate healing of injured tissue. A balanced, "protective" inflammatory response consists of diverse mechanisms and involves activation of both pro- and anti-inflammatory pathways within the innate and the acquired immune system. The immune system can recognize and counteract previously unknown pathogens by initiating different defensive pathways. After successful defense and initiation of healing, the immune system would return to a state of homeostasis and assume a wait-and-see role. All of this is achieved by complex mechanisms that are controlled and balanced by multiple activating and inhibitory feedback loops. Thus, in an appropriate inflammatory response, there is a balance between adequate cytokine production to clear invaders, on the one hand, and avoidance of a hyperinflammatory response, in which an excess of mediators causes clinically significant collateral damage, on the other.

Cytokines play a pivotal role in these control mechanisms by regulating the immune response, which they can thus amplify but also dissolve. By default, their comparatively short biological half-lives prevent remote effects outside the inflammatory foci. In the case of disseminated infections, increased levels of circulating cytokines may also occur, although this is generally considered pathological. However, it is precisely this systemic effect that can lead to collateral damage to various vital organ systems. Numerous pro- and anti-inflammatory factors are involved in the context of a dysregulated inflammatory response as occurs in CS. In addition to cytokines and factors of the complement and coagulation systems, cellular responses—mediated by, e.g., monocytes, macrophages, neutrophils, NK cells, and endothelial cells—also play a role.

A dysregulated inflammatory response can have several causes: excessively high pathogen load in the context of sepsis, inadequate sensing or triggering of the immune system without the presence of a pathogen at all (as occurs with Castleman's disease), or inappropriate inflammasome activation due to genetic disease. Further examples are the inability of the immune system to terminate an initially adequate immune response and return to baseline (e.g., primary hemophagocytic lymphohistiocytosis, HLH) or conditions with uncontrolled infection and persistent immune activation (e.g., macrophage activation syndrome (MAS)-HLH in, e.g., CMV, EBV, or influenza). Common to these syndromes are absence or failure of negative feedback control, which usually would prevent hyperactivation of the inflammatory response. The excessive release of pro-inflammatory factors ultimately leads to systemic damage and even multiorgan failure.

3.3 Inflammation Due to Sepsis

Adaptive and innate immunity relies on a multitude of different soluble, intracellular, and membrane-bound receptors. Pattern recognition receptors (PRRs) recognize pathogen-associated molecular markers (PAMPs, e.g., endo- and exotoxins, DNA, lipids) of foreign invaders, but also endogenous host-derived danger signals (damage-associated molecular patterns, DAMPs).

The interaction of Toll-like receptors (TLRs), a subclass of PRRs located on the membrane surfaces of antigen-presenting cells (APCs) and monocytes, with PAMPs or DAMPs results in the initiation of signaling cascades and the expression of genes involved in inflammation, adaptive immunity, and cellular metabolism like the key transcription factors activator protein-1 (AP-1) and nuclear factor kappa-light-chain-enhancer (NF-κB). This leads to the expression of so-called early activation genes, which include various pro-inflammatory cytokines such as IL-1, IL-12, IL-18, tumor necrosis factor alpha (TNF-α), and interferons (IFNs). This in turn leads to the release of other cytokines (e.g., IFN-γ, IL-6, IL-8) and components of the complement and coagulation systems.

This systemic increase of pro- and anti-inflammatory cytokines in the early phase is considered the classic hallmark of sepsis. The pro-inflammatory components cause inflammation which, if systemic, can lead to progressive tissue damage and to organ dysfunction. Concomitant immune suppression caused by downregulation of activating cell surface molecules, increased apoptosis of immune cells, and depletion of T cells leads to "immune paralysis" in later stages of the disease course, making the organism susceptible to nosocomial infections, opportunistic pathogens, and viral reactivation [5, 6].

Neutrophils are part of the first line of defense against microbes and, as a component of the innate immune system, may contribute to hyperinflammation in sepsis through the release of proteases and reactive oxygen species. Severe bacterial infections cause the release of both mature and immature forms of neutrophils after emergency granulocyte formation from the bone marrow. When activated by PAMPs or DAMPs, they show phagocytosis activity as well as oxidative burst capacity, and additionally they can release neutrophil extracellular traps (NETs).

NETs are diffuse extracellular structures consisting of a network of chromatin fibers, antimicrobial peptides, and proteases such as myeloperoxidase, cathepsin G, and elastase. NETs contribute to antibacterial defenses because of the potential to trap and eliminate a wide range of pathogens, including Gram-positive and Gram-negative bacteria, viruses, yeasts, as well as protozoa and parasites that cannot be phagocytosed [7, 8]. In animal studies, restriction of NET formation led to increased bacteremia and thus to lower survival rate of test animals with sepsis [9]. However, excessive NETosis in sepsis can also be harmful. Large amounts of NETs in tissues or vessels due to excessive release or inadequate removal are associated with hypercoagulation and endothelial damage. NETs are rich in histones, and binding of NETs to endo- or epithelia can lead to cell damage, both directly by NETs and histone mediated. This can lead to the formation of intravascular thrombi and even multiple-organ damage. Release of NETs has also been reported by cytokines, platelet agonists, and antibodies; high concentrations of immature granulocytes in sepsis are also associated with clinical deterioration because of increased spontaneous production and release of NETs [10, 11].

A further essential component of innate immunity is the complement system. In the early phase of hyperinflammation, increased levels of activated complement factors such as the pro-inflammatory anaphylatoxins C3a, C4a, and C5a can be detected [12]. Increased C5a is associated with a worse clinical course due to increased systemic inflammation and apoptosis. C5a plays a role in neutrophil chemotaxis—by binding to the C5a receptor (C5aR), neutrophils gain the ability to migrate and enter inflamed tissue. There, activation occurs through PAMPs and DAMPs with the

3

release of granular enzymes, reactive oxygen species, as well as NETs. Inhibition of fibrinolysis accompanied by increased prothrombotic activity can induce disseminated microvascular thrombosis, leading to overt disseminated intravascular coagulation (DIC) due to consumption of clotting factors. Animal studies have shown higher survival of animals in which C5a or C5aR had been inhibited. In human patients with sepsis, on the other hand, a decreased C5aR level is indicative of a poor outcome if C5a is simultaneously increased.

During evolution, complement system and coagulation systems have developed from a single pathway. The release of the strongly pro-inflammatory anaphylatoxins C3a and C5a in the context of complement activation also causes the recruitment and activation of platelets, endothelial cells, and leukocytes. The activation of the human contact system or intrinsic coagulation in the form of coagulopathy is nowadays also understood as part of the innate immune response [13]. This system is directed against not only exogenous material, but also misfolded proteins and foreign organisms. Coagulation is activated by factor XI or cleavage of kininogen with release of bradykinin and antimicrobial peptides. In various experimental models, it could be shown that the inhibition of coagulation led to an impairment of the antimicrobial defense. In 2013, Engelmann and Massberg introduced the term "immunothrombosis" [14].

In sepsis, as a specific form of hyperinflammation, coagulopathy is also a frequent complication, which can be detected in up to a third of critically ill patients and can lead to the development of multiple-organ failure in severe cases. DIC is described by the International Society on Thrombosis and Haemostasis (ISTH) as a syndrome *"characterized by the intravascular activation of coagulation with loss of localization arising from different causes. It can originate from and cause damage to the microvasculature, which if sufficiently severe can produce organ dysfunction"* [15]. The occurrence of DIC in sepsis represents a consumptive coagulopathy due to suppressed fibrinolysis with concomitant system-wide coagulation activation, which, in conjunction with systemic inflammation, can lead to organ dysfunction. For this, the term sepsis-induced coagulopathy (SIC) has been introduced, which is based on existing organ dysfunction, decreased platelets, and increased PT-INR.

The endothelium and its protective layer of glycoprotein polysaccharides (glycocalyx) play a critical role in disease progression during dysregulated hypercytokinemia. The endothelium and glycocalyx are the sites of action of a variety of mechanisms that lead to an inflammatory response. These include direct, PAMP-associated activation and interactions with microbial products, as well as the effect of DAMPs. Thus, endothelial cells in turn become drivers of coagulopathy—they lose antithrombotic properties, the expression of surface-bound thrombomodulin is reduced, and there is increased expression of tissue factor (TF), which in turn, together with leukocytic microparticles and monocytes that are also TF occupied, leads to coagulation activation. Combined with the release of other pro-inflammatory factors of their own, there is increased recruitment of inflammatory cells, further expression of adhesion molecules, progressive hyperpermeability, and release of cytokines. Physiologically, TF (F III) is a primary trigger of the coagulation cascade, produced by perivascular and subendothelial cells (e.g., epithelial cells, fibroblasts, and pericytes) [16]. Complex formation with coagulation factor VIIa (F VIIa) results in activation of the coagulation cascade via factors IX and

X. Microbes as well as various cytokines and factors of the complement system cause the increased expression of TF on endothelial cells, macrophages, and monocytes [17].

An additional enhancement of the prothrombotic situation occurs through binding of released TF to activated platelets and neutrophils, among others, while at the same time the activity of the antithrombotic effect of antithrombin, the protein C system, and the tissue factor pathway inhibitor (TFPI) is reduced.

3.4 Hypercytokinemia in Sepsis

The most frequent cause of CS is invasive microbial infection. A proportion of infected patients develop a dysregulated immune response and the clinical appearance of sepsis as a life-threatening condition. At present, the Third International Consensus (Sepsis-3) emphasizes the crucial role of the innate and adaptive immune response in the development of the clinical syndrome sepsis by defining it as "organ dysfunction caused by a dysregulated host response to infection" [18]. Sepsis affects approximately 49 million people annually. Estimates suggest that up to 11 million deaths occur annually due to sepsis, representing approximately 19.7% of all global deaths. Although global sepsis mortality rates appear to be decreasing, it is still as high as 25% in septic adults hospitalized in high-income countries [3]. In particularly severe courses with pronounced circulatory, cellular, and metabolic disturbances, known as septic shock, the hospital mortality rate may reach almost 60% [19].

It is difficult to distinguish between adequate cytokine production to fight systemic infection and dysregulated cytokine production. Disseminated microbial infections also induce the production and release of numerous cytokines in the setting of sepsis, which can subsequently lead to fever, blood pressure disturbances, cell death, coagulopathies, and multiple-organ dysfunction. The immune response can be a significantly greater threat to the host through collateral damage to various tissues and organs than the infection itself.

Various Gram-positive bacteria like Streptococci and Staphylococci can produce so-called superantigens [20]. These bacterial superantigens are exceptionally potent mitogens; concentrations of less than 0.1 pg/mL are sufficient to lead to polyclonal T cell activation by cross-linking T cell receptors and the major histocompatibility complex (MHC) [21]. Toxic shock syndrome may be the consequence, which is an immediate threat to the survival of the affected host.

Some patients with an exaggerated immunological response towards infection have defects in pathogen recognition, regulatory mechanisms, or mechanisms responsible for termination/resolution of the inflammatory response. For example, patients with a specific perforin disorder develop HLH-associated hypercytokinemia when infected with cytomegalovirus or Epstein-Barr virus [22]. Perforin usually participates in the termination of the inflammatory response, but the defective form appears to lead to impaired cytolysis, which in turn prolongs the interaction between APC and lymphocytes and influences the clearance of antigen-bearing dendritic cells. This results in a self-sustaining loop of autocrine pro-inflammatory cytokine expression, continuous activation of macrophages and T cells, and sustained hemophagocytosis [23, 24].

3.5 Hypercytokinemia in Post-cardiac Arrest Syndrome

Another example of the onset of a CS is in the context of the post-cardiac arrest syndrome (PCAS). In 2016, the American Health Association registry reported about 350,000 cases of out-of-hospital cardiac arrest (OHCA) and approximately 200,000 cases of in-hospital cardiac arrest (IHCA) in the USA [25]. The rate of return of spontaneous circulation (ROSC) was 45–50%, with high mortality before hospital discharge [26]. The development of PCAS with ischemia-reperfusion injury, hypoxic brain injury, and continued myocardial dysfunction seems to play an important role, in addition to the primary disease [27].

Cardiac arrest leads to global hypoxemia and organ damage due to no flow or low flow. After reperfusion, oxidative damage and formation of free radicals lead to tissue damage, activation of different metabolic cascades, and release of pro-inflammatory cytokines [28]. Endothelial cells release TNF-α and IL-1β, which subsequently promotes further cytokines such as IL-6, IL-8, and IL-10 [29]. The resulting hypercytokinemia causes extensive cardiovascular and brain dysfunction, with elevated levels of IL-6, IL-8, and IL-10 in non-survivors compared to survivors [28]. Systemic levels of IL-6 and IL-8 are associated with neurologic and cardiovascular impairment and mortality.

IL-6 and IL-8 concentrations increase both systemically and in the cerebrospinal fluid (CSF). IL-8 is known to have beneficial effects on neuronal growth and hippocampal neuronal survival, but just like IL-6, it also causes increased blood-brain barrier (BBB) permeability leading to an enlargement of ischemic areas, propagation of cerebral edema, and also activation of the complement system [30]. This in turn leads to further systemic inflammation, endothelial activation, and perpetuation of a persistent hemodynamically unstable state, giving rise to further damage to the heart and brain [31].

Hypercytokinemia associated with PCAS also has a direct impact on cardiac performance. Increasing levels of IL-1β, IL-6, and TNF-α observed shortly after ROSC both decrease systemic vascular resistance and impair myocardial function [32]. TNF-α and IL-6 cause the expression of cell adhesion molecules (CAMs), promoting endothelial inflammation and further organ damage [33]. IL-6-mediated impairment of endothelium and glycocalyx results in progressive vasodilation and capillary leakage with increasing circulatory instability [33, 34]. Syndecan-1 and thrombomodulin are markers of endothelial damage and are associated with the severity of PCAS [31].

3.6 Endotoxin-Induced CS

Lipopolysaccharide (LPS, endotoxin) is one of the most important virulence factors of Gram-negative bacteria and has an extraordinarily high pathogenicity to humans. LPS makes up approximately 75% of the outer membrane of Gram-negative bacteria and is primarily responsible for the activation of innate immunity [35, 36]. It is recognized by specific and highly conserved PRRs, stimulates the release of pro-inflammatory cytokines, and leads to an exuberant pro-inflammatory host response [37].

Chemically, LPS are glycolipid macromolecules consisting of an oligosaccharide core, an outer O-antigen polysaccharide, and a lipid A domain. The latter serves as a hydrophobic attachment to the microbial membrane and is the only LPS region recognized by the innate immune system [38]. Distinct lipid A residues in different pathogens cause different recognition by immune system receptors; for example, lipid A of *Escherichia coli* has a particularly stimulatory effect on the human immune system [39]. Picomolar amounts of this lipid A are sufficient to activate macrophages and induce the expression of pro-inflammatory cytokines such as IL-1β and TNF-α [40, 41]. The primary receptor for recognition of LPS is Toll-like receptor 4 (TLR4) [42]. However, while lipid A is used for recognition, the immune response is primarily directed against the O-antigen portion [43].

LPS binds to LPS-binding protein (LBP) in the circulation and is transferred to the membrane protein CD14 on the surface of leukocytes [44]. After transfer of LPS from CD14 to MD-2, binding to TLR4 occurs [45]. The complex of LPS, TLR4, and MD-2 dimerizes and binds cytoplasmic adapter molecules through the Toll-interleukin-1 receptor domain (TIR) [46]. This initiates the intracellular signaling cascade through either a MyD88-dependent or -independent pathway, leading to the release of pro-inflammatory cytokines, production of NF-κB, and induction of type 1 interferons [47].

3.7 CS After Splenectomy

Another example of a dysregulated immune response in the setting of CS is overwhelming post-splenectomy infection (OPSI). This occurs in splenectomized patients who have an increased susceptibility to infection and are at risk for increased mortality and morbidity. Common pathogens are encapsulated bacteria (bacteria with a poorly opsonized polysaccharide capsule), from which *Streptococcus pneumoniae* infections are by far the most common cause of post-splenectomy infection and are associated with a mortality rate of up to 60% [48]. However, recent studies suggest that *Haemophilus influenzae* (type b) and *Neisseria meningitidis* are other common pathogens in addition to Gram-negative bacteria such as Pseudomonas species and *Escherichia coli* [49]. Although the definition is not standardized, OPSI can be considered a fulminant course of sepsis [50]. After general and nonspecific symptoms such as fever, chills, and gastrointestinal symptoms, the full clinical picture of septic shock with DIC, hypoperfusion, and MOF may be present within 48 h caused by increased vascular permeability and loss of vascular tone (due to high levels of nitric oxide and prostaglandin).

In contrast, levels for C3 and C4 as parameters of the complement system remain largely unremarkable in the context of an OPSI. However, the spleen plays an important role in choline-mediated hypoinflammatory control [51]. In sepsis, splenic macrophages are considered potent producers of TNF-α. Vagal interference results in marked reduction of the expression of TNF-α and other pro-inflammatory cytokines, with concomitant increased release of anti-inflammatory cytokines such as IL-10. This anti-inflammatory influence is absent after splenectomy [52]. Thus, clearance of attacking microbes is impaired because of delayed and impaired production of immunoglobulins and reduced phagocytic function [53]. Opsonization of microbes is also reduced, resulting in an increased risk of infection and a severe course of disease after splenectomy.

3.8 Invasive Meningococcal Disease (IMD)

In about 10% of the healthy population, Gram-negative diplococcus *Neisseria meningitidis* can be detected on the mucosal surface of the nasopharynx as colonization [54]. Only a small proportion of the different strains present cause invasive meningococcal disease (IMD). The disease begins as soon as meningococci enter the bloodstream and replicate. Systemic spread leads to different clinical forms of IMD with central or peripheral manifestations such as meningitis, purpura fulminans, pneumonia, and, less commonly, septic arthritis or pericarditis [37, 55].

Each year, approximately 500,000 people worldwide develop invasive meningococcal disease. Infants and young children are particularly affected because their immune system is not yet fully mature. A second age peak of disease is seen in adolescents [56, 57]. Meningococcal disease of serogroup B, which affects up to 80,000 people worldwide annually, is associated with a high morbidity and mortality of up to 15%. In fulminant cases, death can occur in less than 4 h after infection [58, 59].

Different strains of meningococci have unique virulence factors that promote adhesion, colonization, and invasion of the bloodstream. In serogroup B meningococci, for example, a similarity of the polysaccharide to polysialic acid structures of the human cell adhesion molecule ensures only low immunogenicity. Sialylated lipooligosaccharide (LOS) and factor H-binding protein (fHBP) support bacterial survival in the bloodstream, as they help microbes to resist the host's pro-inflammatory response, e.g., antibody recognition and phagocytosis by innate immune cells [60]. Thus, meningococcal factor H-binding protein circumvents the bactericidal effect of the complement system by inactivating host complement fHBP [55, 61].

A critical factor in the pathogenicity of meningococci is the ability to interact with endothelial cells including those forming the BBB [19]. The close interaction with vascular endothelia is among the reasons for endothelial dysfunction such as vascular leakage, local thrombotic reactions, and necrotic purpura [19] and forms a niche in which the pathogen can replicate, leading to high mortality through continuous bacteremia [62].

On the cell membrane of meningococci, type IV pili (T4P) are localized, which are widely distributed in bacteria and are physiologically involved in different regulatory mechanisms. Known modes of action of this so called *prokaryotic Swiss Army knife* include adhesion to abiotic and biotic surfaces, biofilm formation, motility, aggregation, and DNA uptake [63, 64].

When colonizing human endothelia, meningococcal T4P first interacts with CD147, a surface protein of the immunoglobulin superfamily that is expressed on different cell types and consists of two Ig-like domains extracellularly [65]. CD147 regulates different physiological and pathological mechanisms within the neurological and cardiac system, the T cell-mediated immune response, as well as the progression of different types of cancer [66]. CD147 can strongly stimulate the secretion of pro-inflammatory cytokines as well as further activation of B and T cells through downstream-mediated activity of the JAK/STAT pathway [67, 68].

3.9 COVID-19

"Sepsis should be defined as life-threatening organ dysfunction caused by a dysregulated host response to infection" [18]. The Sepsis-3 definition can be effortlessly applied to COVID-19 since it emphasizes the role of the host response towards an invading pathogen.

The term CS has re-emerged with the occurrence of the pandemic. Although not all mechanisms of SARS-CoV-2 virus-induced lung injury have been fully elucidated to date, CS has almost become synonymous with it, both in the scientific community and in the mass media. Therapeutic agents that interfere with cytokines, such as the monoclonal antibody Tocilizumab or the Janus kinase (JAK) inhibitors Baricitinib and Tofacitinib, are used in the treatment of COVID-19. In each case, the justification is a need to control the dysregulated host response. Furthermore, there is ample evidence that ubiquitous viral spread occurs affecting multiple organ systems [69, 70].

In many cases, pronounced hyperinflammation has been observed in severe courses with often lethal outcome, which resembles the course of other hyperinflammatory syndromes. Especially in patients with an unfavorable clinical course, the typical appearance is an exuberant immune response with hyperactivity of dendritic cells, lymphocytes, macrophages, and other cells, which in the further progression leads to a self-amplifying and self-sustaining pathophysiology. Elevated values of inflammatory mediators and markers such as IL-6, IL-8, IL-10, ferritin, and CRP were frequently found in these patients.

Currently, however, CS as the contemporary hallmark of COVID-19 does not seem to be as ubiquitous as it has been conveyed initially. In an observational study comparing the laboratory and clinical parameters of patients with COVID-19-associated as well as COVID-19-independent ARDS, Sinha et al. showed that IL-6 and other parameters were comparable or higher when the underlying ARDS was not COVID-19 associated [71]. COVID-19 patients with a hyperinflammatory phenotype had about 20% increased mortality compared to those with a hypoinflammatory course, but the latter made up about four-fifths of all patients.

This was supported by other studies which showed that critically ill COVID-19 patients with ARDS had comparable or even lower levels of circulating pro-inflammatory cytokines (e.g., IL-6, IL-8, TNF-α) than patients who had a hyperinflammatory syndrome based on other conditions, such as bacterial induced septic shock, severe trauma, or cardiac arrest [72, 73]. Published trials with severe courses of COVID-19 in which IL-6 levels were collected have been analyzed in a meta-analysis by Leisman et al., and the results were compared with studies including patients with COVID-19-independent conditions such as ARDS, sepsis, and CRS [74]. In summary, they presented that the systemic levels of IL-6 in patients with COVID-19 were about 12 times lower than in ARDS, about 27 times lower than in patients with sepsis, and as much as 100 times lower than in CRS.

Webb et al. have developed a COVID-19-specific hyperinflammation score (cHIS) that uses six parameters to assess the inflammatory situation in COVID-19 [75]: fever, macrophage activation (hyperferritinemia), hematological dysfunction (neutrophil-to-lymphocyte ratio), hepatic injury (lactate dehydrogenase or aspartate aminotransferase), coagulopathy (D-dimer), and cytokinemia (C-reactive protein, interleukin-6, or triglycerides). Applied to a cohort of nearly 300 COVID-19 patients,

3

the score was associated with a 95% sensitivity and 59% specificity predicting the need for mechanical ventilation and 96% sensitivity/49% specificity predicting mortality, making hyperinflammation a potential major factor for poor clinical outcome in COVID-19 patients, in addition to functional immunoparalysis, coagulopathy, and direct viral cell injury. It remains undisputed that severe COVID-19 disease is associated with a hyperinflammatory course, elevated biomarkers, and tissue damage. However, whether we should speak generally of a CS or rather about a cytokine "breeze," as noted by Lippi et al., needs to be debated [76].

3.10 Iatrogenic CS

As a modality of immunotherapy, CAR-T cell therapy is used for certain forms of acute lymphocytic leukemia (ALL) as well as some types of non-Hodgkin lymphoma (NHL) [77, 78]. The patient's own T cells are extracted and equipped with chimeric antigen receptor ex vivo by use of viral vectors. This allows the genome information of the receptors to be maintained even during activation and division of these T cells. The receptors encoded by this consist of an extracellular binding domain, a linker region, as well as a transmembrane domain and an intracellular signal sequence, which do not occur together and give rise to the term "chimeric."

Tumor cells that were previously "invisible" to the immune system are recognized by the binding domain through a specific antigen structure, which leads to adhesion and activation of the CAR-T cells. Due to the intracellular signal sequences, which differ depending on the intended use, the decisive reaction for the therapeutic activity can be different [77].

These highly activated CAR-T cells are mostly directed against the surface protein CD19, which is found on almost all lymphoma cells, but also on natural B lymphocytes. Reimplantation is the trigger of hypercytokinemia with high systemic levels of IFN-γ and IL-6, already a few hours to days after reinfusion [79]. These cytokines lead to activation of further immune cells followed by typical symptoms such as fever, headache, drop in blood pressure, and neurological symptoms up to life-threatening CS with corresponding damage to organ systems. With organ support and anti-inflammatory measures, CS often regresses after a few days and affected organ systems recover.

3.11 After the Storm

Even if patients survive a CS in the context of septic shock, the elimination of pathogens does not guarantee complete convalescence. Rather, after the numerous host-damaging events, the picture of a scorched earth remains. Although the general focus is on the early phase of sepsis, there are important immunosuppressive components that take place in the late phase and may lead to sepsis-induced immune paralysis (◘ Fig. 3.1).

In early phases of the course of sepsis, low B and T lymphocyte counts are often found [81]. The cause of this septic lymphopenia, which is associated with increased mortality if it persists, has not been extensively elucidated, but is apparently based on a variety of mechanisms: In addition to increased apoptosis and tissue migration, there is also decreased production of lymphocytes as a result of emergency hemato-

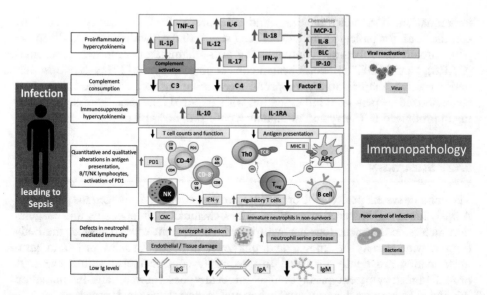

Fig. 3.1 Aspects of immunological dysfunction caused by sepsis with details of the entities involved. *APC* antigen-presenting cell, *BLC* B lymphocyte chemoattractant, *CD* cluster of differentiation, *CNC* critical neutrophil concentration, *IFN-y* interferon y, *Ig* immunoglobulin, *IL* interleukin, *IP-10* IFN-gamma-inducible protein 10, *MCP-1* monocyte chemoattractant protein-1, *MHC II* major histocompatibility complex II, *PD1* programmed death protein 1, *TCR* T cell receptor. (Adapted from Bermejo-Martin JF with permission [80])

poiesis, which prioritizes the production of monocytes and neutrophils and flushes immature myeloid-derived suppressor cells (MDSCs) into the peripheral blood [82, 83]. There, they become functionally active and release anti-inflammatory cytokines (e.g., IL-10 and transforming growth factor-β, TGF-β), resulting in marked immunosuppression. Recently, using single-cell RNA sequencing, different MDSC subsets could be detected, each of which could be used as prognostic factors for the different courses of sepsis-related diseases. This makes MDSC a worthwhile approach in future research of septic mechanisms [84]. Other causative factors of lymphopenia include increased migration into tissues and increased apoptosis.

Another component of immune paralysis is a markedly decreased expression of HLA-DR on the surfaces of monocytes and dendritic cells, which impairs pathogen recognition by decreased opsonization and impedes the Th1 and Th2 response as an essential part of the adaptive immune response. If monocytes fail to restore HLA-DR expression, clinical outcome is likely to be unfavorable [85, 86].

In addition to the reduction in lymphocytes, increased apoptosis of monocytes and APC occurs in a clustered fashion during the later course, which significantly reduces the production of pro-inflammatory cytokines [87]. Controlled apoptosis of innate and adaptive immune cells may initially be beneficial. However, uncontrolled reduction of the inflammatory response leads to incompetence in defense against further invasive microbes. Attempts to suppress immune cell apoptosis in sepsis have been shown to be promising [88].

A significant proportion of sepsis survivors develop persistent critical illness (PCI) with ongoing organ dysfunction and markedly impaired quality of life [89]. A proportion of these PCI patients also develop a clinical syndrome of persistent inflammation, immunosuppression, and catabolism (PICS) described in 2012 by Gentile et al. for patients who had an ICU stay >10 days with a surgical diagnosis [90]. Initially described as "compensatory anti-inflammatory response syndrome" (CARS), "late MOF," or "complicated clinical course," typical PICS develops after major trauma, major surgery, or pronounced inflammatory or septic insult. It is characterized by persistent inflammation with acquired immunosuppression, resulting in prolonged ICU stay and ultimately a poor prognosis [91].

3.12   Summary

The immune system protects the organism from exogenous and endogenous pathogens. A finely tuned and balanced array of cytokines, chemokines, interleukins, and coagulation factors complement together with immunocompetent cells to protect the body from a wide variety of known and unknown invaders. Usually, pro- and anti-inflammation are tightly regulated to adequately counter the infectious event. A pro-inflammatory milieu typically dominates the early phase; however, anti-inflammation is initiated early to reach a new equilibrium and to start tissue repair processes.

Various pathogens, malignant and autoimmune diseases, as well as genetic changes, but also iatrogenic interventions, can disturb this equilibrium and the balanced feedback regulation and thereby negatively affect it, so that excessive release of cytokines can occur. In its severe form, this is referred to as a cytokine storm. As a result, self-reinforcing feedback mechanisms and excessive activation of immune cells occur. The resulting hyperinflammation can lead to a life-threatening condition. Endotheliopathy, disseminated intravascular coagulation, microcirculatory disturbances, and profound hemodynamic alterations occur. Consequently, distal organ damage may develop culminating in multiple-organ failure and death in particularly severe cases. The damage caused by the immune response may be more severe than the damage caused by the pathogen itself. If patients survive, chronic critical illness with high morbidity and high long-term mortality can evolve.

> **Take-Home Messages**
>
> - A cytokine storm is a particularly severe form of hypercytokinemia, from which it differs in its extreme manifestation. Here, the immune system releases high concentrations of inflammation-relevant cytokines, which in turn stimulate leukocytes and endothelial cells to produce further cytokines (positive feedback).
> - Many clinical consequences of infections (bacterial, viral, parasitic) are caused less by the pathogen and more by a dysregulated immune response of the host. This insight could lay the foundation for new therapeutic approaches.
> - Infections are not the only cause of a cytokine storm. Graft-versus-host reactions, CAR-T cell therapy, rituximab, and other hemato-oncologic interventions are among noninfectious triggers.
> - As a consequence, endotheliopathy, disseminated intravascular coagulation, microcirculatory disturbances, and hemodynamic alterations cause distal organ damage and may lead to multiorgan failure and death. In surviving patients, chronic critical illness may develop.

References

1. Ferrara JL, Abhyankar S, Gilliland DG. Cytokine storm of graft-versus-host disease: a critical effector role for interleukin-1. Transplant Proc. 1993;25(1 Pt 2):1216–7.
2. Chatenoud L, Ferran C, Bach JF. The anti-CD3-induced syndrome: a consequence of massive in vivo cell activation. Curr Top Microbiol Immunol. 1991;174:121–34.
3. Rudd KE, Johnson SC, Agesa KM, Shackelford KA, Tsoi D, Kievlan DR, et al. Global, regional, and national sepsis incidence and mortality, 1990-2017: analysis for the global burden of disease study. Lancet. 2020;395(10219):200–11.
4. Kellum JA, Kong L, Fink MP, Weissfeld LA, Yealy DM, Pinsky MR, et al. Understanding the inflammatory cytokine response in pneumonia and sepsis: results of the Genetic and Inflammatory Markers of Sepsis (GenIMS) Study. Arch Intern Med. 2007;167(15):1655–63.
5. Walton AH, Muenzer JT, Rasche D, Boomer JS, Sato B, Brownstein BH, et al. Reactivation of multiple viruses in patients with sepsis. PLoS One. 2014;9(2):e98819.
6. Hotchkiss RS, Monneret G, Payen D. Sepsis-induced immunosuppression: from cellular dysfunctions to immunotherapy. Nat Rev Immunol. 2013;13(12):862–74.
7. Kaplan MJ, Radic M. Neutrophil extracellular traps: double-edged swords of innate immunity. J Immunol. 2012;189(6):2689–95.
8. Lu T, Kobayashi SD, Quinn MT, Deleo FR. A NET outcome. Front Immunol. 2012;3:365.
9. Czaikoski PG, Mota JM, Nascimento DC, Sonego F, Castanheira FV, Melo PH, et al. Neutrophil extracellular traps induce organ damage during experimental and clinical sepsis. PLoS One. 2016;11(2):e0148142.
10. Daix T, Guerin E, Tavernier E, Mercier E, Gissot V, Herault O, et al. Multicentric standardized flow cytometry routine assessment of patients with sepsis to predict clinical worsening. Chest. 2018;154(3):617–27.
11. Cox LE, Walstein K, Vollger L, Reuner F, Bick A, Dotsch A, et al. Neutrophil extracellular trap formation and nuclease activity in septic patients. BMC Anesthesiol. 2020;20(1):15.
12. Ward PA, Gao H. Sepsis, complement and the dysregulated inflammatory response. J Cell Mol Med. 2009;13(10):4154–60.
13. Oehmcke-Hecht S, Kohler J. Interaction of the human contact system with pathogens-an update. Front Immunol. 2018;9:312.
14. Engelmann B, Massberg S. Thrombosis as an intravascular effector of innate immunity. Nat Rev Immunol. 2013;13(1):34–45.
15. Taylor FB Jr, Toh CH, Hoots WK, Wada H, Levi M, Scientific Subcommittee on Disseminated Intravascular Coagulation (DIC) of the International Society on Thrombosis and Haemostasis (ISTH). Towards definition, clinical and laboratory criteria, and a scoring system for disseminated intravascular coagulation. Thromb Haemost. 2001;86(5):1327–30.
16. Grover SP, Mackman N. Tissue factor: an essential mediator of hemostasis and trigger of thrombosis. Arterioscler Thromb Vasc Biol. 2018;38(4):709–25.
17. Ince C, Mayeux PR, Nguyen T, Gomez H, Kellum JA, Ospina-Tascon GA, et al. The endothelium in sepsis. Shock. 2016;45(3):259–70.
18. Singer M, Deutschman CS, Seymour CW, Shankar-Hari M, Annane D, Bauer M, et al. The third international consensus definitions for sepsis and septic shock (Sepsis-3). JAMA. 2016;315(8):801–10.
19. Vincent JL, Jones G, David S, Olariu E, Cadwell KK. Frequency and mortality of septic shock in Europe and North America: a systematic review and meta-analysis. Crit Care. 2019;23(1):196.
20. Alouf JE, Muller-Alouf H. Staphylococcal and streptococcal superantigens: molecular, biological and clinical aspects. Int J Med Microbiol. 2003;292(7–8):429–40.
21. Proft T, Fraser JD. Streptococcal superantigens: biological properties and potential role in disease. In: Ferretti JJ, Stevens DL, Fischetti VA, editors. Streptococcus pyogenes: basic biology to clinical manifestations. Oklahoma City; 2016.
22. Lykens JE, Terrell CE, Zoller EE, Risma K, Jordan MB. Perforin is a critical physiologic regulator of T-cell activation. Blood. 2011;118(3):618–26.
23. Zhang M, Bracaglia C, Prencipe G, Bemrich-Stolz CJ, Beukelman T, Dimmitt RA, et al. A heterozygous RAB27A mutation associated with delayed cytolytic granule polarization and hemophagocytic lymphohistiocytosis. J Immunol. 2016;196(6):2492–503.

24. Terrell CE, Jordan MB. Perforin deficiency impairs a critical immunoregulatory loop involving murine CD8(+) T cells and dendritic cells. Blood. 2013;121(26):5184–91.

25. Benjamin EJ, Virani SS, Callaway CW, Chamberlain AM, Chang AR, Cheng S, et al. Heart disease and stroke statistics-2018 update: a report from the American Heart Association. Circulation. 2018;137(12):e67–e492.

26. Nichol G, Thomas E, Callaway CW, Hedges J, Powell JL, Aufderheide TP, et al. Regional variation in out-of-hospital cardiac arrest incidence and outcome. JAMA. 2008;300(12):1423–31.

27. Nolan JP, Neumar RW, Adrie C, Aibiki M, Berg RA, Bottiger BW, et al. Post-cardiac arrest syndrome: epidemiology, pathophysiology, treatment, and prognostication. A scientific statement from the International Liaison Committee on Resuscitation; the American Heart Association Emergency Cardiovascular Care Committee; the Council on Cardiovascular Surgery and Anesthesia; the Council on Cardiopulmonary, Perioperative, and Critical Care; the Council on Clinical Cardiology; the Council on Stroke. Resuscitation. 2008;79(3):350–79.

28. Adrie C, Adib-Conquy M, Laurent I, Monchi M, Vinsonneau C, Fitting C, et al. Successful cardiopulmonary resuscitation after cardiac arrest as a "sepsis-like" syndrome. Circulation. 2002;106(5):562–8.

29. Peberdy MA, Andersen LW, Abbate A, Thacker LR, Gaieski D, Abella BS, et al. Inflammatory markers following resuscitation from out-of-hospital cardiac arrest-a prospective multicenter observational study. Resuscitation. 2016;103:117–24.

30. Araujo DM, Cotman CW. Trophic effects of interleukin-4, -7 and -8 on hippocampal neuronal cultures: potential involvement of glial-derived factors. Brain Res. 1993;600(1):49–55.

31. Bro-Jeppesen J, Johansson PI, Hassager C, Wanscher M, Ostrowski SR, Bjerre M, et al. Endothelial activation/injury and associations with severity of post-cardiac arrest syndrome and mortality after out-of-hospital cardiac arrest. Resuscitation. 2016;107:71–9.

32. Niemann JT, Rosborough JP, Youngquist S, Shah AP, Lewis RJ, Phan QT, et al. Cardiac function and the proinflammatory cytokine response after recovery from cardiac arrest in swine. J Interf Cytokine Res. 2009;29(11):749–58.

33. Annborn M, Dankiewicz J, Erlinge D, Hertel S, Rundgren M, Smith JG, et al. Procalcitonin after cardiac arrest—an indicator of severity of illness, ischemia-reperfusion injury and outcome. Resuscitation. 2013;84(6):782–7.

34. Chelazzi C, Villa G, Mancinelli P, De Gaudio AR, Adembri C. Glycocalyx and sepsis-induced alterations in vascular permeability. Crit Care. 2015;19:26.

35. Bone RC. Sepsis, the sepsis syndrome, multi-organ failure: a plea for comparable definitions. Ann Intern Med. 1991;114(4):332–3.

36. Morrison DC, Ryan JL. Endotoxins and disease mechanisms. Annu Rev Med. 1987;38:417–32.

37. van Deuren M, Brandtzaeg P, van der Meer JW. Update on meningococcal disease with emphasis on pathogenesis and clinical management. Clin Microbiol Rev. 2000;13(1):144–66, table of contents.

38. Raetz CR, Whitfield C. Lipopolysaccharide endotoxins. Annu Rev Biochem. 2002;71:635–700.

39. Schromm AB, Brandenburg K, Loppnow H, Moran AP, Koch MH, Rietschel ET, et al. Biological activities of lipopolysaccharides are determined by the shape of their lipid A portion. Eur J Biochem. 2000;267(7):2008–13.

40. Dinarello CA. Interleukin-1 and interleukin-1 antagonism. Blood. 1991;77(8):1627–52.

41. Miller SI, Ernst RK, Bader MW. LPS, TLR4 and infectious disease diversity. Nat Rev Microbiol. 2005;3(1):36–46.

42. Medzhitov R, Preston-Hurlburt P, Janeway CA Jr. A human homologue of the drosophila toll protein signals activation of adaptive immunity. Nature. 1997;388(6640):394–7.

43. Bryant CE, Spring DR, Gangloff M, Gay NJ. The molecular basis of the host response to lipopolysaccharide. Nat Rev Microbiol. 2010;8(1):8–14.

44. Cowan JR, Salyer L, Wright NT, Kinnamon DD, Amaya P, Jordan E, et al. SOS1 gain-of-function variants in dilated cardiomyopathy. Circ Genom Precis Med. 2020;13(4):e002892.

45. Wright SD, Ramos RA, Tobias PS, Ulevitch RJ, Mathison JC. CD14, a receptor for complexes of lipopolysaccharide (LPS) and LPS binding protein. Science. 1990;249(4975):1431–3.

46. Feng C, Stamatos NM, Dragan AI, Medvedev A, Whitford M, Zhang L, et al. Sialyl residues modulate LPS-mediated signaling through the toll-like receptor 4 complex. PLoS One. 2012;7(4):e32359.

47. Lu YC, Yeh WC, Ohashi PS. LPS/TLR4 signal transduction pathway. Cytokine. 2008;42(2):145–51.
48. Zandvoort A, Timens W. The dual function of the splenic marginal zone: essential for initiation of anti-TI-2 responses but also vital in the general first-line defense against blood-borne antigens. Clin Exp Immunol. 2002;130(1):4–11.
49. Davies JM, Lewis MP, Wimperis J, Rafi I, Ladhani S, Bolton-Maggs PH, et al. Review of guidelines for the prevention and treatment of infection in patients with an absent or dysfunctional spleen: prepared on behalf of the British Committee for Standards in Haematology by a working party of the Haemato-Oncology Task Force. Br J Haematol. 2011;155(3):308–17.
50. Luu S, Spelman D, Woolley IJ. Post-splenectomy sepsis: preventative strategies, challenges, and solutions. Infect Drug Resist. 2019;12:2839–51.
51. Rosas-Ballina M, Ochani M, Parrish WR, Ochani K, Harris YT, Huston JM, et al. Splenic nerve is required for cholinergic antiinflammatory pathway control of TNF in endotoxemia. Proc Natl Acad Sci U S A. 2008;105(31):11008–13.
52. Huston JM, Ochani M, Rosas-Ballina M, Liao H, Ochani K, Pavlov VA, et al. Splenectomy inactivates the cholinergic antiinflammatory pathway during lethal endotoxemia and polymicrobial sepsis. J Exp Med. 2006;203(7):1623–8.
53. Cameron PU, Jones P, Gorniak M, Dunster K, Paul E, Lewin S, et al. Splenectomy associated changes in IgM memory B cells in an adult spleen registry cohort. PLoS One. 2011;6(8):e23164.
54. Lyczko K, Borger J. Meningococcal prophylaxis. Treasure Island: StatPearls; 2021.
55. Coureuil M, Bourdoulous S, Marullo S, Nassif X. Invasive meningococcal disease: a disease of the endothelial cells. Trends Mol Med. 2014;20(10):571–8.
56. Deghmane AE, Taha S, Taha MK. Global epidemiology and changing clinical presentations of invasive meningococcal disease: a narrative review. Infect Dis. 2021;54:1–7.
57. Gabutti G, Stefanati A, Kuhdari P. Epidemiology of Neisseria meningitidis infections: case distribution by age and relevance of carriage. J Prev Med Hyg. 2015;56(3):E116–20.
58. Sridhar S, Greenwood B, Head C, Plotkin SA, Safadi MA, Saha S, et al. Global incidence of serogroup B invasive meningococcal disease: a systematic review. Lancet Infect Dis. 2015;15(11):1334–46.
59. Reher D, Fuhrmann V, Kluge S, Nierhaus A. A rare case of septic shock due to Neisseria meningitidis serogroup B infection despite prior vaccination in a young adult with paroxysmal nocturnal haemoglobinuria receiving eculizumab. Vaccine. 2018;36(19):2507–9.
60. Coureuil M, Join-Lambert O, Lecuyer H, Bourdoulous S, Marullo S, Nassif X. Pathogenesis of meningococcemia. Cold Spring Harb Perspect Med. 2013;3(6):a012393.
61. Bille E, Ure R, Gray SJ, Kaczmarski EB, McCarthy ND, Nassif X, et al. Association of a bacteriophage with meningococcal disease in young adults. PLoS One. 2008;3(12):e3885.
62. Capel E, Barnier JP, Zomer AL, Bole-Feysot C, Nussbaumer T, Jamet A, et al. Peripheral blood vessels are a niche for blood-borne meningococci. Virulence. 2017;8(8):1808–19.
63. Berry JL, Pelicic V. Exceptionally widespread nanomachines composed of type IV pilins: the prokaryotic Swiss Army knives. FEMS Microbiol Rev. 2015;39(1):134–54.
64. Dos Santos SI, Ziveri J, Bouzinba-Segard H, Morand P, Bourdoulous S. Meningococcus, this famous unknown. C R Biol. 2021;344(2):127–43.
65. Bernard SC, Simpson N, Join-Lambert O, Federici C, Laran-Chich MP, Maissa N, et al. Pathogenic Neisseria meningitidis utilizes CD147 for vascular colonization. Nat Med. 2014;20(7):725–31.
66. Knutti N, Huber O, Friedrich K. CD147 (EMMPRIN) controls malignant properties of breast cancer cells by interdependent signaling of Wnt and JAK/STAT pathways. Mol Cell Biochem. 2019;451(1–2):197–209.
67. Xiong L, Edwards CK 3rd, Zhou L. The biological function and clinical utilization of CD147 in human diseases: a review of the current scientific literature. Int J Mol Sci. 2014;15(10):17411–41.
68. Morris R, Kershaw NJ, Babon JJ. The molecular details of cytokine signaling via the JAK/STAT pathway. Protein Sci. 2018;27(12):1984–2009.
69. Puelles VG, Lutgehetmann M, Lindenmeyer MT, Sperhake JP, Wong MN, Allweiss L, et al. Multiorgan and renal tropism of SARS-CoV-2. N Engl J Med. 2020;383(6):590–2.
70. Lopes-Pacheco M, Silva PL, Cruz FF, Battaglini D, Robba C, Pelosi P, et al. Pathogenesis of multiple organ injury in COVID-19 and potential therapeutic strategies. Front Physiol. 2021;12:593223.
71. Sinha P, Matthay MA, Calfee CS. Is a "cytokine storm" relevant to COVID-19? JAMA Intern Med. 2020;180(9):1152–4.

3

72. Zhou F, Yu T, Du R, Fan G, Liu Y, Liu Z, et al. Clinical course and risk factors for mortality of adult inpatients with COVID-19 in Wuhan, China: a retrospective cohort study. Lancet. 2020;395(10229):1054–62.

73. Stolarski AE, Kim J, Zhang Q, Remick DG. Cytokine drizzle-the rationale for abandoning "cytokine storm". Shock. 2021;56(5):667–72.

74. Leisman DE, Ronner L, Pinotti R, Taylor MD, Sinha P, Calfee CS, et al. Cytokine elevation in severe and critical COVID-19: a rapid systematic review, meta-analysis, and comparison with other inflammatory syndromes. Lancet Respir Med. 2020;8(12):1233–44.

75. Webb BJ, Peltan ID, Jensen P, Hoda D, Hunter B, Silver A, et al. Clinical criteria for COVID-19-associated hyperinflammatory syndrome: a cohort study. Lancet Rheumatol. 2020;2(12):e754–63.

76. Lippi G, Plebani M. Cytokine "storm", cytokine "breeze", or both in COVID-19? Clin Chem Lab Med. 2020;59(4):637–9.

77. Gauthier J, Yakoub-Agha I. Chimeric antigen-receptor T-cell therapy for hematological malignancies and solid tumors: clinical data to date, current limitations and perspectives. Curr Res Transl Med. 2017;65(3):93–102.

78. Grupp SA, Kalos M, Barrett D, Aplenc R, Porter DL, Rheingold SR, et al. Chimeric antigen receptor-modified T cells for acute lymphoid leukemia. N Engl J Med. 2013;368(16):1509–18.

79. Porter DL, Hwang WT, Frey NV, Lacey SF, Shaw PA, Loren AW, et al. Chimeric antigen receptor T cells persist and induce sustained remissions in relapsed refractory chronic lymphocytic leukemia. Sci Transl Med. 2015;7(303):303ra139.

80. Bermejo-Martin JF, Andaluz-Ojeda D, Almansa R, Gandia F, Gomez-Herreras JI, Gomez-Sanchez E, et al. Defining immunological dysfunction in sepsis: a requisite tool for precision medicine. J Infect. 2016;72(5):525–36.

81. Hotchkiss RS, Tinsley KW, Swanson PE, Schmieg RE Jr, Hui JJ, Chang KC, et al. Sepsis-induced apoptosis causes progressive profound depletion of B and CD4+ T lymphocytes in humans. J Immunol. 2001;166(11):6952–63.

82. Park SH, Park BG, Park CJ, Kim S, Kim DH, Jang S, et al. An extended leukocyte differential count (16 types of circulating leukocytes) using the cytodiff flow cytometric system can provide informations for the discrimination of sepsis severity and prediction of outcome in sepsis patients. Cytometry B Clin Cytom. 2013.

83. Monserrat J, de Pablo R, Diaz-Martin D, Rodriguez-Zapata M, de la Hera A, Prieto A, et al. Early alterations of B cells in patients with septic shock. Crit Care. 2013;17(3):R105.

84. Darden DB, Bacher R, Brusko MA, Knight P, Hawkins RB, Cox MC, et al. Single cell RNA-SEQ of human myeloid derived suppressor cells in late sepsis reveals multiple subsets with unique transcriptional responses: a pilot study. Shock. 2021;55(5):587–95.

85. Shankar-Hari M, Datta D, Wilson J, Assi V, Stephen J, Weir CJ, et al. Early PREdiction of sepsis using leukocyte surface biomarkers: the ExPRES-sepsis cohort study. Intensive Care Med. 2018;44(11):1836–48.

86. Pena OM, Hancock DG, Lyle NH, Linder A, Russell JA, Xia J, et al. An endotoxin tolerance signature predicts sepsis and organ dysfunction at initial clinical presentation. EBioMedicine. 2014;1(1):64–71.

87. Bhardwaj N, Mathur P, Kumar S, Gupta A, Gupta D, John NV, et al. Depressed monocytic activity may be a predictor for sepsis. J Lab Phys. 2015;7(1):26–31.

88. van der Poll T, van de Veerdonk FL, Scicluna BP, Netea MG. The immunopathology of sepsis and potential therapeutic targets. Nat Rev Immunol. 2017;17(7):407–20.

89. Deutschman CS, Tracey KJ. Sepsis: current dogma and new perspectives. Immunity. 2014;40(4):463–75.

90. Gentile LF, Cuenca AG, Efron PA, Ang D, Bihorac A, McKinley BA, et al. Persistent inflammation and immunosuppression: a common syndrome and new horizon for surgical intensive care. J Trauma Acute Care Surg. 2012;72(6):1491–501.

91. Lord JM, Midwinter MJ, Chen YF, Belli A, Brohi K, Kovacs EJ, et al. The systemic immune response to trauma: an overview of pathophysiology and treatment. Lancet. 2014;384(9952):1455–65.

Hemophagocytic Lymphohistiocytosis

Gunnar Lachmann and Frank Brunkhorst

Contents

© The Author(s), under exclusive license to Springer Nature Switzerland AG 2023
Z. Molnar et al. (eds.), *Management of Dysregulated Immune Response in the Critically Ill*,
Lessons from the ICU, https://doi.org/10.1007/978-3-031-17572-5_4

4

● Learning Objectives
This chapter provides a broad overview of hemophagocytic lymphohistiocytosis
(HLH) and the importance of its knowledge for intensive care physicians. It shows
recent advances in epidemiology, triggers, pathophysiological mechanisms, and differential diagnoses. The detailed presentation of the clinical picture will help to identify
HLH patients in clinical practice and to distinguish them from sepsis. Internalization
of current diagnostic and therapeutic recommendations will lead to high diagnostic
vigilance and timely treatment to ultimately save lives.

4.1 Introduction

If patients with multiple-organ failure (MOF) or sepsis do not respond adequately
to anti-infective therapy or if no infectious cause can be identified, they may have
developed hemophagocytic lymphohistiocytosis (HLH). HLH is a life-threatening
syndrome of immune dysregulation and hyperinflammation due to excessive
immune activation of T cells and macrophages, which leads to a cytokine storm
and is associated with MOF and high mortality. The clinical course is widely similar to sepsis, and, therefore, HLH is very difficult to recognize for intensive care
physicians and also for specialists in medicine (hematology, oncology, infectious
diseases, immunology, rheumatology, gastroenterology, neurology, emergency and
general medicine). Due to multiple etiologies, variations in clinical presentation,
and rapid deterioration in most patients, management of HLH is challenging.
The rate of undiagnosed cases is consequently high, which is why HLH is assumed
to be an undetected cause of death in critically ill patients. HLH requires—different from sepsis—immunosuppressive treatment; together with early recognition
and aggressive supportive care, it currently constitutes the best care for HLH
patients. If the diagnosis is delayed, HLH frequently is fatal due to irreversible
MOF. A high diagnostic vigilance with timely initiation of immunosuppressive
therapy is decisive for the prognosis. Every intensive care physician should be
familiar with the diagnosis and therapy of this challenging disorder, which is
essential for the survival of patients [1, 2].

▶ **Example**
A 30-year-old, previously healthy patient is admitted to the intensive care unit (ICU)
after a 3-month trip to Asia and South America with an unclear fever and respiratory failure. A broad infectious and autoimmunological diagnostic workup does not
produce any pathological findings. Further diagnostics do not reveal any evidence of
neoplasia either. The patient does not improve despite broad anti-infective therapy.
Persistent fever, high ferritin and triglyceride levels, splenomegaly, and increased soluble interleukin-2 receptor (sIL-2R) are noticeable. In the further course, hemophagocytosis appears in the bone marrow smear. After the diagnosis of HLH, the patient is
treated with dexamethasone, immunoglobulins, and IL-1 receptor antagonist anakinra.
After a total of 12 days, the patient can be discharged home after a full recovery. It has
to be assumed that this patient had an unidentified infectious trigger, leading to the full
picture of HLH [3]. ◀

HLH is a life-threatening syndrome of immune dysregulation and hyperinflammation with excessive immune activation and associated high mortality. Knowledge of diagnosis and therapy is crucial for the survival of patients.

4.2 Types

The first report on HLH dates from 1939 [4]. In general, distinction is made on the basis of its pathogenesis between a primary, genetically determined form in early childhood and a secondary, acquired form in adults associated with an underlying trigger, which can affect every patient at any time during life (■ Table 4.1). The primary form, which has been well studied in children, is based on a known genetic defect and therefore usually occurs at an early age. Much less is known about secondary HLH (sHLH), which is more common in adults, but with only limited scientific analyses done, yet. During the last 15 years, case reports of adult patients with sHLH without a family history of primary HLH (pHLH) or a known HLH-associated biallelic genetic mutation have been increasing, suggesting that sHLH in adults is increasingly frequently diagnosed. In the secondary form, which is predominantly relevant in ICUs for adult patients, an infectious, autoimmune/autoinflammatory, or malignancy-related trigger is assumed to be the cause of the syndrome leading to a pathological activation of the immune system with hyperinflammation, severe cytokine storm, and immune-mediated organ damage. Immunosuppression is an important cause for infection-associated HLH [6]. Current knowledge of sHLH in adults is mainly learned from pediatricians treating

■ **Table 4.1** Causes of primary and secondary HLH [5]

Primary HLH	Secondary HLH
– *Cytotoxicity defects*: PRF1, UNC13D, STX11, STXBP2, Griscelli syndrome type 2, Chediak-Higashi syndrome, Hermansky-Pudlak syndrome type 2, X-linked lymphoproliferative disease type 1 – *Inflammasome defects*: NLRC4, X-linked lymphoproliferative disease type 2	– *Infections*: EBV, HIV, CMV, influenza, SARS-CoV-2, tuberculosis, other bacteria, parasites, fungi – *Malignancies*: Lymphoma, leukemia, multiple myeloma, MDS – *Autoimmune/autoinflammatory*: SLE, sJIA, AOSD, rheumatoid arthritis, systemic vasculitis, inflammatory bowel disease – History of transplantation – *Immunosuppression*: Chemotherapy, long-term immunosuppressive therapy – *Novel immunotherapies*: CART, BiTE, checkpoint inhibitors – Drugs, vaccination, surgery, burn injuries, pregnancy

Genetic defects of pHLH and frequent triggers and underlying conditions of sHLH

AOSD adult-onset Still's disease, *BiTE* bispecific T cell engager, *CART* chimeric antigen receptor modified T cells, *CMV* cytomegalovirus, *EBV* Epstein-Barr virus, *HIV* human immunodeficiency virus, *MDS* myelodysplastic syndrome, *sJIA* systemic onset juvenile idiopathic arthritis, *SLE* systemic lupus erythematosus

pHLH, though triggers, cohorts, comorbidities, and clinical presentations are fundamentally different. The success of the treatment protocols HLH-94 and HLH-2004 in children with pHLH have led to their adaption for sHLH in adults with positive effects on survival, but validation studies are pending [7]. Reports and studies on both pHLH and sHLH are still increasing.

> HLH comprises two forms: the primary form in children due to genetic defects and the secondary form in adults induced by various triggers. The latter form is mainly relevant in adult critically ill patients.

4.3 Epidemiology

HLH is a rare syndrome with an estimated incidence of about 1 in 800,000 people over all ages per year in Japan [8] and 1 in 3000 inpatient admissions in a children hospital in the USA [9]. In Sweden, pHLH was seen in 1.2 of 1,000,000 children per year. One child per 50,000 live births developed pHLH [10]. Turkey reported an incidence of pHLH of 7.5 in 10,000 births [11]. Incidences of HLH in children were 1.5 of 100,000 children per year in the USA [12] and 0.12 of 100,000 children per year in Italy [13]. Various genetic factors, triggers, and underlying conditions, particularly infections, result in regional differences, which is a key epidemiological characteristic of HLH [6].

A Chinese registry comprising 1445 HLH patients reported that 34.6% of HLH cases occurred in adults [14]. Of 30 children with HLH, 17 patients required admission to an ICU (56.7%) [15], whereas 2313 of 7420 adult sHLH patients (31.2%) were critically ill [16]. sHLH can affect every age with a mean of 49 years in the total cohort of adult sHLH patients (63% male) [6] and 47 years (61% male) in adult critically ill sHLH patients [17]. The exact incidence of sHLH is unknown, exemplified in a study where sHLH remained undiagnosed in seven of nine adult critically ill patients [1]. A retrospective study found an incidence of sHLH of 40 among 116,310 (0.0344%) adult critically ill patients in a mixed ICU cohort [18]. In the same authors' cohort of 2623 adult critically ill patients with hyperferritinemia (≥ 500 µg/L), sHLH incidence was 1.52%. Another retrospective study reported the diagnosis of sHLH in 102 of 5027 (2.03%) adult critically ill patients in a medical ICU [19]. There is the general belief that sHLH is a relevant but underdiagnosed cause of death in ICU with higher incidences than reported [20]. Only 20% of adult critically ill sHLH patients were diagnosed prior to ICU admission, which emphasizes the importance of HLH for intensive care physicians [21].

> HLH is a rare syndrome with regional different incidences. A relevant portion of critically ill patients develop HLH, with a high rate of undiagnosed cases.

4.4 Triggers and Underlying Conditions

Triggers and underlying conditions are heterogeneous, depending on regional differences and age [6]. pHLH-associated inflammation is often triggered by infections such as herpes viruses, but can also occur in the absence of any detectable infection [22]. The main triggers of sHLH are infections, malignancies, and autoimmune/autoinflammatory diseases, which can either initiate sHLH or increase the risk of developing sHLH (◘ Table 4.1). In adult sHLH patients, infections (50.4%) and malignancies (47.7%) were the most frequent triggers, followed by autoimmune/autoinflammatory diseases (12.6%), transplantations and other conditions (8.4%), and unknown triggers (3.7%). More than a third of all sHLH had more than one trigger [6]. In adult critically ill patients, sHLH was triggered by infections (49.9%), malignancies (28.0%), autoimmune/autoinflammatory diseases (12.1%), unknown triggers (9.4%), and drugs (0.6%) [17]. HLH can be the first manifestation of autoimmune/autoinflammatory diseases or malignancies, or arise from progression of these [23]. Distribution of sHLH triggers in adult critically ill patients is shown in ◘ Fig. 4.1.

Viral infections (34.7% of all sHLH triggers) with Epstein-Barr virus (EBV), cytomegalovirus (CMV), or human immunodeficiency virus (HIV) are the most common infectious triggers. 43.3% were due to EBV, 22.7% due to HIV, and 9.1% due to CMV. Global-regional differences are noteworthy: While HIV-induced sHLH was frequently reported in Europe, EBV was the leading virus trigger in the USA and

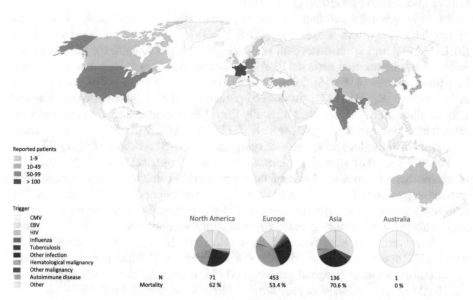

◘ **Fig. 4.1** Distribution of secondary HLH triggers in adult critically ill patients, taken from [17]. *CMV* cytomegalovirus, *EBV* Epstein-Barr virus, *HIV* human immunodeficiency virus

Asia. The immunosuppression developing in sepsis patients can lead to reinfection or reactivation of these viruses in critically ill patients. Other virus triggers are hepatitis viruses, herpes viruses, influenza, SARS-CoV-2, and parvovirus B19. sHLH can also be triggered by bacteria, protozoa, and fungi. Bacterial infections were reported to be responsible for about 9.4% of all sHLH, of which 37.9% were caused by tuberculosis, 8.3% by rickettsia, 7.3% by staphylococcus, and 5.3% by *Escherichia coli*. Leishmania, plasmodium, toxoplasma, histoplasma, candida, and cryptococcus are common protozoal and fungal triggers, respectively [6, 24]. Infectious triggers can occur either alone, with underlying opportunistic or superinfections, malignancies, or autoimmune/autoinflammatory diseases [6, 24]. In a cohort of adult critically ill sHLH patients, most frequent infectious triggers were EBV (24.8%), bacterial infection (20.3%), and CMV (6.7%) [17].

Among malignancy-triggered sHLH, hematological neoplasms (93.7%) are more common than solid tumors (3.1%). Risk of malignancy-triggered sHLH increases with age. Most frequent malignant triggers are T cell or natural killer (NK) cell lymphoma (35.2%), B-cell lymphoma (31.8%), leukemia (6.4%), Hodgkin lymphoma (5.8%), and Castleman's disease (2.1%) [6]. In these cases, infections due to immunodeficiency, excessive cytokine secretion, or tumor cells themselves may be triggers [25]. Concomitant viral infection, particularly EBV, is often present [26]. It is estimated that 1% of patients with hematological neoplasms develop sHLH [27], with increased incidences in malignant lymphoma (2.8%) [28], and acute myeloid leukemia (AML) after intensive induction chemotherapy (10%) [29]. In adult critically ill sHLH patients, most frequent malignant triggers were lymphoma (76.2%), leukemia (7.6%), and multiple myeloma (1.6%) [17].

In autoimmune/autoinflammatory triggered sHLH—traditionally known as macrophage activation syndrome (MAS-HLH)—systemic lupus erythematosus (SLE) (48.2%) and adult-onset Still's disease (AOSD) (19.6%) are the main triggers, followed by rheumatoid arthritis (6.5%), systemic vasculitis (4.0%), and inflammatory bowel disease (4.0%) [6]. 5.1% of patients with SLE and 11.5% of patients with AOSD developed sHLH [30]. In 46% of patients with SLE, sHLH occurred as the first manifestation [31]. In adult critically ill sHLH patients, most frequent autoimmune/autoinflammatory triggers were SLE (38.8%), AOSD (21.3%), and drug reaction with eosinophilia and systematic symptom (DRESS) syndrome (7.5%) [17].

Patients during or after transplantations for hematological or solid malignancies or chemotherapy are also at risk of developing sHLH due to infections caused by immunosuppression (fungal, bacterial, central line-associated), or without a tangible trigger [6]. In a large analysis of adult sHLH patients, 4.3% of sHLH patients were after transplantations for hematological or solid malignancies [6]. 0.4% of renal transplant recipients were reported to develop sHLH [32]. 50% of adult sHLH patients [33] and 75% of adult critically ill sHLH patients [21] had prior immunosuppression. In immunosuppressed patients, sHLH is often related to severe opportunistic infections such as *Pneumocystis jiroveci*, *Toxoplasma gondii*, and fungi [24].

Various other conditions can also trigger sHLH: drugs, vaccination, surgery, burn injuries, and pregnancy [6]. Novel immunotherapies for hematological malignancies, including chimeric antigen receptor-modified T cells (CART), bispecific T cell engager (BiTE) antibodies, and checkpoint inhibitors, can induce a cytokine release syndrome (CRS) that may evolve into sHLH [31].

Triggers and underlying conditions of sHLH depend on regional differences and age. sHLH is mainly triggered by infections, malignancies, and autoimmune/autoinflammatory diseases. Infections are the most frequent triggers in adult critically ill patients. A relevant amount of sHLH patients had prior immunosuppression.

4.5 Pathobiology

pHLH has been the subject of extensive research in pediatric medicine, resulting in an advanced understanding of its pathogenesis and pathophysiology. Key feature of HLH is an overactivated immune system directed against the own body, comparable to an autoinflammatory disease. Biallelic genetic defects (■ Table 4.1) in the granule-dependent cytotoxic pathway (PRF1, UNC13D, STX11, STXBP2, Griscelli syndrome type 2, Chediak-Higashi syndrome, Hermansky-Pudlak syndrome type 2) affect cytotoxic granule exocytosis and lymphocyte cytotoxicity [5, 34, 35]. Impaired release of perforin or perforin mutations prevent apoptotic cell death of target cells such as malignant cells or pathogens or autoimmune/autoinflammatory processes, but also of antigen-presenting and T cells, resulting in failed termination of the immune response. Consequently, persistent antigen presentation leads to constant activation of T cells and macrophages with uncontrolled massive release of pro-inflammatory and anti-inflammatory cytokines. High amounts of interferon gamma (IFN-γ) are released by cytotoxic T cells, activating Toll-like receptors of macrophages with consecutive release of interleukin (IL)-1, IL-6, IL-10, IL-18, and tumor necrosis factor alpha (TNF-α). However, no single cytokine appears to drive HLH pathophysiology [5, 36]. Activated cytotoxic T cells and macrophages infiltrate the spleen, liver, lymph nodes, brain, and bone marrow, and cause severe MOF. Hemophagocytosis occurs in the bone marrow and other organs of the mononuclear phagocytic system, i.e., ingestion of red and white blood cells or platelets by activated macrophages (■ Fig. 4.2). In most cases, the infiltration leads to hepatosplenomegaly, often accompanied by elevated transaminases and hyperbilirubinemia, and to MOF, life-threatening cytopenias and secondarily to sepsis [5, 23, 36, 38–40]. Periportal lymphohistiocytic infiltrates with biliary duct obstruction cause liver damage and result in jaundice and biliary tract sclerosis [41]. Macrophages release plasminogen activator, which promotes fibrinolysis and leads to hypofibrinogenemia. Heme oxygenase of macrophages is increased, which raises ferritin levels [42]. Pancytopenia and hypertriglyceridemia result from excessive increase in TNF-α and IFN-γ, which inhibit hematopoiesis and lipoprotein lipase, and may induce hemophagocytosis of hematopoietic stem cells. Persistent fever is due to high levels of IL-1 and IL-6. Ultimately, the cytokine storm leads to tissue damage and progressive MOF with fatal outcome [5, 36, 38, 39, 43].

The underlying pathogenesis of sHLH is postulated to be complex and multifactorial: genetic polymorphisms of the immune response and heterozygous mutations in genes of pHLH, inflammasome disorders, autoinflammatory processes, tissue damage, impaired cytolytic degranulation, acquired defects of the adaptive immune system, T cell exhaustion (host factors), immune evasion strategies, and prevention

4

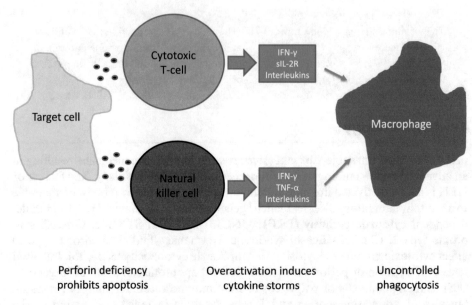

Perforin deficiency   Overactivation induces   Uncontrolled
prohibits apoptosis   cytokine storms   phagocytosis

Fig. 4.2 Simplified illustration of the pathophysiology of HLH (modified from [37])

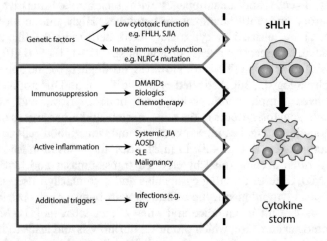

Fig. 4.3 Threshold model of sHLH, modified from [40]. Various predisposing factors and triggers contribute to reaching the threshold of developing sHLH with a consecutive cytokine storm. Different forms of severity (not all are required) lead to a wide spectrum of clinical presentations. *AOSD* adult-onset Still's disease, *DMARDs* disease modifying anti-rheumatic drugs, *EBV* Epstein-Barr virus, *FHLH* primary hemophagocytic lymphocytosis, *sHLH* secondary hemophagocytic lymphohistiocytosis, *SJIA* systemic onset juvenile idiopathic arthritis, *SLE* systemic lupus erythematosus

of apoptosis by viruses and malignant cells are conditions that increase the risk of developing sHLH (non-host factors) [44–48]. The pathophysiological mechanisms of sHLH are assumed to be similar to those of pHLH: In response to triggers, underlying conditions, and pathogenesis (□ Fig. 4.3), it comes to a reversible acquired inability of cytotoxic T and NK cells to adequately restrict stimulatory effects. In analogue to pHLH, the result is a cytokine storm and MOF [34, 40, 49]. Chronic antigen stimulation is believed to lead to malfunction of these cells [23]. In 14% of adult sHLH patients, hypomorphic gene mutations in the HLH-associated genes PRF1, MUNC13–4, and STXBP2, with an assumed threshold function after antigen exposure, have been described [50, 51]. However, biallelic mutations are rare [50], and the influence of genetic variants on the occurrence of sHLH in adults has been questioned [52]. In a study of adult sHLH patients, highly activated NK cells without cytotoxicity defects were seen, in combination with lymphopenia and reduced IFN-ɣ production, which indicates that sHLH pathophysiology cannot completely be explained by cytotoxicity defects, but rather by immune overactivation [53]. Another aspect may be a relative cytotoxic dysfunction as a result of decreased numbers of cytotoxic T or NK cells [5, 54], or possibly polymorphisms in genes responsible for the immune response or mono-allelic mutations of HLH-associated genes [51]. Cytotoxic dysfunction or failed apoptosis may also be induced by viral infections such as EBV, herpes simplex virus (HSV), and influenza [45–47].

In pHLH, underlying genetic defects impair cytotoxicity and induce a cytokine storm and macrophage activation. Pathogenesis of sHLH is multifactorial and comprises host factors such as genetic cytotoxicity defects and genetic polymorphisms, autoinflammatory processes, and non-host factors such as viral and malignancy-associated evasion strategies leading to a dysregulated immune response.

4.6 Clinical Presentation

The effects of the cytokine storm determine the clinical picture and laboratory features with a wide spectrum of initial presentations. Hyperinflammation results in tachycardia, fever, fatigue, dyspnea, jaundice, diarrhea, vomiting, edema, rashes, disseminated intravascular coagulation (DIC), high triglyceride levels with possible pancreatitis, inhibition of hematopoiesis, and end-organ damage with multiple-organ failure in severe forms of HLH. In many cases, kidney, liver, lung, and circulatory failure as well as neurological deficits occur. Infiltration in the bone marrow and hypercytokinemia lead to hemophagocytosis and life-threatening cytopenias with consequent severe bleeding and sepsis. The expansion of immune cells in spleen and liver leads to hepatosplenomegaly, and in the CNS to central nervous symptoms. Macrophage activation causes the release of large amounts of ferritin. Although individual symptoms can vary in severity, the clinical picture in most cases is very similar to sepsis [55, 56]. However, characteristic feature of sHLH is the triad of fever, bicytopenia, and splenomegaly, along with high levels of ferritin (◘ Fig. 4.4).

The cardinal symptoms are persistent high fever, hepatosplenomegaly, lymphadenopathy, and symptoms associated with bicytopenia or pancytopenia (fatigue, infections, bleeding) [58]. In most cases, these patients respond insufficiently to anti-infective therapies or no infectious focus is detectable [59]. The eponymous hemophagocytosis can only be detected in some HLH patients [60]. Depending on the severity of the individual symptoms, the clinical picture can vary with different leading symptoms such as febrile liver failure, febrile sepsis, or febrile neurological symptoms. HLH patients show variable time periods between initial symptoms and complete presentation of HLH, but they can rapidly deteriorate [2, 7].

4

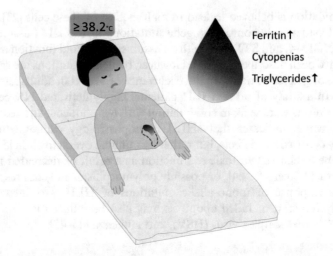

Fig. 4.4 Clinical presentation of HLH, modified from [57]

Due to the diversity of clinical findings, there are many similarities to other inflammatory diseases such as sepsis and septic shock. Thus, they may be difficult to differentiate. A patient with sepsis or septic shock and an unusually protracted course should therefore always initiate diagnostics for sHLH [35].

In adult sHLH patients, fever occurred in 96%, splenomegaly in 69%, and hepatomegaly in 67% of patients [6]. In extreme cases, macrophage invasion can lead to non-traumatic splenic rupture [61]. Thrombocytopenia and anemia were found in about 80% and leukopenia in 69% of cases. Hyperferritinemia ($\geq$500 µg/L) was seen in 90% of patients. 60% of sHLH patients had coagulation disorders due to impaired liver function. Hypofibrinogenemia and increased D-dimers occurred in 50% of all cases. DIC was found in 40% of all patients and is associated with a high mortality rate. There is a high risk of spontaneous bleeding due to hyperinflammation, coagulopathy, and thrombocytopenia. About 80% of patients had changes in their liver function values, including transaminitis, (often direct) hyperbilirubinemia and hypoalbuminemia, up to fulminant liver failure. Cell destruction led to an increase of lactate dehydrogenase (LDH) in 78% of patients. Hyponatremia in 78% of patients may be caused by the syndrome of inappropriate antidiuretic hormone (SIADH) secretion. Hypertriglyceridemia occurred in 69%. Increased acute-phase proteins (erythrocyte sedimentation rate or C-reactive protein (CRP) concentration) were seen in up to 90% of patients [6, 19, 62].

Neurological symptoms in 25% of patients were impaired consciousness, seizures, psychosis, meningitis, encephalomyelitis, thrombosis, or cerebral bleeding. Elevated cerebrospinal fluid (CSF) cell and protein content, activated macrophages, and hemophagocytes can be found in CSF examination, whereas de- or impaired myelination and multifocal inflammation can be seen in radiologic scans. Pulmonary involvement including cough, dyspnea, respiratory failure, and acute respiratory distress syndrome (ARDS) was seen in 42% of patients, particularly in sHLH due to respiratory viruses [6, 62, 63]. Critically ill sHLH patients often require organ support in the form of mechanical ventilation, vasopressors, renal replacement therapy, and multiple blood products (fresh frozen plasma, platelets,

▢ Table 4.2 Characteristics of 40 adult critically ill secondary HLH patients, based on [21]

Age (years)	47 (33–62)	Max. core body temperature at diagnosis (°C)	38.6 (37.7–39.2)
Body mass index (kg/m^2)	23.0 (21.0–26.5)	Septic shock (n) (%)	23 (57.5%)
Male sex (n) (%)	26 (65.0%)	Hepatomegaly (n) (%)	23 (57.5%)
Transfusions (n) (%)	36 (90.0%)	Splenomegaly (n) (%)	26 (65.0%)
Mechanical ventilation (n) (%)	34 (85.0%)	Hemophagocytosis (n) (%), n = 31	16 (51.6%)
Hemodialysis (n) (%)	29 (72.5%)	ICU admission SOFA score	9 (6–13)
ECLA/ECMO (n) (%)	6 (15.0%)	Maximum SOFA score	17 (12–19)
Vasopressors (n) (%)	36 (90.0%)		

Diagnostic parameters with n representing the number of patients with available data. Continuous quantities in median with quartiles

ECLA extracorporeal lung assist, *ECMO* extracorporeal membrane oxygenation, *ICU* intensive care unit, *SOFA* sequential organ failure assessment

packed red blood cells, coagulation factors) [64]. Ultimately, symptoms can also be induced by the underlying diseases. Characteristics of adult critically ill sHLH patients are shown in ▢ Table 4.2.

The effects of the cytokine storm determine the clinical picture, with a wide spectrum of initial presentations, but mostly very similar to sepsis. Characteristic feature of sHLH is the triad of fever, bicytopenia, and splenomegaly, along with high levels of ferritin.

4.7 Diagnosis

For adult intensive care physicians, sHLH diagnosis is a challenge due to the non-specific symptoms, the various initial presentations, and the sepsis-like clinical picture. sHLH is, therefore, often misdiagnosed as sepsis in most cases. An early diagnosis with initiation of appropriate immunosuppressive therapy is crucial for survival in order to avoid irreversible organ damage with fatal outcome [1]. Patients frequently develop HLH characteristics over time, and a delay in diagnosis may harm patients. Familiarity with HLH is, therefore, of outstanding importance for intensive care physicians. The combination of initial laboratory results and clinical examination should raise suspicion of HLH. The clinical picture consists of complex clinical, laboratory, and histopathological findings, although none of them alone are pathognomonic. First signs are fever, cytopenias, and high ferritin levels. Hepato- and/or splenomegaly can also be present. HLH should always be considered in all patients with fever, cytopenias, organomegalies, and signs of multiple-organ involvement, ideally prior to decompensation. All critically ill patients with an unclear or prolonged septic picture, rapidly evolving MOF, unclear cytopenias, inappropriate response to adequate treatment, aggressive supportive and anti-infective therapy, need diagnostic workup for HLH [7].

Diagnostic and therapeutic decisions for sHLH in adults are mostly based on clinical experience and expert opinion, which led to official diagnostic and treatment recommendations for adult sHLH patients in 2019 [7] and for adult critically ill sHLH patients in 2021 [64]. The currently recommended diagnostic standard for both pHLH and sHLH comprises most widespread and accepted HLH-2004 diagnostic criteria (◨ Table 4.3), which are based on expert opinion in studies of children with pHLH, published in 1991 by the Histiocyte Society [65] and revised in 2007 within the HLH-2004 protocol [58]. Although sensitivity and specificity have only been prospectively studied in children and were never validated in the adult population, the pediatric HLH-2004 diagnostic criteria are officially recommended in conjunction with clinical judgement and the patient's history. They are widely used in adults [7].

HLH-2004 diagnostic criteria require a molecular diagnosis consistent with HLH (biallelic mutations in PRF1, UNC13D, STX11, STXBP2, LYST, RAB27A, XIAP, SH2D1A, or NLCR4) or at least 5 out of 8 positive criteria for diagnosis of pHLH and sHLH [58, 64]. General genetic testing is recommended in all pHLH patients for HLH-associated gene mutations [64]. In adult sHLH patients, routine genetic testing is not recommended—except for patients with relapsing disease of unknown cause, pathologic NK functional tests, or recurrent EBV infections—since abnormalities in HLH-associated genes in adults are rare [7]. Since not all findings are initially apparent but may develop over a short time period, patients with suspected sHLH need regular reevaluation. HLH is characterized by a progressive course, where three fulfilled HLH-2004 diagnostic criteria can quickly become five. In cases of high suspicion, sHLH-directed treatment may be initiated, even though five HLH-2004 diagnostic criteria are not fulfilled, yet, to avoid irreversible organ damage and fatal outcome [7]. In a retrospective study of 40 sHLH patients among 2623 adult critically ill patients with hyperferritinemia ($\geq$500 µg/L), a cutoff of four fulfilled HLH-2004 diagnostic criteria showed 95.0% sensitivity and 93.6% specificity [66]. When

◨ **Table 4.3**   HLH-2004 diagnostic criteria based on Henter et al. [58]

HLH-2004 diagnostic criteria: molecular diagnosis consistent with HLH or $\geq$5 criteria must be fulfilled

– Ferritin $\geq$500 µg/L
– Fever ($\geq$38.2 °C)
– Splenomegaly
– Cytopenias in $\geq$2 lines (hemoglobin <9 g/dL, plateltes <100/nL, neutrophils <1.0/nL)
– Hypertriglyceridemia and/or hypofibrinogenemia (fasting triglycerides $\geq$265 mg/dL, fibrinogen <1.5 g/L)
– Hemophagocytosis in bone marrow or spleen or lymph nodes
– Low or absent NK cell activity
– Soluble IL-2 receptor $\geq$2400 U/mL

adjusting cutoffs of fever to 38.2 °C and hyperferritinemia to 3000 µg/L in this cohort, the cutoff of four fulfilled HLH-2004 diagnostic criteria reached 97.5% sensitivity and 96.1% specificity. Of note, fever may be masked in critically ill patients by use of antipyretics, hemodialysis, and extracorporeal life support (ECLS).

In order to understand HLH, it is important to note that none of the HLH-2004 diagnostic criteria is sufficient to diagnose HLH. HLH is rather defined through the overall clinical picture and the combination of HLH-2004 diagnostic criteria, which makes the diagnosis so challenging. No single criterion—including hemophagocytosis—is specific for HLH, and can also be found in sepsis patients and other conditions. Therefore, the combination of HLH-2004 diagnostic criteria is valuable for HLH diagnosis, and critically ill patients with at least four fulfilled HLH-2004 diagnostic criteria represent patients with uncontrolled inflammation, i.e., HLH phenotype [66].

Ferritin as one HLH-2004 diagnostic criterion is a quick, cheap, and widely available marker in everyday clinical practice and plays a decisive role in the differentiation from other inflammatory systemic syndromes or diseases such as systemic inflammatory response syndrome (SIRS), sepsis, or septic shock [67]. A cutoff of 2000 µg/L had 68% sensitivity and 68% specificity in a retrospective study of pHLH patients [68]. Another retrospective study of 40 sHLH patients among 2623 adult critically ill patients with hyperferritinemia (≥500 µg/L) investigated ferritin levels between sHLH, septic shock, sepsis, and other diagnoses and found significant differences between all groups (◘ Fig. 4.5) [18]. In this cohort, a ferritin cutoff of 9083 µg/L had 92.5% sensitivity and 91.9% specificity for sHLH diagnosis underscoring the value of ferritin as a screening parameter of sHLH in the adult population. In a prospective study in adult critically ill patients, ferritin showed best performance in the diagnosis of sHLH compared to IFN-γ, CXCL9, glycosylated ferritin, IL-18, sIL-2R, sCD14, IL-10, and sCD163 [69]. Therefore, ferritin should be a standard parameter in all sepsis patients, at least in unusual courses. Initiation of further HLH

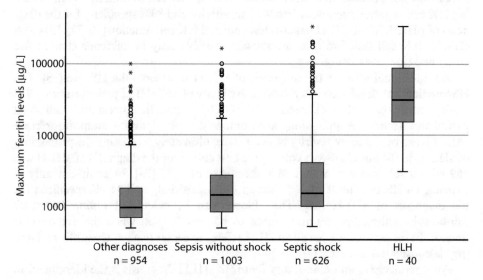

◘ Fig. 4.5 Maximum ferritin levels between adult critically ill patients with secondary HLH, septic shock, sepsis, and other diagnoses, taken from [18]

4

diagnostic workup is required in case of hyperferritinemia. Ferritin is known to be also increased in various other clinical conditions such as liver diseases, rheumatological diseases, and hemochromatosis or in patients after transfusions [70]. In critically ill patients, no significant increase of ferritin was seen in patients with hemodialysis, ECLS, and transfusions. However, ferritin was positively correlated with increased transaminases [71]. Of note, half-life of serum ferritin is 30 hours [72].

In addition to ferritin, the T cell activation marker sIL-2R is one criterion for HLH diagnosis with less specificity compared to ferritin. In adult patients, a cutoff of 2515 U/mL had 100% sensitivity and 72.5% specificity for the diagnosis of sHLH [73]. In adult critically ill patients, best sIL-2R cutoff was 4621 U/mL with 66.7% sensitivity and 76.6% specificity [18]. Of note, sIL-2R is mostly available only in reference centers, is costly and time consuming. Pending results must not delay lifesaving therapy [7].

Even though eponymous, hemophagocytosis had a sensitivity of only 83% and a specificity of 60% for the diagnosis of HLH in a mixed pediatric/adult cohort [74]. Hemophagocytosis can also be present in transfused patients, after surgery, and in hemolysis, infections, autoimmune/autoinflammatory diseases, sepsis and, therefore, does not prove or disprove HLH [59]. In 20% of all initial bone marrow biopsies of HLH patients, no hemophagocytosis was seen [75]. In adult critically ill sHLH patients, hemophagocytosis had only 51.6% sensitivity and 93.2% specificity [18]. Thus, hemophagocytosis is neither sensitive, specific nor necessary for HLH diagnosis. A bone marrow biopsy nevertheless needs to be done to look for hemophagocytosis and, importantly, to search for underlying triggers such as malignancies and infections, e.g., lymphoma and leishmaniasis. As of low bleeding risk, coagulopathy or DIC does not exclude bone marrow biopsies [7].

Decreased or absent NK cell function is suggestive of HLH, but normal tests in both pHLH and sHLH are possible. Better markers may be CD107a mobilization and perforin expression with higher sensitivity and specificity for diagnosis of pHLH. Of note, steroid treatment can also lead to NK cell dysfunction [76]. A resting NK cell degranulation <5% had 96% sensitivity and 88% specificity for the diagnosis of pHLH. Most sHLH patients have normal NK cell function [76, 77]. Likewise sIL-2R, NK cell function tests are mostly available only in reference centers, are costly and time consuming.

An additional tool for the diagnosis of sHLH represents the HScore [78]. The HScore that was developed in a retrospective study of 162 sHLH patients among 312 adult patients (▢ Table 4.4). Parts of HLH-2004 diagnostic criteria and additional parameters (immunosuppression, hepatomegaly, and aspartate aminotransferase (ASAT)) are weighted by severity of symptoms, ultimately estimating the probability of sHLH. In the initial HScore cohort, the best cutoff for the diagnosis of sHLH was 169 with a sensitivity of 93% and a specificity of 86% [78]. In adult critically ill patients, an HScore cutoff of 168 showed 100% sensitivity and 94.1% specificity for the diagnosis of sHLH [66]. The HScore can be calculated online (▸ http://saintantoine.aphp.fr/score/) and proves to be very helpful when the diagnosis is unclear. In these cases, advice by an HLH reference center (e.g., ▸ www.hlh-registry.org) is considered as useful [7].

Another decisive and mandatory factor in sHLH diagnosis is the identification of the underlying trigger (▢ Table 4.1), since adequate trigger treatment may con-

⬛ Table 4.4 HScore based on Fardet et al. [78]

HScore: calculated by scoring criteria of each parameter (▶ http://saintantoine.aphp.fr/score/)

Known underlying immunosuppression (no|yes)
Temperature (<38.4 °C|38.4–39.4 °C|>39.4 °C)
Organomegaly (no|hepato- or splenomegaly|hepatosplenomegaly)
Cytopenias (1|2|3, hemoglobin ≤9.2 g/dL, leukocytes ≤5000/µL, platelets ≤110,000/µL)
Ferritin (<2000 µg/L|2000–6000 µg/L/>6000 µg/L)
Triglycerides (<1.5 mM|1.5–4 mM|>4 mM)
Fibrinogen (>2.5 g/L|≤2.5 g/L)
Aspartate aminotransferase (<30 U/L|≥30 U/L)
Hemophagocytosis in bone marrow aspirate (no|yes)

tribute to HLH remission. Search for underlying triggers needs to be continued during HLH treatment until trigger identification. Travel (viral diseases of endemic regions) and medication history (immunosuppression, novel immunotherapies) are important. Patients with unclear trigger need an extensive trigger search with a broad infectious and rheumatologic workup, including viral triggers and CSF studies, and a profound cancer workup with repeated tissue biopsies if necessary, particularly considering Hodgkin and all subtypes of non-Hodgkin lymphomas (NHL). T cell or Hodgkin lymphomas can often only be detected through follow-up examinations due to corticosteroid treatment [7, 79]. An increased sIL-2R/ferritin ratio (>2) may indicate a possible underlying lymphoma [80]. PET-CT scan is recommended to reveal occult diseases in still unclear cases with a diagnostic accuracy of 71.4% [7, 81, 82]. sHLH triggered by malignancy always requires an infectious workup as concomitant infections are frequent [26]. In suspected leishmaniasis—particularly in travelers or inhabitants of Mediterranean countries—early PCR from bone marrow is recommended [7].

Diagnosis of HLH should be based on HLH-2004 diagnostic criteria. The HScore is helpful in initially unclear cases. Ferritin is a sensitive screening parameter and should be determined in critically ill patients with unclear septic picture to possibly initiate HLH diagnostic workup. Identification of the underlying trigger is mandatory.

4.8 Treatment

The HLH-94 [83] and HLH-2004 [58] treatment protocols as HLH cornerstones include immunosuppressive therapy and chemotherapy as key therapeutic approach for HLH patients less than 18 years. HLH-94 consists of a short-term approach ("bridging to transplant") to control hyperinflammation, i.e., delete overactivated T cells and inhibit inflammatory cytokine production, with an 8-week induction and following maintenance therapy with dexamethasone (penetrates CSF), etoposide, cyclosporine A (CSA), and intrathecal methotrexate in case of progressive neurological symptoms (⬛ Fig. 4.6). In the long-term, allogeneic hematopoietic stem cell

4

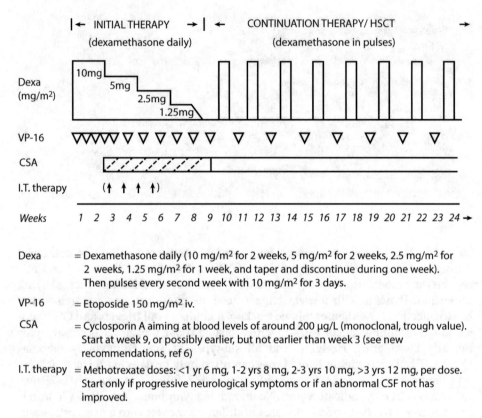

Dexa = Dexamethasone daily (10 mg/m² for 2 weeks, 5 mg/m² for 2 weeks, 2.5 mg/m² for 2 weeks, 1.25 mg/m² for 1 week, and taper and discontinue during one week). Then pulses every second week with 10 mg/m² for 3 days.

VP-16 = Etoposide 150 mg/m² iv.

CSA = Cyclosporin A aiming at blood levels of around 200 µg/L (monoclonal, trough value). Start at week 9, or possibly earlier, but not earlier than week 3 (see new recommendations, ref 6)

I.T. therapy = Methotrexate doses: <1 yr 6 mg, 1-2 yrs 8 mg, 2-3 yrs 10 mg, >3 yrs 12 mg, per dose. Start only if progressive neurological symptoms or if an abnormal CSF not has improved.

☐ **Fig. 4.6**   HLH-94 treatment protocol, taken from [7]

transplantation (HSCT) is necessary to replace the defective immune system for cure in children with pHLH and rarely also in childhood sHLH. Remission of HLH prior to HSCT results in better survival [84]. Though survival for children increased from 4 to 54% with the HLH-94 protocol [62], its efficacy in adults has not been investigated in studies. Mortality in EBV-driven HLH in children was 14 times higher, when etoposide was not given within 4 weeks after diagnosis [85].

The second protocol, HLH-2004 [58], intended to optimize induction treatment of HLH-94 by adding CSA to etoposide and dexamethasone up front. Additionally, intravenous immunoglobulins (IVIG) were recommended as a supportive therapy. As mortality was not significantly reduced compared to HLH-94 [86] and due to potential side effects of CSA, treatment according to HLH-2004 is no longer recommended [7, 64]. 0.4% of children developed treatment-related AML after HLH-94 treatment [62]. Cytopenias, cholestasis, or liver dysfunction secondary to HLH must not prevent initiation of etoposide therapy as they may improve with timely HLH-directed therapy. Of note, CSA was associated with increased risk of death in a systematic review with pooled analysis in adult critically ill sHLH patients, but without adjustment for disease severity [17].

There are no randomized controlled trials of sHLH in adults. Diagnostic and therapeutic decisions for sHLH in adults are mostly based on clinical experience and expert opinion. However, diagnostic and treatment recommendations are available as expert consensus for adult sHLH patients [7] and for adult critically ill sHLH patients [64].

The following simultaneous steps are decisive for acute sHLH therapy in critically ill patients:

1. Circulatory stabilization and supportive intensive care (e.g., vasopressors, mechanical ventilation, hemodialysis, transfusions, and coagulation factors)
2. Elimination of the trigger (specific pathogen- or malignancy-directed therapy) to remove the stimuli for uncontrolled immune activation
3. Immunomodulatory, immunosuppressive, or cytotoxic therapy to inhibit hyperinflammation and cell proliferation of uncontrolled cytotoxic T and NK cells

Immediate initiation of HLH-directed immunomodulatory/-suppressive treatment and therapy against the underlying trigger is essential. Adequate treatment of the underlying trigger (◻ Table 4.1) is mandatory for optimal HLH therapy and can lead to remission or prevent a relapse after discontinuation of immunosuppressive therapy. In a systematic review with pooled analysis in adult critically ill sHLH patients, 23.3% of all patients with infectious-triggered HLH were treated without immunosuppression, of whom 49.4% survived. This underscores the importance of an adequate anti-infective trigger treatment [17].

Treatment of sHLH differs from pHLH as adults may suffer from multiple comorbidities leading to a higher vulnerability of the cytokine storm and higher toxicity of immunosuppressive therapy. Therefore, the widely used pediatric HLH-94 treatment protocol needs adaption to avoid harm in adults due to toxicity and long-term immunosuppression (◻ Fig. 4.7). Type, dosage and duration of immunosuppressive treatment must be decided individually [7].

IVIG as a supportive therapy were initially included into the HLH-2004 treatment protocol and are still part of current recommendations with a total dose of up to 1.6 g/kg in split doses over three days [7, 64, 87]. IVIG have anti-inflammatory

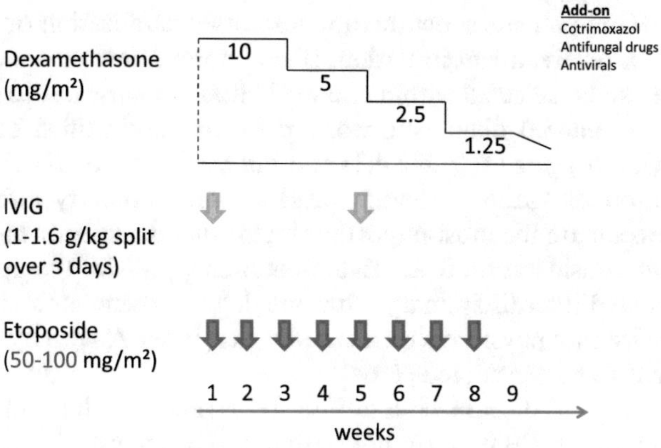

◻ **Fig. 4.7** Exemplary therapy for secondary HLH (etoposide in severe cases), modified from [37]. *IVIG* intravenous immunoglobulins

effects by blocking antibody Fc fragments and macrophage Fc receptors, inhibiting complement activation and neutralizing cytokines. Additionally, they support defective humoral immunity during deficiency of immunoglobulins, e.g., under HLH-specific immunosuppression [88]. A systematic review with pooled analysis in adult critically ill sHLH patients found an improved survival after addition of IVIG [17].

Length and intensity of immunosuppressive treatment of adult critically ill sHLH patients should be tailored to disease severity, considering underlying triggers, comorbidities, and treatment response. Addition of etoposide—to target activated T cells and reversal of defective apoptosis—in adult sHLH patients depends on the severity of illness and initial therapy response to corticosteroids within 48 h.

In mild sHLH—no evidence of organ dysfunctions—rather trigger than immunosuppressive treatment is required unless there is deterioration. In moderate sHLH—evidence of moderate organ dysfunction—corticosteroid treatment according to HLH-94 is indicated, together with supportive IVIG. In severe sHLH—evidence of severe organ dysfunction, non-response, relapse, or progression—treatment according to the HLH-94 protocol with renal- and age-adjusted etoposide dosage (reduced hematopoietic reserve in adults: 75 mg/m^2 once weekly for adults, 50 mg/m^2 once weekly for elderly) is recommended. In sHLH with CNS involvement, immediate etoposide treatment is advised to prevent deleterious effects. Importantly, disease severity can dramatically increase within hours [64]. Intrathecal therapy may be considered in patients with persisting neurologic symptoms, CSF abnormalities, and pathological MRI findings [7].

Importantly, due to the autoaggressive inflammatory process, most patients with infection-triggered sHLH require therapeutic intervention both against the trigger and immunosuppressive treatment. The latter may seem to be anti-intuitive and contraproductive, but is mandatory to prevent inflammatory lymphoproliferation, macrophage activation, and consecutive irreversible organ damage, MOF, and death [7, 64]. The major therapeutic challenge is the balance between immunosuppressive treatment inhibiting uncontrolled inflammation and desired immune reconstitution to resolve infections [89].

Normally, sHLH patients show therapy response (stabilization or improvement) within 48 hours after treatment initiation. If no improvement or deterioration after initial response can be detected within one week, non-response has to be considered. This necessitates renewed diagnostic workup for an unidentified or insufficiently treated underlying triggers (◙ Table 4.1) and intensification of HLH-directed therapy (e.g., addition of "salvage therapy"). However, secondary infections due to immunosuppression are the most important factor that determines mortality, necessitating cautious consideration to escalate immunosuppressive therapy. These cases should be evaluated interdisciplinary with oncologists, rheumatologists, infectiologists, and intensive care physicians on a case-by-case basis. Advice by an HLH reference center needs to be considered [7, 64].

For monitoring of disease course and HLH activity, ferritin, sIL-2R, cell counts, and copies of EBV-DNA are valuable parameters [7]. A retrospective study of 40 adult critically ill sHLH patients found higher ferritin values at diagnosis and during treatment in non-survivors [21]. In this study, a minimum fer-ritin of 4083 μg/L after diagnosis was predictive for 30-day mortality. CRP and fever may be early indicators of secondary infections during immunosuppressive therapy, while increases in ferritin and sIL-2R suggest relapse. Based on disease monitoring and clinical course, immunosuppressive treatment needs to be tapered as soon as possible to prevent prolonged immunosuppression and secondary infections. However, close monitoring for relapse and secondary infections is mandatory [7].

In patients with EBV-associated HLH, addition of rituximab (CD20-specific antibody to target B cells) may be effective to inhibit EBV replication in B cells [90]. Patients with continuously rising or high levels of EBV-DNA, e.g., chronic active EBV, particularly in association with relapsing lymphoma, should be evaluated for HSCT [7, 91]. A new approach in refractory EBV-associated HLH is nivolumab therapy, which led to remission in 5 out of 7 adult sHLH patients until 16-month follow-up [92]. Patients with sHLH due to intracellular infections such as tuberculo-sis, leishmaniasis, or rickettsia disease usually respond well to specific antimicrobial treatment, e.g., liposomal amphotericin as specific therapy for leishmaniasis [7, 93]. Immunosuppressive therapy is recommended in refractory cases only [7]. In sHLH due to novel immunotherapies such as CART, BiTE, and checkpoint inhibitors, HLH-specific therapy with dexamethasone should be sufficient. Patients with severe organ dysfunction may need tocilizumab. In refractory cases, etoposide is recom-mended [7].

In patients with malignancy-triggered HLH, immunosuppression with dexa-methasone and etoposide, supplemented by IVIG, as an intensified pre-phase therapy, must often precede the actual chemotherapy in order to reverse the threatening organ failure. As soon as the organ dysfunction is resolved or the patient has improved, specific malignancy-directed therapy is advocated [7, 94]. A prospective study of adult HLH patients, including pHLH and sHLH due to lymphoma or EBV, who were refractory to the HLH-94 treatment protocol, found a 76.2% response rate after salvage therapy with doxorubicin, etoposide, and methylprednisolone [95]. Of note, etoposide can be added to CHOP- or CHOP-like protocols [87]. In HLH patients with unknown trigger, splenomegaly, and high suspicion of lymphoma, splenectomy may be considered to detect hidden lymphomas in the spleen or perisplenic tissues [7]. In a retrospective study of 18 patients with refractory HLH and splenomegaly, splenectomy increased survival and confirmed lymphoma in 7 patients [96].

Further salvage therapy options include anakinra, ruxolitinib, tocilizumab, plasmapheresis, cytokine adsorption, emapalumab, CHOP-like protocols plus eto-poside, and HSCT. However, consideration of the underlying trigger is necessary [7]. The IL-1 receptor antagonist anakinra was successfully used in combination with dexamethasone and IVIG in a retrospective study [97]. Mortality of sepsis patients with features of sHLH was reduced by 47% after anakinra treatment in a reanalysis of a randomized controlled trial [98]. Variable dosages of anakinra were used within the reports: up to 10 mg/kg/day subcutaneously or intravenously, and 2 mg/kg/h as a continuous infusion over 72 h. In critically ill patients, resorption of

4

subcutaneous anakinra under high doses of catecholamines was questioned, whereas intravenous application was considered safe and effective [99]. Targeted inhibition of Janus kinase (JAK) signaling with ruxolitinib 15 mg twice daily resulted in 100% survival after 2 months in 5 adult sHLH patients [100]. A retrospective study found good therapeutic success of tocilizumab in adult sHLH patients [101]. Plasmapheresis as well as cytokine adsorption were described in case reports as effective therapeutic options [102–104]. In a prospective study, the anti-IFN-γ antibody emapalumab was an efficacious targeted therapy for relapsing and refractory pHLH and for patients with pHLH intolerant to previous HLH therapy. It is approved in the USA for the therapy of relapsing pHLH [105]. In a retrospective study, HSCT was performed in patients with malignancy-triggered sHLH. 2-year overall survival was 50.0% [84].

> Immediate initiation of therapy is decisive and should be based on the HLH-94 treatment protocol using dexamethasone and etoposide. In sHLH patients, immunosuppressive therapy needs adaption based on the triggers and underlying conditions. Most sHLH patients require dexamethasone, IVIG, and specific therapy of the underlying trigger. Etoposide should be restricted to severe sHLH. Anakinra is often used alternatively to etoposide.

4.9 Macrophage activation syndrome (MAS-HLH)

sHLH triggered by autoimmune/autoinflammatory diseases, such as systemic onset juvenile idiopathic arthritis (sJIA), AOSD, SLE, dermatomyositis, Kawasaki's disease, and rheumatoid arthritis, is historically called MAS-HLH, though official nomenclature is sHLH [7, 106]. In children with suspected sJIA, MAS-HLH can be diagnosed by separate diagnostic criteria for MAS-HLH complicating sJIA in patients not fulfilling HLH-2004 diagnostic criteria (◘ Table 4.5) [107]. Up to 10% of sJIA patients develop MAS-HLH [108]. MAS-HLH patients need a profound infectious trigger workup as they often have a prior history of immunosuppression [7]. Treatment of MAS-HLH differs from other types of sHLH: high-dose pulse methylprednisolone (30 mg/kg/day with maximum of 1 g/day, for 3–5 consecutive days) with IVIG (up to 1.6 g/kg in split doses over three days) as initial treatment. In case of insufficient response, addition of CSA (2–7 mg/kg/day) and/or anakinra (2–6–10 mg/kg/day subcutaneously) is recommended. Etoposide should only be considered in severe and refractory cases [7].

> sHLH triggered by autoimmune/autoinflammatory diseases is historically called MAS-HLH. Treatment differs from other types of sHLH. High-dose pulse methylprednisolone with IVIG is the initial treatment of choice. Anakinra or CSA instead of etoposide is recommended in case of insufficient response.

Table 4.5 Diagnostic criteria for MAS-HLH complicating sJIA [107]

Suspected or confirmed diagnosis of sJIA

Fever

Ferritin >684 µg/L

AND two of the below:

  Platelets ≤181/nL

  Aspartate aminotransferase >48 U/L

  Triglycerides >156 mg/dL

  Fibrinogen ≤3.6 g/L

Systemic onset juvenile idiopathic arthritis

4.10 HLH and Sepsis

Sepsis is characterized by an initial pro-inflammatory activation with dysregulated anti-inflammatory response, followed by immune failure and consecutive further organ dysfunctions [109]. Pathogenetic and physiological mechanisms differ between sHLH and sepsis. Both, however, share the same cause: a systemic immune dysregulation due to a specific stimulus [109]. In this context, it is important to note that both HLH and sepsis constitute syndromes, not independent diseases. "Hyperinflammatory sepsis," "hyperferritinemic sepsis," and "MAS-like sepsis" refer to sepsis patients with signs of hyperinflammation, who do not completely fulfill HLH-2004 diagnostic criteria for the diagnosis of sHLH, but have a high risk of death [110]. Whether these patients also need sHLH therapy is under investigation. Close reevaluation and aggressive sepsis therapy against the stimulus are necessary, as they can quickly develop sHLH as a sign of progressive immune failure [111]. Phenotypes of sHLH and sepsis are overlapping. Therefore, sHLH is often misdiagnosed as sepsis or evolving sHLH is not diagnosed in sepsis patients [1]. Importantly, sHLH can evolve in sepsis patients. In fact, sHLH can be triggered by the pathogen itself or the consecutive immunosuppression caused by sepsis [64, 111]. This may lead to reinfection or reactivation of viruses in sepsis patients. Patients with sHLH and underlying sepsis usually insufficiently respond to sepsis therapy, which makes immunomodulatory/-suppressive HLH treatment necessary simultaneously to sepsis therapy [64, 111]. Hyperferritinemia between 500 and 1000 µg/L is frequent in sepsis patients, but higher values require diagnostic workup for sHLH. Compared to sHLH patients, splenomegaly usually does not occur in sepsis patients under anti-infective treatment [111]. If possible, etoposide and other chemotherapeutics as sHLH therapy should be avoided in patients with coincidental bacterial sepsis [89]. An alternative may be anakinra, which showed reduced mortality of sepsis patients with features of sHLH in a reanalysis of a randomized controlled trial [64, 98]. When patients are receiving continuous intravenous hydrocortisone 200 mg/day as part of sepsis therapy, corticosteroid treatment needs to be switched to dexamethasone, or hydrocortisone dosage needs to be increased in equivalent to dexamethasone to treat sHLH [111].

sHLH can evolve in sepsis patients. It can be triggered by the pathogen itself or the consecutive immunosuppression caused by sepsis. Clinical presentations of sHLH and sepsis are overlapping. Therefore, sHLH is often misdiagnosed as sepsis or sHLH is not diagnosed in sepsis patients. Hyperferritinemia is frequent in sepsis patients. High ferritin values require diagnostic workup for sHLH and close reevaluation. Etoposide and other chemotherapeutics should be avoided in patients with coincidental bacterial sepsis. Anakinra may be an alternative.

4.11 Prognosis

Early detection and initiation of HLH-specific therapy is most relevant for prognosis. Without therapy, pHLH is invariably fatal with a median survival rate of 1–2 months [112]. The HLH-94 treatment protocol increased survival to 54%. The initial response rate was >80%. However, some patients relapsed before HSCT and post-transplant mortality was more than 30% [62]. Occurrence of MOF in the early phase of the syndrome, infections and drug side effects in the late phase—when the early phase was survived—determine the prognosis. This makes HLH one of the most critical and complicated syndromes and diseases in adults [6]. Despite HLH-specific treatment, mortality was 41% in adult sHLH patients [6] and 57.8% in adult critically ill sHLH patients [17]. In the latter cohort, differences in mortality occurred between subgroups of triggers: autoimmune/autoinflammatory diseases (26.3%), infections (56.4%), malignancies (63.2%), drug-induced (75.0%), and unknown trigger (75.8%). Relapse of HLH occurred in 25.0% of patients who initially responded, of whom 75.0% died [21]. Overall, mortality remains high for both pHLH and sHLH. To reduce mortality and improve prognosis, awareness of HLH still needs to be increased, since most of the diagnoses are delayed or missed [1]. A more rapid diagnostic workup together with investigation of pathophysiological mechanisms and novel therapy concepts may reduce immunosuppressive effects with consecutive secondary complications, which will finally improve survival in this most complex syndrome.

Early detection and initiation of HLH-specific therapy are most relevant for the prognosis. Despite HLH-specific therapy, mortality remains high for both pHLH and sHLH. A more rapid diagnostic workup together with investigation of pathophysiological mechanisms and novel therapy concepts is warranted for reduction of mortality.

4.12 Summary

HLH is a life-threatening syndrome of immune dysregulation and hyperinflammation with excessive immune activation and associated high mortality. HLH is rare with regionally different incidences. Knowledge of diagnosis and therapy is crucial for survival of patients. A relevant number of critically ill patients develops sHLH, with a high rate of undiagnosed cases due to the sepsis-like clinical presentation. The primary form in children is due to genetic defects, while the secondary form in adults is induced by trigger diseases. Underlying genetic defects impair cytotoxicity and induce hyperinflammation. Pathogenesis of sHLH is multifactorial, leading to impaired cytotoxicity and immune overactivation with a consecutive cytokine storm. The effects of the cytokine storm and the infiltration of various organs by lymphocytes and macrophages determine the clinical picture, with a wide spectrum of initial presentations, but mostly very similar to sepsis. The characteristic feature of sHLH is the triad of fever, bicytopenia, and splenomegaly, along with high levels of ferritin. Triggers and underlying conditions of sHLH depend on regional differences and age. sHLH is mainly triggered by infections, malignancies, and autoimmune/autoinflammatory diseases. A relevant number of sHLH patients are priorly immunosuppressed. Infections are the most frequent triggers in adult critically ill patients. sHLH can also evolve in sepsis patients. It can be triggered by the pathogen itself or the consecutive immunosuppression caused by sepsis. Identification of the underlying trigger is mandatory. Early detection and initiation of HLH-specific therapy is most relevant for the prognosis. Ferritin is a sensitive screening parameter and should be determined in critically ill patients with unclear septic picture to possibly initiate HLH diagnostic workup. Diagnosis of HLH should be based on HLH-2004 diagnostic criteria. HLH-2004 diagnostic criteria safely discriminate between sHLH and differential diagnoses such as sepsis. The HScore is helpful in initially unclear cases (◘ Fig. 4.8). Immediate initiation of therapy is decisive and

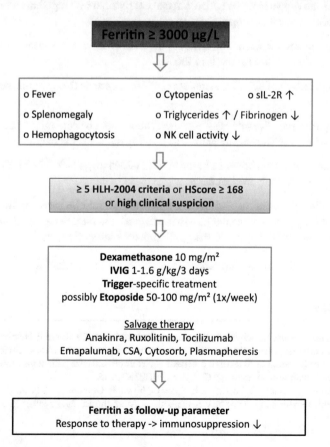

◘ **Fig. 4.8** Suggested diagnostic and therapeutic flow of sHLH, modified from [57]. *IVIG* intravenous immunoglobulins, *CSA* cyclosporine A

should be based on the HLH-94 treatment protocol, using dexamethasone and etoposide in severe cases. In sHLH patients, immunosuppressive therapy needs adaption based on the triggers and underlying conditions. Most sHLH patients require dexamethasone, IVIG, and specific therapy of the underlying trigger. Despite HLH-specific therapy, mortality remains high for both pHLH and sHLH. A high diagnostic vigilance and a more rapid diagnostic workup, together with investigation of biological mechanisms and novel therapy concepts, are warranted for reduction of mortality.

4

> **Take-Home Messages**
>
> — sHLH is a life-threatening syndrome of immune dysregulation and hyperinflammation with excessive immune activation and associated high mortality.
>
> — sHLH has a high rate of undiagnosed cases in adult critically ill patients due to the sepsis-like clinical presentation.
>
> — sHLH is mainly triggered by infections, malignancies, and autoimmune/autoinflammatory diseases. A relevant number of sHLH patients had prior immunosuppression. Identification of the underlying trigger is mandatory.
>
> — sHLH can evolve in sepsis patients. It can be triggered by the pathogen itself or the consecutive immunosuppression caused by sepsis.
>
> — The characteristic feature of sHLH is the triad of fever, bicytopenia, and splenomegaly, along with high levels of ferritin.
>
> — Early detection of sHLH and initiation of HLH-specific therapy are most relevant for survival.
>
> — Ferritin is a sensitive screening parameter and should be determined in critically ill patients with unclear septic picture to possibly initiate HLH diagnostic workup.
>
> — Diagnosis of HLH should be based on HLH-2004 diagnostic criteria. The HScore is helpful in initially unclear cases.
>
> — Immediate initiation of therapy is decisive and should be based on the HLH-94 treatment protocol with adaption to the triggers and underlying conditions. Dexamethasone and IVIG are the drugs of choice for initial therapy.

References

1. Lachmann G, Spies C, Schenk T, Brunkhorst FM, Balzer F, La Rosee P. Hemophagocytic lymphohistiocytosis: potentially underdiagnosed in intensive care units. Shock. 2018;50(2):149–55.
2. Machowicz R, Janka G, Wiktor-Jedrzejczak W. Your critical care patient may have HLH (hemophagocytic lymphohistiocytosis). Crit Care. 2016;20(1):215.
3. Lachmann G, Knaak C, La Rosee P, Spies C, Nyvlt P, Oberender C, et al. [Hemophagocytic lymphohistiocytosis in unspecific virus infection]. Anaesthesist. 2019;68(9):626–32.

4. Scott DW, Miller WH Jr, Tasker JB, Schultz RD, Meuten DJ. Lymphoreticular neoplasia in a dog resembling malignant histiocytosis (histiocytic medullary reticulosis) in man. Cornell Vet. 1979;69(3):176–97.

5. Brisse E, Wouters CH, Matthys P. Advances in the pathogenesis of primary and secondary hae-mophagocytic lymphohistiocytosis: differences and similarities. Br J Haematol. 2016;174(2):203–17.

6. Ramos-Casals M, Brito-Zeron P, Lopez-Guillermo A, Khamashta MA, Bosch X. Adult haemo-phagocytic syndrome. Lancet. 2014;383(9927):1503–16.

7. La Rosee P, Horne A, Hines M, von Bahr Greenwood T, Machowicz R, Berliner N, et al. Recommendations for the management of hemophagocytic lymphohistiocytosis in adults. Blood. 2019;133(23):2465–77.

8. Ishii E, Ohga S, Imashuku S, Yasukawa M, Tsuda H, Miura I, et al. Nationwide survey of hemo-phagocytic lymphohistiocytosis in Japan. Int J Hematol. 2007;86(1):58–65.

9. Allen CE, Yu X, Kozinetz CA, McClain KL. Highly elevated ferritin levels and the diagnosis of hemophagocytic lymphohistiocytosis. Pediatr Blood Cancer. 2008;50(6):1227–35.

10. Henter JI, Elinder G, Soder O, Ost A. Incidence in Sweden and clinical features of familial hemo-phagocytic lymphohistiocytosis. Acta Paediatr Scand. 1991;80(4):428–35.

11. Gurgey A, Gogus S, Ozyurek E, Aslan D, Gumruk F, Cetin M, et al. Primary hemophagocytic lymphohistiocytosis in Turkish children. Pediatr Hematol Oncol. 2003;20(5):367–71.

12. Biank VF, Sheth MK, Talano J, Margolis D, Simpson P, Kugathasan S, et al. Association of Crohn's disease, thiopurines, and primary epstein-barr virus infection with hemophagocytic lym-phohistiocytosis. J Pediatr. 2011;159(5):808–12.

13. Arico M, Danesino C, Pende D, Moretta L. Pathogenesis of haemophagocytic lymphohistiocy-tosis. Br J Haematol. 2001;114(4):761–9.

14. Yao S, Wang Y, Sun Y, Liu L, Zhang R, Fang J, et al. Epidemiological investigation of hemo-phagocytic lymphohistiocytosis in China. Orphanet J Rare Dis. 2021;16(1):342.

15. Gupta AA, Tyrrell P, Valani R, Benseler S, Abdelhaleem M, Weitzman S. Experience with hemo-phagocytic lymphohistiocytosis/macrophage activation syndrome at a single institution. J Pediatr Hematol Oncol. 2009;31(2):81–4.

16. Kumar G, Hererra M, Patel D, Nanchal R, Guddati AK. Outcomes of adult critically ill patients with hemophagocytic lymphohistiocytosis in united states-analysis from an administrative data-base from 2007 to 2015. Am J Blood Res. 2020;10(6):330–8.

17. Knaak C, Schuster FS, Nyvlt P, Spies C, Feinkohl I, Beutel G, et al. Treatment and mortality of hemophagocytic lymphohistiocytosis in adult critically ill patients: a systematic review with pooled analysis. Crit Care Med. 2020;48(11):e1137–46.

18. Lachmann G, Knaak C, Vorderwulbecke G, La Rosee P, Balzer F, Schenk T, et al. Hyperferritinemia in critically ill patients. Crit Care Med. 2020;48(4):459–65.

19. Buyse S, Teixeira L, Galicier L, Mariotte E, Lemiale V, Seguin A, et al. Critical care management of patients with hemophagocytic lymphohistiocytosis. Intensive Care Med. 2010;36(10):1695–702.

20. Okabe T, Shah G, Mendoza V, Hirani A, Baram M, Marik P. What intensivists need to know about hemophagocytic syndrome: an underrecognized cause of death in adult intensive care units. J Intensive Care Med. 2012;27(1):58–64.

21. Knaak C, Schuster FS, Spies C, Vorderwulbecke G, Nyvlt P, Schenk T, et al. Hemophagocytic lymphohistiocytosis in critically ill patients. Shock. 2020;53(6):701–9.

22. Zhang K, Astigarraga I, Bryceson Y, Lehmberg K, Machowicz R, Marsh R, et al. Familial hemo-phagocytic lymphohistiocytosis. In: Adam MP, Ardinger HH, Pagon RA, Wallace SE, Bean LJH, Mirzaa G, et al, editors. GeneReviews((R)). Seattle; 1993.

23. Tothova Z, Berliner N. Hemophagocytic syndrome and critical illness: new insights into diagno-sis and management. J Intensive Care Med. 2015;30(7):401–12.

24. Rouphael NG, Talati NJ, Vaughan C, Cunningham K, Moreira R, Gould C. Infections associ-ated with haemophagocytic syndrome. Lancet Infect Dis. 2007;7(12):814–22.

25. Emmenegger U, Schaer DJ, Larroche C, Neftel KA. Haemophagocytic syndromes in adults: cur-rent concepts and challenges ahead. Swiss Med Wkly. 2005;135(21–22):299–314.

26. Lehmberg K, Sprekels B, Nichols KE, Woessmann W, Muller I, Suttorp M, et al. Malignancy-associated haemophagocytic lymphohistiocytosis in children and adolescents. Br J Haematol. 2015;170(4):539–49.

27. Machaczka M, Vaktnas J, Klimkowska M, Hagglund H. Malignancy-associated hemophagocytic lymphohistiocytosis in adults: a retrospective population-based analysis from a single center. Leuk Lymphoma. 2011;52(4):613–9.

28. Sano H, Kobayashi R, Tanaka J, Hashino S, Ota S, Torimoto Y, et al. Risk factor analysis of non-Hodgkin lymphoma-associated haemophagocytic syndromes: a multicentre study. Br J Haematol. 2014;165(6):786–92.

29. Delavigne K, Berard E, Bertoli S, Corre J, Duchayne E, Demur C, et al. Hemophagocytic syndrome in patients with acute myeloid leukemia undergoing intensive chemotherapy. Haematologica. 2014;99(3):474–80.

30. Fukaya S, Yasuda S, Hashimoto T, Oku K, Kataoka H, Horita T, et al. Clinical features of haemophagocytic syndrome in patients with systemic autoimmune diseases: analysis of 30 cases. Rheumatology (Oxford). 2008;47(11):1686–91.

31. Sadaat M, Jang S. Hemophagocytic lymphohistiocytosis with immunotherapy: brief review and case report. J Immunother Cancer. 2018;6(1):49.

32. Karras A, Thervet E, Legendre C, Groupe Coopératif de transplantation d'Ile de France. Hemophagocytic syndrome in renal transplant recipients: report of 17 cases and review of literature. Transplantation. 2004;77(2):238–43.

33. Riviere S, Galicier L, Coppo P, Marzac C, Aumont C, Lambotte O, et al. Reactive hemophagocytic syndrome in adults: a retrospective analysis of 162 patients. Am J Med. 2014;127(11):1118–25.

34. Brisse E, Wouters CH, Matthys P. Hemophagocytic lymphohistiocytosis (HLH): a heterogeneous spectrum of cytokine-driven immune disorders. Cytokine Growth Factor Rev. 2015;26(3):263–80.

35. Jordan MB, Allen CE, Weitzman S, Filipovich AH, McClain KL. How I treat hemophagocytic lymphohistiocytosis. Blood. 2011;118(15):4041–52.

36. Behrens EM, Koretzky GA. Review: cytokine storm syndrome: looking toward the precision medicine era. Arthritis Rheumatol. 2017;69(6):1135–43.

37. Lachmann G, La Rosee P, Schenk T, Brunkhorst FM, Spies C. [Hemophagocytic lymphohistiocytosis: a diagnostic challenge on the ICU]. Anaesthesist. 2016;65(10):776–786.

38. Rosado FG, Kim AS. Hemophagocytic lymphohistiocytosis: an update on diagnosis and pathogenesis. Am J Clin Pathol. 2013;139(6):713–27.

39. Arceci RJ. When T cells and macrophages do not talk: the hemophagocytic syndromes. Curr Opin Hematol. 2008;15(4):359–67.

40. Carter SJ, Tattersall RS, Ramanan AV. Macrophage activation syndrome in adults: recent advances in pathophysiology, diagnosis and treatment. Rheumatology (Oxford). 2019;58(1):5–17.

41. de Kerguenec C, Hillaire S, Molinie V, Gardin C, Degott C, Erlinger S, et al. Hepatic manifestations of hemophagocytic syndrome: a study of 30 cases. Am J Gastroenterol. 2001;96(3):852–7.

42. Knutson MD, Vafa MR, Haile DJ, Wessling-Resnick M. Iron loading and erythrophagocytosis increase ferroportin 1 (FPN1) expression in J774 macrophages. Blood. 2003;102(12):4191–7.

43. Kuriyama T, Takenaka K, Kohno K, Yamauchi T, Daitoku S, Yoshimoto G, et al. Engulfment of hematopoietic stem cells caused by down-regulation of CD47 is critical in the pathogenesis of hemophagocytic lymphohistiocytosis. Blood. 2012;120(19):4058–67.

44. Janka G. Biology and treatment of hemophagocytic lymphohistiocytosis. Iran J Blood Cancer. 2018;10(4):108–13.

45. Chuang HC, Lay JD, Hsieh WC, Wang HC, Chang Y, Chuang SE, et al. Epstein-Barr virus LMP1 inhibits the expression of SAP gene and upregulates Th1 cytokines in the pathogenesis of hemophagocytic syndrome. Blood. 2005;106(9):3090–6.

46. Jenkins MR, Rudd-Schmidt JA, Lopez JA, Ramsbottom KM, Mannering SI, Andrews DM, et al. Failed CTL/NK cell killing and cytokine hypersecretion are directly linked through prolonged synapse time. J Exp Med. 2015;212(3):307–17.

47. Mao H, Tu W, Qin G, Law HK, Sia SF, Chan PL, et al. Influenza virus directly infects human natural killer cells and induces cell apoptosis. J Virol. 2009;83(18):9215–22.

48. Duncan JA, Canna SW. The NLRC4 inflammasome. Immunol Rev. 2018;281(1):115–23.

49. Janka GE, Lehmberg K. Hemophagocytic syndromes—an update. Blood Rev. 2014;28(4):135–42.

50. Zhang K, Jordan MB, Marsh RA, Johnson JA, Kissell D, Meller J, et al. Hypomorphic mutations in PRF1, MUNC13-4, and STXBP2 are associated with adult-onset familial HLH. Blood. 2011;118(22):5794–8.

51. Wang Y, Wang Z, Zhang J, Wei Q, Tang R, Qi J, et al. Genetic features of late onset primary hemophagocytic lymphohistiocytosis in adolescence or adulthood. PLoS One. 2014;9(9):e107386.

52. Miller PG, Niroula A, Ceremsak JJ, Gibson CJ, Taylor MS, Birndt S, et al. Identification of germline variants in adults with hemophagocytic lymphohistiocytosis. Blood Adv. 2020;4(5):925–9.

53. Carvelli J, Piperoglou C, Farnarier C, Vely F, Mazodier K, Audonnet S, et al. Functional and genetic testing in adults with HLH reveals an inflammatory profile rather than a cytotoxicity defect. Blood. 2020;136(5):542–52.

54. Grom AA, Villanueva J, Lee S, Goldmuntz EA, Passo MH, Filipovich A. Natural killer cell dysfunction in patients with systemic-onset juvenile rheumatoid arthritis and macrophage activation syndrome. J Pediatr. 2003;142(3):292–6.

55. Barba T, Maucort-Boulch D, Iwaz J, Bohe J, Ninet J, Hot A, et al. Hemophagocytic lymphohistiocytosis in intensive care unit: a 71-case strobe-compliant retrospective study. Medicine (Baltimore). 2015;94(51):e2318.

56. Zoller EE, Lykens JE, Terrell CE, Aliberti J, Filipovich AH, Henson PM, et al. Hemophagocytosis causes a consumptive anemia of inflammation. J Exp Med. 2011;208(6):1203–14.

57. Lachmann G. Hämophagozytische Lymphohistiozytose bei Patienten mit COVID-19. Intensiv-News. 2021;25(1/21):15–7. Abdruck mit freundlicher Genehmigung der Medicom Verlags GmbH.

58. Henter JI, Horne A, Arico M, Egeler RM, Filipovich AH, Imashuku S, et al. HLH-2004: diagnostic and therapeutic guidelines for hemophagocytic lymphohistiocytosis. Pediatr Blood Cancer. 2007;48(2):124–31.

59. Price B, Lines J, Lewis D, Holland N. Haemophagocytic lymphohistiocytosis: a fulminant syndrome associated with multiorgan failure and high mortality that frequently masquerades as sepsis and shock. S Afr Med J. 2014;104(6):401–6.

60. Lehmberg K, Ehl S. Diagnostic evaluation of patients with suspected haemophagocytic lymphohistiocytosis. Br J Haematol. 2013;160(3):275–87.

61. Bell MD, Wright RK. Fatal virus-associated hemophagocytic syndrome in a young adult producing nontraumatic splenic rupture. J Forensic Sci. 1992;37(5):1407–17.

62. Trottestam H, Horne A, Arico M, Egeler RM, Filipovich AH, Gadner H, et al. Chemoimmunotherapy for hemophagocytic lymphohistiocytosis: long-term results of the HLH-94 treatment protocol. Blood. 2011;118(17):4577–84.

63. Horne A, Wickstrom R, Jordan MB, Yeh EA, Naqvi A, Henter JI, et al. How to treat involvement of the central nervous system in hemophagocytic lymphohistiocytosis? Curr Treat Options Neurol. 2017;19(1):3.

64. Hines MR, von Bahr Greenwood T, Beutel G, Beutel K, Hays JA, Horne A, et al. Consensus-based guidelines for the recognition, diagnosis, and management of hemophagocytic lymphohistiocytosis in critically ill children and adults. Crit Care Med. 2022;50(5):860–72.

65. Henter JI, Elinder G, Ost A. Diagnostic guidelines for hemophagocytic lymphohistiocytosis. The FHL Study Group of the Histiocyte Society. Semin Oncol. 1991;18(1):29–33.

66. Knaak C, Nyvlt P, Schuster FS, Spies C, Heeren P, Schenk T, et al. Hemophagocytic lymphohistiocytosis in critically ill patients: diagnostic reliability of HLH-2004 criteria and HScore. Crit Care. 2020;24(1):244.

67. Knovich MA, Storey JA, Coffman LG, Torti SV, Torti FM. Ferritin for the clinician. Blood Rev. 2009;23(3):95–104.

68. Lehmberg K, McClain KL, Janka GE, Allen CE. Determination of an appropriate cut-off value for ferritin in the diagnosis of hemophagocytic lymphohistiocytosis. Pediatr Blood Cancer. 2014;61(11):2101–3.

69. Debaugnies F, Mahadeb B, Nagant C, Meuleman N, De Bels D, Wolff F, et al. Biomarkers for early diagnosis of hemophagocytic lymphohistiocytosis in critically ill patients. J Clin Immunol. 2021;41(3):658–65.

70. Sackett K, Cunderlik M, Sahni N, Killeen AA, Olson AP. Extreme hyperferritinemia: causes and impact on diagnostic reasoning. Am J Clin Pathol. 2016;145(5):646–50.

71. Knaak C, Schuster FS, Nyvlt P, Heeren P, Spies C, Schenk T, et al. Influence of transfusions, hemodialysis and extracorporeal life support on hyperferritinemia in critically ill patients. PLoS One. 2021;16(7):e0254345.

72. Cullis JO, Fitzsimons EJ, Griffiths WJ, Tsochatzis E, Thomas DW, British Society for Haematology. Investigation and management of a raised serum ferritin. Br J Haematol. 2018;181(3):331–40.

73. Hayden A, Lin M, Park S, Pudek M, Schneider M, Jordan MB, et al. Soluble interleukin-2 receptor is a sensitive diagnostic test in adult HLH. Blood Adv. 2017;1(26):2529–34.

74. Goel S, Polski JM, Imran H. Sensitivity and specificity of bone marrow hemophagocytosis in hemophagocytic lymphohistiocytosis. Ann Clin Lab Sci. 2012;42(1):21–5.

75. Henter JI, Samuelsson-Horne A, Arico M, Egeler RM, Elinder G, Filipovich AH, et al. Treatment of hemophagocytic lymphohistiocytosis with HLH-94 immunochemotherapy and bone marrow transplantation. Blood. 2002;100(7):2367–73.

76. Rubin TS, Zhang K, Gifford C, Lane A, Bleesing JJ, Marsh RA. Perforin and CD107a testing are superior to NK cell function testing for screening patients for genetic HLH. Blood. 2017;129(22):2993–9.

77. Bryceson YT, Pende D, Maul-Pavicic A, Gilmour KC, Ufheil H, Vraetz T, et al. A prospective evaluation of degranulation assays in the rapid diagnosis of familial hemophagocytic syndromes. Blood. 2012;119(12):2754–63.

78. Fardet L, Galicier L, Lambotte O, Marzac C, Aumont C, Chahwan D, et al. Development and validation of the HScore, a score for the diagnosis of reactive hemophagocytic syndrome. Arthritis Rheumatol. 2014;66(9):2613–20.

79. Bains A, Mamone L, Aneja A, Bromberg M. Lymphoid malignancy-associated hemophagocytic lymphohistiocytosis: search for the hidden source. Ann Diagn Pathol. 2017;28:37–42.

80. Tsuji T, Hirano T, Yamasaki H, Tsuji M, Tsuda H. A high sIL-2R/ferritin ratio is a useful marker for the diagnosis of lymphoma-associated hemophagocytic syndrome. Ann Hematol. 2014;93(5):821–6.

81. Yuan L, Kan Y, Meeks JK, Ma D, Yang J. 18F-FDG PET/CT for identifying the potential causes and extent of secondary hemophagocytic lymphohistiocytosis. Diagn Interv Radiol. 2016;22(5):471–5.

82. Kim J, Yoo SW, Kang SR, Bom HS, Song HC, Min JJ. Clinical implication of F-18 FDG PET/CT in patients with secondary hemophagocytic lymphohistiocytosis. Ann Hematol. 2014;93(4):661–7.

83. Henter JI, Arico M, Egeler RM, Elinder G, Favara BE, Filipovich AH, et al. HLH-94: a treatment protocol for hemophagocytic lymphohistiocytosis. HLH study Group of the Histiocyte Society. Med Pediatr Oncol. 1997;28(5):342–7.

84. Fu L, Wang J, Wei N, Wu L, Wang Y, Huang W, et al. Allogeneic hematopoietic stem-cell transplantation for adult and adolescent hemophagocytic lymphohistiocytosis: a single center analysis. Int J Hematol. 2016;104(5):628–35.

85. Imashuku S, Kuriyama K, Teramura T, Ishii E, Kinugawa N, Kato M, et al. Requirement for etoposide in the treatment of Epstein-Barr virus-associated hemophagocytic lymphohistiocytosis. J Clin Oncol. 2001;19(10):2665–73.

86. Bergsten E, Horne A, Arico M, Astigarraga I, Egeler RM, Filipovich AH, et al. Confirmed efficacy of etoposide and dexamethasone in HLH treatment: long-term results of the cooperative HLH-2004 study. Blood. 2017;130(25):2728–38.

87. La Rosee P. Treatment of hemophagocytic lymphohistiocytosis in adults. Hematology Am Soc Hematol Educ Program. 2015;2015:190–6.

88. Emmenegger U, Spaeth PJ, Neftel KA. Intravenous immunoglobulin for hemophagocytic lymphohistiocytosis? J Clin Oncol. 2002;20(2):599–601.

89. Janka GE, Lehmberg K. Hemophagocytic lymphohistiocytosis: pathogenesis and treatment. Hematology Am Soc Hematol Educ Program. 2013;2013:605–11.

90. Chellapandian D, Das R, Zelley K, Wiener SJ, Zhao H, Teachey DT, et al. Treatment of Epstein Barr virus-induced haemophagocytic lymphohistiocytosis with rituximab-containing chemo-immunotherapeutic regimens. Br J Haematol. 2013;162(3):376–82.

91. Sawada A, Inoue M, Kawa K. How we treat chronic active Epstein-Barr virus infection. Int J Hematol. 2017;105(4):406–18.

92. Liu P, Pan X, Chen C, Niu T, Shuai X, Wang J, et al. Nivolumab treatment of relapsed/refractory Epstein-Barr virus-associated hemophagocytic lymphohistiocytosis in adults. Blood. 2020;135(11):826–33.

93. Bode SF, Bogdan C, Beutel K, Behnisch W, Greiner J, Henning S, et al. Hemophagocytic lymphohistiocytosis in imported pediatric visceral leishmaniasis in a nonendemic area. J Pediatr. 2014;165(1):147–153.e1.

94. Daver N, McClain K, Allen CE, Parikh SA, Otrock Z, Rojas-Hernandez C, et al. A consensus review on malignancy-associated hemophagocytic lymphohistiocytosis in adults. Cancer. 2017;123(17):3229–40.

95. Wang Y, Huang W, Hu L, Cen X, Li L, Wang J, et al. Multicenter study of combination DEP regimen as a salvage therapy for adult refractory hemophagocytic lymphohistiocytosis. Blood. 2015;126(19):2186–92.

96. Jing-Shi W, Yi-Ni W, Lin W, Zhao W. Splenectomy as a treatment for adults with relapsed hemophagocytic lymphohistiocytosis of unknown cause. Ann Hematol. 2015;94(5):753–60.

97. Wohlfarth P, Agis H, Gualdoni GA, Weber J, Staudinger T, Schellongowski P, et al. Interleukin 1 receptor antagonist anakinra, intravenous immunoglobulin, and corticosteroids in the management of critically ill adult patients with hemophagocytic lymphohistiocytosis. J Intensive Care Med. 2019;34(9):723–31.

98. Shakoory B, Carcillo JA, Chatham WW, Amdur RL, Zhao H, Dinarello CA, et al. Interleukin-1 receptor blockade is associated with reduced mortality in sepsis patients with features of macrophage activation syndrome: reanalysis of a prior phase III trial. Crit Care Med. 2016;44(2):275–81.

99. Mehta P, Cron RQ, Hartwell J, Manson JJ, Tattersall RS. Silencing the cytokine storm: the use of intravenous anakinra in haemophagocytic lymphohistiocytosis or macrophage activation syndrome. Lancet Rheumatol. 2020;2(6):e358–67.

100. Ahmed A, Merrill SA, Alsawah F, Bockenstedt P, Campagnaro E, Devata S, et al. Ruxolitinib in adult patients with secondary haemophagocytic lymphohistiocytosis: an open-label, single-centre, pilot trial. Lancet Haematol. 2019;6(12):e630–7.

101. Dufranc E, Del Bello A, Belliere J, Kamar N, Faguer S, TAIDI (Toulouse Acquired Immune Deficiency and Infection) Study Group. IL6-R blocking with tocilizumab in critically ill patients with hemophagocytic syndrome. Crit Care. 2020;24(1):166.

102. Nusshag C, Morath C, Zeier M, Weigand MA, Merle U, Brenner T. Hemophagocytic lymphohistiocytosis in an adult kidney transplant recipient successfully treated by plasmapheresis: a case report and review of the literature. Medicine (Baltimore). 2017;96(50):e9283.

103. Frimmel S, Schipper J, Henschel J, Yu TT, Mitzner SR, Koball S. First description of single-pass albumin dialysis combined with cytokine adsorption in fulminant liver failure and hemophagocytic syndrome resulting from generalized herpes simplex virus 1 infection. Liver Transplant. 2014;20(12):1523–4.

104. Greil C, Roether F, La Rosee P, Grimbacher B, Duerschmied D, Warnatz K. Rescue of cytokine storm due to HLH by hemoadsorption in a CTLA4-deficient patient. J Clin Immunol. 2017;37(3):273–6.

105. Locatelli F, Jordan MB, Allen C, Cesaro S, Rizzari C, Rao A, et al. Emapalumab in children with primary hemophagocytic lymphohistiocytosis. N Engl J Med. 2020;382(19):1811–22.

106. Ramanan AV, Baildam EM. Macrophage activation syndrome is hemophagocytic lymphohistiocytosis—need for the right terminology. J Rheumatol. 2002;29(5):1105; author reply

107. Ravelli A, Minoia F, Davi S, Horne A, Bovis F, Pistorio A, et al. 2016 classification criteria for macrophage activation syndrome complicating systemic juvenile idiopathic arthritis: a European League Against Rheumatism/American College of Rheumatology/Paediatric Rheumatology International Trials Organisation Collaborative Initiative. Arthritis Rheumatol. 2016;68(3):566–76.

108. Behrens EM, Beukelman T, Paessler M, Cron RQ. Occult macrophage activation syndrome in patients with systemic juvenile idiopathic arthritis. J Rheumatol. 2007;34(5):1133–8.

109. Rubio I, Osuchowski MF, Shankar-Hari M, Skirecki T, Winkler MS, Lachmann G, et al. Current gaps in sepsis immunology: new opportunities for translational research. Lancet Infect Dis. 2019;19(12):e422–36.

110. Kyriazopoulou E, Leventogiannis K, Norrby-Teglund A, Dimopoulos G, Pantazi A, Orfanos SE, et al. Macrophage activation-like syndrome: an immunological entity associated with rapid progression to death in sepsis. BMC Med. 2017;15(1):172.
111. Machowicz R, Janka G, Wiktor-Jedrzejczak W. Similar but not the same: differential diagnosis of HLH and sepsis. Crit Rev Oncol Hematol. 2017;114:1–12.
112. Janka GE. Familial hemophagocytic lymphohistiocytosis. Eur J Pediatr. 1983;140(3):221–30.

4

Extracorporeal Circulation-Related Immune Response

Katrina K. Ki, Silver Heinsar, Daman Langguth, and John F. Fraser

Contents

- To describe the immune dysregulation associated with extracorporeal circulations, notably renal replacement therapy (RRT) and extracorporeal membrane oxygenation (ECMO)
- To explain the factors that contribute to immune dysregulation related to RRT and ECMO
- To appreciate the need for increased immunological knowledge to prompt measures that deliver risk-stratified, targeted and patient-centred care

5.1 Introduction

Extracorporeal circulation (ECC) refers to artificial devices carrying blood outside of the body to temporarily assume an organ's function. In the intensive care unit (ICU), patients can be exposed to various ECCs such as **renal replacement therapy (RRT)**, **extracorporeal membrane oxygenation (ECMO)**, extracorporeal carbon dioxide removal ($ECCO_2R$) and blood purification procedures. Recent developments in ECC technologies have improved the management of critically ill patients. Yet, while life-saving, the long-term outcomes of patients treated with these modalities remain suboptimal and they suffer from high re-hospitalisation and mortality rates. Importantly, initiation of ECC devices elicits dysregulation of the physiological immune response, predisposing patients to complications such as systemic inflammatory response syndrome (SIRS), infections, secondary organ dysfunction, bleeding, and thrombosis. Alteration of the humoral and cellular immune response is triggered when blood interfaces with the foreign and non-endothelialised surfaces of the extracorporeal circuits. Notably, ECC provokes:
1. Activation of contact and complement systems
2. Activation of peripheral pro-inflammatory responses
3. Modulation of closely regulated blood leukocyte subsets and their interactions with platelets and endothelial cells

All of the above play a significant role in maintaining immune homeostasis.

In addition to ECC-related immunomodulatory effects, the underlying disease and other medical interventions all influence the delicate balance of the immune response in ICU patients. This complicates the ability to quantify the magnitude of immune modulation attributable to a specific ECC. Given that immune homeostasis is paramount to defending the host from disease, better characterisation of the immunological signatures related to these procedures could facilitate patient risk stratification and prognosis. Additionally, by optimising circuit design, pump strategies and materials, we may lessen their immunomodulatory effects, thus limiting complications and improving patient outcomes.

This chapter provides an overview of the current pathophysiological understanding of the immune response related to two of the most commonly used ECCs in the ICU, RRT and ECMO. It also discusses how different ECC designs and materials, as well as other factors (clinical therapies and ECC-related stressors), can influence immune modulation. It highlights how changes in the immune system imposed by ECC can affect patient outcomes in the ICU. Finally, shortcomings in the literature and priorities for future research are addressed.

5.2   Extracorporeal Circulations in ICU Practice

Amongst the different forms of ECC used in intensive care management, RRT and ECMO are the most common. These interventions are used to replace the function of vital organs when other therapeutic resources have been exhausted. While RRT is used to replace the normal blood-filtering function of the kidneys, ECMO can provide gas exchange and/or sustain organ perfusion, depending on whether the lungs, heart or both are in refractory failure.

5.2.1   Renal Replacement Therapy

Modern RRT originates from the works of Scottish chemist Thomas Graham, the inventor of a so-called dialyser—a device with the ability to separate colloids from crystalloids. Following persistent efforts to improve the technology, RRT has now emerged as a frontline therapy for treating critically ill patients with acute kidney injury (AKI) [1]. Patients with AKI may require RRT if they experience an acute decrease in glomerular filtration rate and have developed, or are at risk of developing, a clinically significant solute imbalance/toxicity or volume overload. As RRT has become more available, population demographics have changed (ageing population) and the prevalence of type 2 diabetes has increased, use of RRT has increased exponentially [2, 3], with ~14% of critically ill patients admitted to ICUs receiving RRT [4–6].

The RRT system is connected to a double-lumen wide-bore central venous catheter and comprises an extracorporeal circuit, including a roller pump to adjust blood flow velocity and a semi-permeable hollow fibre polysulphone membrane (◘ Fig. 5.1). The latter ensures selective transport of waste solutes and fluid while maintaining intravascular compartmentalisation of blood cells and proteins.

Of the approximately 60% of patients within the ICU who develop AKI, two-thirds require RRT. The latter can be achieved in one of the three ways:

- Continuous renal replacement therapy (CRRT)
- Intermittent haemodialysis (IHD)
- Peritoneal dialysis (PD, seldom used in adults)

Most procedures (75%) are performed with a continuous modality (CRRT), which includes any RRT that is planned to be used for 24 h per day in the ICU [6]. CRRT is particularly beneficial for haemodynamically unstable patients as it allows for slow (100–200 mL/min) and isotonic removal of large volumes of fluid. Nevertheless, CRRT has its limitations as it requires anticoagulation and is associated with increased cost. Depending on the patient requirements and clinician preferences, several CRRT modalities are available. Continuous venovenous haemofiltration

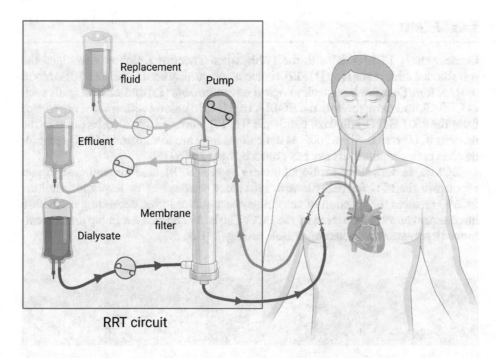

□ Fig. 5.1 Components of the renal replacement therapy (RRT) circuit. Blood is accessed via a central venous catheter with two wide-bore lumens, pumped into the membrane filter and returned into the patient through the second lumen. The RRT circuit can include dialysate, replacement fluid or both. (Figure created with ► BioRender.com)

uses convection, where high ultrafiltration rates force solutes and plasma water across the semi-permeable membrane, while a pump infuses replacement fluid into the blood. Alternatively, in continuous venovenous haemodialysis, solutes and plasma can move from the semi-permeable membrane into the dialysate compartment of the filter by means of diffusion. Finally, solutes and plasma can be removed by a combination of diffusion, convection and ultrafiltration in continuous haemodiafiltration.

IHD is an alternative to CRRT for more haemodynamically stable patients and provides rapid (300–400 mL/min) and effective removal of fluid and solutes within 3–5 h. While IHD is cost effective, does not require anticoagulation and decreases the risk of bleeding, it can cause significant haemodynamic instability in critically ill patients. Due to the preferential use of CRRT in haemodynamically unstable patients and limited availability of IHD in all centres, high-quality evidence comparing CRRT and IHD is limited [7]. The shortcomings of CRRT and IHD have led to an increasing use of sustained low-efficiency daily dialysis, a variant of IHD which can be used between 8 and 12 h per day with lower blood-pump speeds (200 mL/min) and slower solute clearance [8]. It is associated with less haemodynamic instability than IHD and provides excellent solute control [9, 10]. In summary, RRT can be achieved by several complementary modalities, determined by the clinical condition of the patient and resources within the ICU.

5.2.2 ECMO

Contemporary ECMO dates to the 1970s, when Theodor Kolobow developed the spiral coiled membrane lung [11, 12], replacing previously used bubble and disc blood oxygenators. Decades later, technological advancements [13] and clinical trials such as CESAR and more recently the EOLIA trial [14, 15], along with clinical experience from the 2009 H1N1 influenza pandemic [16, 17], have consolidated its place in the modern ICU arsenal. Since 2009, as indications have broadened and ECMO technology has been simplified, its use has grown by over 300% [18].

5

ECMO is a derivate of cardiopulmonary bypass (CPB), used for temporary organ support in the ICU for patients with refractory cardiac and/or respiratory failure. ECMO replaces the function of the native heart and/or lungs, depending on disease involvement and configuration of the ECC. The latter comprises a pump and a membrane oxygenator connected by flexible tubing (◘ Fig. 5.2).

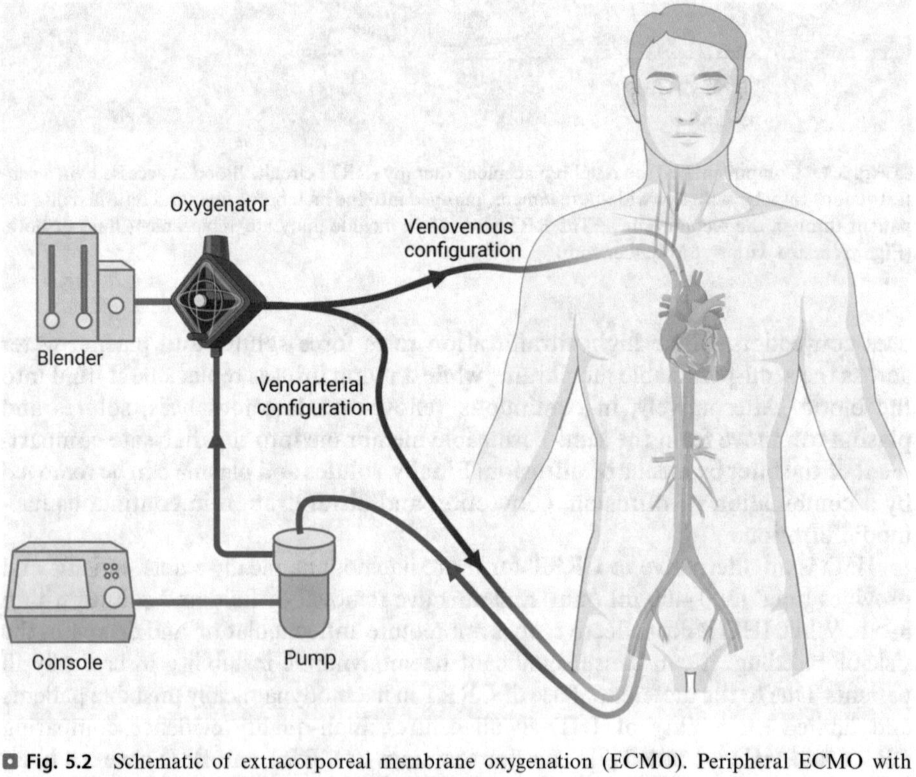

◘ **Fig. 5.2** Schematic of extracorporeal membrane oxygenation (ECMO). Peripheral ECMO with femoral vein drainage. ECMO pump drives blood movement through a membrane oxygenator, ensuring gas exchange (oxygenation and CO_2 removal) via a semi-permeable membrane. Oxygenated blood can then be returned to the body via the arterial (venoarterial ECMO) or venous (venovenous ECMO) system, depending on heart and lung involvement. (Figure created with ► BioRender.com)

In essence, ECMO drains blood from a major vein, pumps it through a membrane oxygenator and returns it into the body through a large vein (venovenous or VV ECMO) or artery (venoarterial or VA ECMO). The former is used for isolated refractory lung failure, as the membrane oxygenator provides gas exchange (blood oxygenation and CO_2 removal), after which blood is returned to the venous system [19, 20]. In venoarterial configuration, ECMO establishes a parallel circulation, with most of the circulation bypassing the heart and lungs to reinstate organ perfusion through a major artery distal to the heart. Hence, VA ECMO is predominantly indicated for refractory cardiogenic shock (with or without pulmonary failure), a state of decreased cardiac output due to low contractility with resultant end-organ hypoperfusion refractory to conventional measures. In comparison with RRT, typical ECMO pump speeds achieve a blood flow of 4–5 L/min, an approximately 20 times higher recirculation volume applied continuously throughout the day.

While RRT and ECMO are life-saving modalities, both have been associated with an increased risk of infections [21–23], bleeding and thrombosis [18, 24–27] and development of secondary organ dysfunction [18, 28], with clear links to alteration of the physiological immune response. Despite impressive progress in ECC technologies and clinical management, these complications remain frequent and modify patient outcomes. To improve patient outcomes, there is an urgent need to expand our understanding of the immune mechanisms underpinning the complications associated with ECC.

5.3 Extracorporeal Circulation-Related Immune Response and the Clinical Implications

Initiation of ECCs is known to elicit secondary humoral and cellular immune responses on top of the patient's primary disease burden (◻ Fig. 5.3). It is triggered when blood interfaces with the foreign and non-endothelialised surfaces of the extracorporeal circuits, leading to aberrant modulations of the:
- Contact and complement system
- Inflammatory cytokine and chemokine response
- Leukocytes and their interactions with platelets and endothelial cells

Dysregulation of these vital responses exerts a domino effect that creates a self-activation feedback loop. This results in amplification of the immune processes, which can predispose patients to infections, bleeding and thrombosis and development of secondary organ dysfunction (e.g. AKI).

5

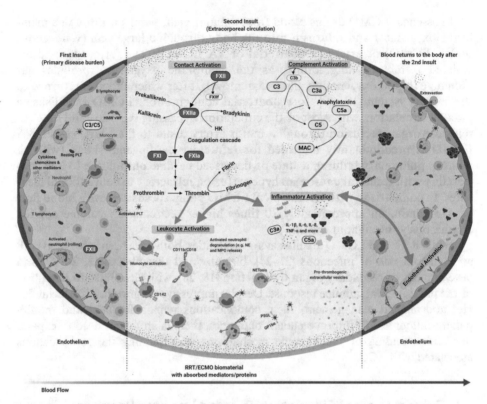

◘ Fig. 5.3 Model of extracorporeal circulation as a second immune insult: Basic representation of immune modulation associated with renal replacement therapy (RRT) and extracorporeal membrane oxygenation (ECMO). *First insult:* Immune modulation derived from the patient's primary disease burden. *Second insult:* Activation of the contact pathway (factor XII (FXII), prekallikrein (PK), high-molecular-weight kininogen (HK)), coagulation cascade and complement system, and the inflammatory response to extracorporeal circulation is proposed to activate upon contact of blood with the non-endothelialised surfaces of the circuits and is further amplified by the surrounding non-physiological conditions. Extracorporeal circulation-mediated promotion of pro-inflammatory cytokines and chemokines and activation of other mediators (e.g. complement products) can lead to additional activation of leukocyte subpopulations. Innate immune neutrophils and monocytes are the first to activate with an increased expression of surface integrins cluster differentiation (CD)11b and CD18. The modulated integrin expression potentiates an increase in leukocyte adhesion to the membrane filter/oxygenator, as well as to activated endothelium (e.g. increased intercellular adhesion molecule (ICAM)-1) expression) and platelets (PLT, e.g. increased P-selectin glycoprotein ligand-1 (PSGL) and glycoprotein Ib alpha polypeptide (GPIbα) expression). Neutrophil degranulation, neutrophil extracellular trap (NET)osis, monocyte tissue factor expression, pro-thrombogenic extracellular vesicle release and modulation of downstream lymphocytes are also promoted as blood continues to circulate extracorporeally. If such dysregulation is unresolved, it can contribute to the development of systemic inflammatory response syndrome (SIRS), secondary infections and end-organ damage, but also bleeding and thrombosis in the critically ill patients who require RRT and ECMO. (Figure created with ▶ BioRender.com)

5.3.1 Contact and Complement System

Contact System

RRT and ECMO are known to alter the contact system, a cascade structure that interfaces between inflammation, immunity and coagulation. Close interaction of blood with ECC provokes intrinsic activation of the pro-inflammatory kallikrein-kinin system and the pro-coagulation pathway, governed by various serine proteases. In particular, the active form of serine protease factor XII (factor XIIa) is assumed to be immediately generated and converts plasma prekallikrein (PK) and high-molecular-weight kininogen (HK) into their respective pro-inflammatory active forms, kallikrein and bradykinin. Production of these factors stimulates systemic inflammatory response and activates neutrophils [29–32], which contributes to the SIRS in ECMO patients. Studies have reported a rapid peak in factor XIIa and kallikrein activities following ECMO initiation [29, 31, 32]. However, the relevance of the same concept remains debatable in RRT [33, 34]. While bradykinin activity has yet to be investigated in ECMO, it is known to increase in CPB and stimulate tumour necrosis factor (TNF)-α, interleukin (IL)-10 and nitric oxide release [35, 36]. As for RRT, studies suggest that endogenous bradykinin contributes to increased production of monocyte chemoattractant protein 1 (MCP-1) and plasminogen activator inhibitor 1 (PAI-1) antigen, which further enhances the production of bradykinin and decreases its degradation, hence amplifying the inflammatory response to RRT [37].

In parallel, ECC-mediated contact activation also triggers intrinsic (surface activation) and extrinsic (tissue factor) activation of coagulation pathways, resulting in thrombin generation and clotting [38, 39]. In turn, increased thrombin production can provoke leukocyte and platelet activation and adherence as it upregulates surface expression of adhesion molecules on endothelial cells. It also mediates the release of platelet-activating factor (PAF) that potentiates leukocyte and platelet activation with degranulation. Clinically, the impaired haemostasis and cellular activation associated with ECCs may have, in part, contributed to the reported 5.6- to 12-fold increased risk for thrombotic events in RRT patients [40], as well as the 40% thrombosis rate in ECMO patients [18, 24]. In addition, this hypercoagulable state is known to simultaneously deplete platelets and clotting factors. Hence, patients treated with these modalities have an increased risk of bleeding owing to the interference in the delicate equilibrium of haemostasis [41]. This is critical since RRT and ECMO patients are often on local or systemic anticoagulation to suppress clot formation and subjected to haemodilution, which reduces platelet numbers and can result in excessive bleeding. In such conditions, whole-blood coagulation assays are highly beneficial for monitoring this delicate balance between thrombosis and bleeding as they also account for the cellular interactions in the coagulation cascade.

Complement System

The completement system is another humoral cascade system that is modulated during RRT and ECMO. If its activation is unregulated, it can hinder the host innate immune response. In parallel with the production of kallikrein during ECC-related contact activation, continuous production of anaphylatoxins complement component (C)3a and C5a and activation of the membrane attack complex (MAC) are triggered. For ECCs, dysregulation in complement activity stems from the lack of endothelial cells on the biomaterial lining of the extracorporeal circuits, which usually act as surface inhibitors of complement component hydrolysis. Consequently, these changes stimulate clot formation and can lead to thrombotic events. In addition to precipitating thrombosis, generation and degradation of C3a and C5a during ECC can have an immunomodulatory anaphylactic effect as they promote recruitment and activation of leukocytes. This induces the synthesis of pro-inflammatory cytokines and chemokines [42, 43].

Modulation of the complement system occurs immediately upon initiation of ECMO [31, 44–49], similarly in CPB [50], plasmapheresis [51] and immunoadsorption [52]. For RRT, while some studies observed a similar increase, others did not [44, 47–49, 53, 54]. Variance in the outcomes of these studies can be associated with differences in the modality of RRT (CRRT vs. IHD), type of membrane and patient cohort.

5.3.2 Inflammatory Cytokine and Chemokine Response

Cytokines and chemokines are key mediators in the systemic inflammatory response to ECCs. If local control is lost, these proteins can initiate a reciprocal cycle of immune activation, SIRS and further immune dysregulation. Several IL cytokines and chemokines have been frequently implicated in the acute-phase reaction during supportive procedures. As reported for CPB [55], the main ILs involved in the inflammatory response to RRT and ECMO are IL-1β, IL-6, IL-8 and IL-10.

Of the IL-1 family, IL-1β is one of the most widely studied subtypes with potent inflammatory effect. After initiation of RRT and ECMO, upregulation of plasma IL-1β [56] with increased gene expression in leukocytes has been reported [57]. Consequently, this provokes leukocytes and endothelial cells to synthesise IL-6 and IL-8.

IL-6 is one of the most pleotropic cytokines and serves as both a pro- and an anti-inflammatory mediator. During ECMO, IL-6 concentration rapidly increases within the first 2–3 h, consistently reported across a mixture of clinical [31, 58–60], ex vivo [56] and animal studies [61–63]. A similar observation has been reported for RRT [64, 65]. As expected for a key acute-phase reactant, its production is also closely coupled to C-reactive protein (CRP) concentrations in RRT and ECMO [58, 66]. Both have been inversely associated with survival [58].

Unlike IL-1β and IL-6, IL-8 is a chemokine, a potent activator and attractor for neutrophils. Levels of IL-8 increase rapidly after initiation of ECMO in ex vivo and animal models [62, 67]. This surge is detected within 15 min of initiation of RRT and ECMO in neonates [60, 68]. It can increase neutrophil activation with subsequent recruitment to tissues, triggering an overwhelming activation of the immune response with resultant secondary organ damage.

In conjunction with previously described IL cytokines and chemokines, elevated levels of TNF-α have been reported during RRT and ECMO [56, 62, 63, 69]. TNF-α is a multifaceted cytokine tasked with a critical role of mediating the inflammatory and immune response via paracrine and endocrine signalling. However, when leukocytes of ECMO patients were stimulated with endotoxin in vitro to perform a function test, suppressed production of TNF-α was reported [70]. This is consistent with Beshish and colleagues' definition of innate immunoparalysis (serum TNF-α concentration <200 pg/mL after in vitro LPS induction) induced by ECMO [71], which has been associated with infections.

Furthermore, it must be noted that the immunomodulatory effects of RRT, unlike ECMO, have not been associated with the aberrant unidirectional increase of cytokines and chemokines. On the contrary, in some studies, RRT has been shown to be beneficial with lower levels of various pro-inflammatory mediators in patients with sepsis, uraemia, AKI and chronic kidney disease [72–75], as well as when integrated within the ECMO circuit in vivo [76–79]. Its capacity to reduce tissue damage, inflammatory response and complement activation and mitochondrial injury has been demonstrated in both clinical and pre-clinical studies [54, 76–80]. These effects preserve immune homeostasis and prevent secondary organ dysfunction development. Given that the central function of RRT is to remove fluids and solutes, this is not surprising. Conflicting reports about the advantages and disadvantages of RRT are likely caused by the differences of the RRT modality, sieving coefficient, dose and membrane type in combination with differences in the patients' underlying disease burden.

5.3.3 Leukocytes

Aside from modulated humoral responses, ECCs also trigger cellular changes in the immune system. Cellular immunity is mainly mediated by leukocytes, which are crucial to the communication between the innate and adaptive immune responses. They also play a multifaceted role in the regulation and stimulation of inflammatory responses and immune tolerance [81] and contribute to coagulation through interaction with platelets and endothelial cells [82–86]. The sequelae linked to ECC-mediated inappropriate leukocyte modulation, resulting in a secondary immunological insult, can be detrimental in critically ill patients [87–92]. This section will focus on the four closely regulated and interdependent major peripheral leukocyte subsets of innate and adaptive immunity: neutrophils, monocytes and T and B lymphocytes.

Impact on the Innate Immune Leukocytes: Neutrophils and Monocytes

In RRT and ECMO, neutrophils and monocytes are the most studied peripheral leukocytes, likely due to their abundant expression and critical role in initiating rapid immune responses and determining the direction of downstream adaptive immunity. Studies investigating RRT and ECMO have consistently reported a dramatic drop in neutrophil and monocyte counts, which can occur within 2 h after initiation [93–99]. These may, in part, result from haemodilution and increased neutrophil and monocyte adhesion to the circuit membrane [100], platelets and endothelium [82–86] as they become activated during ECCs. Slow or delayed recovery of monocytes has been associated with worse prognosis and mortality in both VA and VV ECMO patients [99]. In particular, low number of cluster of differentiation (CD)14$^+$CD16$^+$ and CD14$^+$ toll-like receptor (TLR)4$^+$ monocyte subsets correlates with mortality [99]. A similar reduction trend for monocyte counts has been reported in RRT patients [101], and different subpopulations are found to be affected at different rates.

Impact on Neutrophil Phenotype and Function

In addition to numeric alterations, previous research has characterised several alterations of leukocyte phenotypes in association with RRT and ECMO. Activation of neutrophils during ECMO is largely triggered by increased surface expression of CD11b and CD18 [60, 62, 63, 67, 97, 102–104]. They are essential integrins which regulate adhesion and migration of leukocytes that mediate the inflammatory response. The expression of these integrins is also upregulated during RRT [105, 106]. CD11b upregulation increases after commencement of RRT and shows similar patterns when blood is stimulated with C5a in vitro, suggesting the role of artificial membrane-induced complement activation [106]. Analogous phenotypic modulation of neutrophils has been reported for other ECC patients such as those on CPB [107, 108], but their expression begins to downregulate 3–4 h after initiation of ECMO, and this inhibition can persist for a prolonged duration [60, 62, 102]. Neutrophil functional changes with reduced phagocytic activity are seen as early as in 30 min of RRT, resulting in increased susceptibility to infections during early RRT support [109]. However, neutrophil phagocytic function tends to recover after 24 h of RRT. Similar patterns have been observed for other innate immune cells [102], which could be linked to an upregulation of adhesion molecules or binding with ligands as part of the enhanced activation process during RRT and ECMO. Such activation can hinder a crucial host immune defence process of leukocyte/neutrophil transendothelial and trans-epithelial migration to areas of inflammation, leading to secondary organ injuries if uncontrolled [61, 110].

Another sign of neutrophil activation is the significant degranulation of neutrophil elastase (NE), myeloperoxidase (MPO) and various pro-inflammatory mediators within hours of ECC [56, 62, 102, 104, 111, 112]. These pro-inflammatory mediators are activated for clearance of Gram-negative bacteria and mediate antimicrobial activities [113].

In addition to infections, activated leukocytes can also elicit thrombosis, as they tend to adhere to two of the key players of coagulation: platelets and endothelial cells. In particular, leukocyte integrin interaction with platelet adhesion molecules (P-selectin glycoprotein ligand-1 and glycoprotein Ib alpha polypeptide) is known to provoke thrombosis [82]. Furthermore, both RRT and ECMO cause excessive production of complement mediators and alter complement receptor expressions on leukocytes, all of which can trigger pro-thrombotic events [114]. Such aberrant immunologic activation can result in hyperdynamic states that precipitate AKI [115], but also pulmonary dysfunction [61–63].

Impact on Monocyte Phenotype and Function

Apart from neutrophils, RRT and ECMO can also alter monocyte phenotype and function. Reduced monocyte human leukocyte antigen (HLA)-DR expression and concomitant TNF-α production have been reported in ECMO patients following endotoxin stimulation [70]. HLA complex analysis is used to assess innate immune function and leukocyte activation. During an infective episode, the surface expression of HLA-DR is upregulated on monocytes in anticipation of presenting antigens to lymphocytes, prompting an immune response. This process is suggested to be dampened after initiation of ECMO. Of note, low TLR4 expression on monocytes has been observed in non-survivors during early support and may play an important role in the decreased response, as it is a key pattern recognition receptor for endotoxin [99]. It has been speculated that this is caused by intensive endocytosis of CD14/TLR4 due to high levels of damage-associated molecular pattern (DAMP) molecules from the underlying disease burden (e.g. ARDS/pneumonia) and is further exacerbated by the immunological imbalance mediated by ECCs. These profiles are similarly observed in infected and septic patients [89, 92] and have been associated with increased mortality in these patients [99, 116]. In addition, the responsiveness of non-classical $CD14^+CD16^{++}$ and intermediate $CD14^{++}CD16^+$ monocyte subpopulations has been reported to markedly decrease when challenged with LPS after RRT initiation [96].

The risk of infection increases universally when extracorporeal modalities are initiated, regardless of the aetiology of the primary disease. These studies further highlight that in addition to large vascular access, ECC-acquired immunoparalysis is a contributor to the high infection rate reported with these devices. Such immunological changes may be attributable to the 3.5–64% infection rate in ECMO patients [21, 117] and contribute as one of the leading causes of morbidity and mortality in RRT-supported patients [118, 119]. This risk is proposed to be greater with CRRT in comparison with IHD, possibly due to prolonged exposure to artificial surfaces [120].

Impact on the Adaptive Immune Leukocytes: T and B Lymphocytes

T and B lymphocytes together constitute a distinct branch of the adaptive immune system. If they become dysregulated, the capacity of the immune system to distinguish self from foreign and provide specialised immune defence can be hindered. Decrease in the overall lymphocyte numbers during ECMO and their delayed recovery post-weaning are associated with mortality in patients [98, 121–123]. A subset of T lymphocytes (T regulatory lymphocyte), paired with high levels of anti-inflammatory IL-10, has been further identified to significantly decrease by day 3 of ECMO [99]. A similar reduction was evident in $CD8^+$ cytotoxic T lymphocytes after initiation of RRT, while an increase in the $CD4^+$ T helper lymphocytes was observed [68]. This is likely attributed to the enhanced proliferation capacity of $CD4^+$ lymphocytes after RRT, yet it does not necessarily imply increased functionality.

Additionally, recent publications have examined the potential of neutrophil-to-lymphocyte ratio (NLR) as a predictor of poor prognosis and survival in patients with post-cardiotomy shock supported with ECMO and end-stage kidney failure supported with RRT [124–126]. RRT and ECMO support are reported to increase NLR values, and patients with high NLR have an increased risk for death. ECMO patients with high NLR also showed an increased risk for renal complications [124], potentially necessitating RRT.

Impact on T and B Lymphocyte Phenotype and Function

Both RRT and ECMO have been shown to alter lymphocyte phenotype and function. Patients are reported with suppressed adaptive immunity, contributing to their increased susceptibility to infection. In particular, following in vitro phytohaemagglutinin stimulation, blood from ECMO patients has been reported to exhibit suppressed production of IFN-γ and IL-10 by T lymphocytes [70]. Similarly to ECMO, signs of decreased T lymphocyte response have been reported with RRT. Compared to pre-RRT patients and healthy controls, the CD4+ lymphocytes of those treated with RRT had a reduced expression of co-stimulatory molecule CD28, as well as activation markers CD25 and CD69 after in vitro stimulation with immobilised anti-CD3 antibodies [127].

Lymphocytes are also vital for mediating immune tolerance, hence protecting patients from autoimmune reactions with resultant host tissue damage. Ortega and colleagues have associated acquired brain injury and impaired cerebral autoregulation in ECMO patients with elevated autoreactivity of cytotoxic T lymphocytes and B lymphocytes to central nervous system peptides with a tenfold increase in IL-8 levels [128]. These changes may be a contributor to frequently encountered neurological complications documented by the Extracorporeal Life Support Organization registry [18].

5.4 Causes of Extracorporeal Circulation-Related Immune Response

5.4.1 RRT and ECMO Technology (ECC Circuit Designs and Materials)

Direct interface of blood with the artificial surface of ECC circuits is widely acknowledged as a cause of significant alterations in blood physiology. Despite efforts in advancing the biocompatibility of circuits and dampening the activation of the coagulation system, changes in immune responses persist, potentially contributing to the development of SIRS, secondary infections and organ dysfunction, bleeding and thrombosis. While RRT and ECMO have different functions, they also share similarities in their basic composition: pumps, complex membrane structures and connecting tubing.

Blood Pumps

For most ECCs, pumps are paramount to drive blood movement through the circuit. Most commonly, RRT modalities achieve this with a roller pump. The latter was also the standard in ECMO for decades until the relatively recent introduction of centrifugal pumps—proposed to be less destructive to blood components than roller pumps [129–131].

Yet, there has been no direct comparative investigation performed for ECMO in the context of immune modulation to provide an accurate assessment of differences between pump designs. Similarly, the technological evolution of blood pumps for RRT has not been accompanied by comparative scientific assessment. The putative benefits of newer modified centrifugal pumps over roller pumps have mainly been investigated in studies using CPB. Cardiac surgery with CPB using centrifugal pumps exhibits enhanced preservation of leukocytes and reduced elevation of IL-6, C3a, procalcitonin and haemolysis [130, 131], compared to CPB with roller pumps. Shorter ventilation times and hospital stays were also observed in the centrifugal pump groups. For ECMO, roller pumps are still occasionally encountered in clinical practice and research, as the topic remains controversial due to conflicting results by various studies [132–136].

Membranes

RRT Filter Membranes

The contemporary arsenal of filter membranes for RRT is heterogenous, consisting of different materials with varied pore sizes. Conventionally, these membranes have been broadly classified as cellulosic or non-cellulosic (synthetic), based on their composition, as well as low or high flux, on the basis of water permeability [137].

The previously used cellulose-based cellophane and cuprophane membranes are known to incite significant biological activation during blood contact, triggering rapid leukocytopenia and an inflammatory response with activation of the complement system, production of neutrophil superoxide and release of various cytokines (such as IL-1 and TNF) [93–96, 138, 139]. In contrast, usage of a synthetic membrane RRT showed a trend towards reduced activation and aggregation throughout the course of treatment for granulocytes [93, 105, 140].

To reduce humoral and cellular immune activation, advances in the engineering of more biocompatible membranes have continued over the last decades, ushering RRT into a new technological era. Modified cellulosic membranes and synthetic membranes (e.g. polysulphone, polyethersulphone, AN-69 and polymethylmethacrylate) have greater biocompatibility and are now predominately used in clinical practice [105, 141, 142]. In addition, the use of polymer blending in synthetic membranes has enhanced the biocompatibility and performance of RRTs. While some studies exhibited similarities on efficiency in removing solutes, others reported significant differences [73, 143–146]. These have, in part, led to the development of membranes with specialised characteristics and refined properties that calls for reconsideration of past membrane classification systems.

Given the multitude of variations in RRT modalities, membrane types and clinical practices, the degree of immune changes induced is likely variable and should be considered when performing comparative analyses.

ECMO Membrane Oxygenator

In addition to the introduction of centrifugal pumps, the use of polymethylpentene (PMP) hollow-fibre oxygenator membranes is another notable technological evolution of ECMO post-2008. Enhancements seen with hollow-fibre PMP membranes include dampened activation of neutrophils characterised by lower expression of adhesion molecule CD11b and release of NE and superoxide anion [147, 148]. However, various immunomodulatory effects of ECMO are still observed, despite the enhanced biocompatibility of newer oxygenators. Rungatscher and colleagues have highlighted the role of oxygenator-associated immunomodulation using a rat model of ECC with and without a hollow-fibre oxygenator [63]. Significant upregulation in two major inflammatory signalling pathways of leukocytes, p38 mitogen-activated protein kinase (MAPK) and nuclear factor kappa B (NF-κB) phosphorylation was observed during early ECC with an oxygenator. Studies have also reported high rate of cellular and coagulation factor deposits on PMP membrane oxygenators [100, 149, 150]. To further reduce deposition onto the membrane, further optimisation of the membrane coating by using other non-thrombogenic polymer brushes is an area of intense ongoing research [151].

Although PMP hollow-fibre membrane oxygenators are now ubiquitous in clinical settings, many different systems and manufacturers are available. Obvious variance in leukocyte adhesion and Willebrand factor deposition on PMP hollow-fibre oxygenator membranes between commercially available circuits has been observed [100]. Differences in how an ECMO membrane is folded within the oxygenator can influence blood flow rates and lead to varied cellular and humoral responses, in accordance with RRT and CPB experiences [137, 152]. For this reason, it is anticipated that the level of ECMO-mediated leukocyte and other cellular modulations can be variable between centres and countries.

5.4.2 Non-physiological Conditions

Apart from technological factors, other common causes associated with RRT- and ECMO-related immunomodulatory influence have been proposed. These include extracorporeal circulatory flow rates and the associated non-physiological shear stress generated. During continuous extracorporeal blood flow, wall shear stress within the rigid RRT and ECMO circuit increases to supra-physiological levels as blood flow increases. Variation in flow rate and shear stress can influence the phenotype, function, migration and deformability of immune cells and the humoral response in different ways.

Two ex vivo studies have reported ECMO flow rates and the mediated non-physiological shear stress as potential factors influencing the immune response [56, 153]. Using an ex vivo circuit, Ki et al. reported that higher ECMO flow rates (4 L/min) were associated with a rapid increase in acute inflammatory cytokines and chemokines resembling SIRS and plasma neutrophil granules within 6 h of ECMO, compared to lower (1.5 L/min) flow rates [56]. In parallel, neutrophil activation increased significantly, characterised by a rise in plasma neutrophil granules (NE and MPO). In neonates, Meyer et al. reported a differential influence on leukocyte-derived extracellular vesicles at different ECMO flow rates. In addition, a greater degree of tissue factor antigen was expressed on these extracellular vesicles and leukocytes at higher flow rates, further contributing to ECMO-related inflammation and thrombosis. However, for RRT, no observed differences between high and low flow rates were detected in experimental settings for leukocyte activation phenotype [56], nor in clinical settings [154], possibly related to the smaller variability in flow rates employed. In addition, for each oxygenator design and size, there is likely an optimal flow for different cellular components that differentially minimises non-physiological shear stress and damage [153]. Further animal and clinical investigations are required to validate these effects in vivo.

Another contributor to the excessive non-physiological shear stress with contemporary ECMO pumps is the inability to generate pulsatile propagation of blood, an evolutionary trait present in all mammal circulations. The benefits of physiological pulsatile flow pattern were first explored in CPB, where pulsatility yielded lower levels of pro-inflammatory molecules such as IL-2, IL-6, IL-8, endotoxin and lower levels of anti-inflammatory IL-10 [155–158]. More recently, an experimental model using healthy beagles reported lower levels of TNF-α and IL-1β and higher levels of tumour growth factor (TGF)-β1 with pulsatile flow [159]. Yet, no difference was observed when the systemic inflammatory response was assessed ex vivo, possibly due to interaction of blood components without an "active" immune response [160]. Considering the effects seen in clinical studies using CPB, future studies in pulsatile ECMO should investigate the immune response in animals with injury, before confirming these changes in patient populations.

Notably, the critically ill populations that require RRT and ECMO support are heterogenous. In addition to their differences in RRT and ECMO support, medications, temperature, anticoagulant strategies and comorbidities, patients are also exposed to diverse stressors and therapies, making stratification of their immune modulatory influence complex, with no clear targets for interventions.

5.5 Priorities for Future Research: Potential Therapeutic Interventions in ECC-Associated Immune Response

The importance of the humoral and cellular immune mediators as biomarkers of inflammation, predictors of mortality and/or poor patient outcomes has been highlighted across a spectrum of critical illnesses [58, 87, 89, 161–163]. However, there is still no effective bedside testing available to measure immune dysregulation such as inflammation, other than non-specific tests such as CRP and full blood count. Despite that inflammation and coagulation are two sides of the same coin, current point-of-care testing exists only for coagulation, such as use of activated clotting times and rotational thromboelastometry. In addition, available literature on immune modulation in the context of ECMO is particularly scarce compared to RRT.

A more comprehensive profiling of leukocyte phenotypic expression and function, interrogation into the impact of RRT and ECMO on the extracellular vesicle generation, contact and complement systems, and leukocyte-platelet and -endothelial cell interaction will be important to fill the current gaps in knowledge. Future studies should also consider addressing two major challenges of the current research in RRT- and ECMO-related immune modulation: (1) technological disparity and (2) our incomplete understanding about the cumulative effect of these supportive modalities and the disease process itself. Of note, both challenges are likely to stem from variations in country- or centre-specific practices in the application of RRT and ECMO.

5.5.1 Knowing the Technological Disparities

Between the early times of their inception and the twenty-first century, RRT and ECMO technologies continue to undergo rapid evolution. For RRT, the immunological impact of the different systems and membrane biomaterials is more widely recognised as several comparative studies have been conducted. This phenomenon is less studied in ECMO. While the biomaterials and centrifugal pumps for different ECMO systems are now relatively homogenous, the membrane configuration of different oxygenators still varies. These differences can yield a diverse modulation of the immune profile. However, this area of research has yet to be thoroughly investigated. While they have their drawbacks, benchmark studies of membranes used in ECMO would be a start to help address the discrepancies of the modern-era ECMO devices (post-2007).

Amongst all published immunological ex vivo, animal and clinical ECMO studies, a number of differences in immune modulation associated with specific pumps, biomaterials and oxygenators have already been identified. Yet, to assist systematic assessment of immunologic effects, there is a clear need for more consistent reporting of biomaterials for future publications in the emerging field of ECMO. In addition, ECMO technologies should be disclaimed when performing comparative meta-analyses. These steps will enable fair comparisons between studies and will help to build a more comprehensive library of immune profiles for ECCs.

5.5.2 Understanding Factors Contributing to RRT- and ECMO-Related Immune Modulation

Critically ill patients admitted into ICU are often resource intense due to their underlying disease burden which necessitated RRT and/or ECMO. Not only are the patients exposed to the aforementioned non-physiological stressors of changing flow rates and the associated shear stress generated within the circuit, but they are also frequently subjected to other immunomodulatory therapies. These may include multiple blood transfusions when treating bleeding complications [164], systemic heparinisation [165–167] and supranormal administration of supplemental oxygen for hypoxia [168]. This provides an impetus for the development of a comprehensive mechanistic knowledge of immunobiology and pathophysiology for these modalities in order to optimise the current understanding and clinical outcomes.

5.5.3 Potential Interventions and Targets for RRT- and ECMO-Related Immune Modulation

Given that one of the primary instigators of the modulated immune response is the direct interface between blood and non-endothelial surfaces of the circuits, components with the capacity to reduce activation of contact and complement system, inflammatory response, leukocyte activation and interaction, or to boost pathogenic function, may be beneficial.

To control the acute-phase reaction, combined use with additional extracorporeal devices has been proposed such as CytoSorb® (CytoSorbents Inc., New Jersey, USA) blood purification to effectively absorb excessive inflammatory mediators [169], or the use of CRRT in parallel with ECMO [28, 76–79]. For the latter, extensive evidence has suggested that early intervention may enhance haemodynamic stabilisation and improvement in major organ functions. In addition, use of supplemental nitric oxide has been proposed to enhance the anti-inflammatory capacity of the immune system [170–172]. Of note, some suggest that administering nitric oxide into the membrane oxygenator of the CPB could improve outcomes of cardiac surgery patients, by inhibition of platelet and leukocyte adhesion, activation and aggregation [173, 174]. Finally, adoption of immune-modulating mesenchymal stem cells (MSCs) has also been proposed and reported with anti-inflammatory properties [175, 176]. However, local delivery is required to avoid adhesion of MSCs onto the membrane oxygenators.

Alternatively, the use of specific leukocyte targets may prove to be more effective (e.g. using inhibitors to dampen or temporarily eliminate the inflammatory response mediated by leukocyte activation and adhesion/interaction). Inhibition of β_2-integrin and its downstream processes is suggested to alleviate patients from sustained manifestations of neutrophil activity and regulate inflammation, interaction with endothelial cells and migration to the tissue with resultant multiple-organ dysfunction [177]. Additionally, efficacy in blocking adhesion surface molecules of lymphocytes using antibodies and antagonists has been demonstrated in various inflammatory diseases [178]. A targeted reduction or inhibition of these surface antigens on leukocytes using antibodies may provide an additional path to help reduce the incidence of thrombosis [177, 178]. Furthermore, the use of leukocyte inhibition modules could be useful for RRT and ECMO patients by limiting neutrophil proliferation and the resultant inflammatory response, as demonstrated in cardiac surgery patients [179–181]. To better understand the mechanisms underpinning ECC-related immune dysregulation, future studies may benefit from further investigations into the interaction of neutrophils and monocytes with platelets and endothelial cells, as well as the thrombotic and inflammatory phenotype of extracellular vesicles.

Summary

The understanding of the complex pathophysiological processes and clinical factors of ECC-related immune dysregulation has continued to grow steadily over the last 50 years, as the frequency of their usage has rapidly increased. However, there is less clarity surrounding this dysregulation in patients treated with newer RRT modalities and ECMO compared to ECCs such as CPB. Research and clinical observations are of the utmost importance, specifically in ECMO where the disease that necessitates its support is commonly associated with a grossly deranged physiology. As we move forward, further studies providing a greater understanding and characterisation in RRT- and ECMO-related immune modulation could generate meaningful data to aid delineation of the immunologic signatures between primary disease burden and RRT or ECMO to enable prognostic enrichment and identify suitable targets for therapeutic intervention. Finally, a careful selection of primary parameters and an appropriately powered clinical study design are essential in determining the impact of these biological perturbations on patient outcomes.

> **Take-Home Messages**
>
> ▪ Initiation of RRT and ECMO during ICU trigger immune dysregulation in critically ill: This is a consequence of blood coming into contact with the foreign and non-endothelialised extracorporeal surfaces as well as being exposed to the non-physiological conditions (e.g. flow rate).
> ▪ Critically ill patients suffer from increased morbidity and mortality if RRT- and ECMO-related immune dysregulation is unchecked or unresolved.
> ▪ Current evidence reports that patients exhibit variable immunologic profiles, influenced by the structural and functional differences of distinct ECCs. An understanding and characterisation of the full spectrum of the immune dysregulation related to RRT and ECMO may help in the development of tools necessary for prognostic enrichment to enable targeted care.
> ▪ Future studies should also aim to address two major challenges of current research: ECC technological disparity and lack of understanding in the compound effect with other clinical stressors and therapies.
> ▪ The understanding of ECMO-associated immune dysregulation may yield not only better patient outcomes but also better resource allocation such as lesser use of blood products and shorter time in the ICU and hospital.

References

1. Karkar A. Advances in hemodialysis techniques. 2013 [cited Oct 2021, date last access)]. In: Hemodialysis [Internet]. http://www.intechopen.com/books/hemodialysis/advances-in-hemodialysis-techniques. IntechOpen, [cited Oct 2021, date last access)].
2. Himmelfarb J, Vanholder R, Mehrotra R, Tonelli M. The current and future landscape of dialysis. Nat Rev Nephrol. 2020;16(10):573–85.
3. Damasiewicz MJ, Polkinghorne KR. Global dialysis perspective: Australia. Kidney360. 2020;1(1):48–51.
4. Prowle JR, Bellomo R. Continuous renal replacement therapy: recent advances and future research. Nat Rev Nephrol. 2010;6(9):521–9.
5. Hsu RK, McCulloch CE, Dudley RA, Lo LJ, Hsu CY. Temporal changes in incidence of dialysis-requiring AKI. J Am Soc Nephrol. 2013;24(1):37–42.
6. Hoste EA, Bagshaw SM, Bellomo R, Cely CM, Colman R, Cruz DN, et al. Epidemiology of acute kidney injury in critically ill patients: the multinational AKI-EPI study. Intensive Care Med. 2015;41(8):1411–23.
7. Ahmed AR, Obilana A, Lappin D. Renal replacement therapy in the critical care setting. Crit Care Res Pract. 2019;2019:6948710.
8. Marshall MR, Ma T, Galler D, Rankin APN, Williams AB. Sustained low-efficiency daily diafiltration (SLEDD-f) for critically ill patients requiring renal replacement therapy: towards an adequate therapy. Nephrol Dial Transplant. 2004;19(4):877–84.
9. Kihara M, Ikeda Y, Shibata K, Masumori S, Fujita H, Ebira H, et al. Slow hemodialysis performed during the day in managing renal failure in critically ill patients. Nephron. 1994;67(1):36–41.
10. Marshall MR, Golper TA, Shaver MJ, Alam MG, Chatoth DK. Sustained low-efficiency dialysis for critically ill patients requiring renal replacement therapy. Kidney Int. 2001;60(2):777–85.
11. Trahanas JM, Kolobow MA, Hardy MA, Berra L, Zapol WM, Bartlett RH. "Treating lungs": the scientific contributions of Dr. Theodor Kolobow. ASAIO J. 2016;62(2):203–10.
12. Kolobow T. The promise of the membrane artificial lung. Int J Artif Organs. 1978;1(1):15–20.

13. Lequier L, Horton SB, McMullan DM, Bartlett RH. Extracorporeal membrane oxygenation circuitry. Pediatr Crit Care Med. 2013;14(5 Suppl 1):S7–S12.
14. Peek GJ, Elbourne D, Mugford M, Tiruvoipati R, Wilson A, Allen E, et al. Randomised controlled trial and parallel economic evaluation of conventional ventilatory support versus extracorporeal membrane oxygenation for severe adult respiratory failure (CESAR). Health Technol Assess. 2010;14(35):1–46.
15. Combes A, Hajage D, Capellier G, Demoule A, Lavoue S, Guervilly C, et al. Extracorporeal membrane oxygenation for severe acute respiratory distress syndrome. N Engl J Med. 2018;378(21):1965–75.
16. Davies A, Jones D, Bailey M, Beca J, Bellomo R, Blackwell N, et al. Extracorporeal membrane oxygenation for 2009 influenza A(H1N1) acute respiratory distress syndrome. JAMA. 2009;302(17):1888–95.
17. Zangrillo A, Biondi-Zoccai G, Landoni G, Frati G, Patroniti N, Pesenti A, et al. Extracorporeal membrane oxygenation (ECMO) in patients with H1N1 influenza infection: a systematic review and meta-analysis including 8 studies and 266 patients receiving ECMO. Crit Care. 2013;17(1):R30.
18. Extracorporeal Life Support Organization. ECLS registry report: international summary 2019. Ann Arbor; 2019.
19. Fraser JF, Shekar K, Diab S, Dunster K, Foley SR, McDonald CI, et al. ECMO—the clinician's view. ISBT Sci Ser. 2012;7(1):82–8.
20. Makdisi G, Wang IW. Extra corporeal membrane oxygenation (ECMO) review of a lifesaving technology. J Thorac Dis. 2015;7(7):E166–76.
21. MacLaren G, Schlapbach LJ, Aiken AM. Nosocomial infections during extracorporeal membrane oxygenation in neonatal, pediatric, and adult patients: a comprehensive narrative review. Pediatr Crit Care Med. 2020;21(3):283–90.
22. Li PK-T, Chow KM. Infectious complications in dialysis—epidemiology and outcomes. Nat Rev Nephrol. 2012;8(2):77–88.
23. Parienti J-J, Dugué AE, Daurel C, Mira J-P, Mégarbane B, Mermel LA, et al. Continuous renal replacement therapy may increase the risk of catheter infection. Clin J Am Soc Nephrol. 2010;5(8):1489–96.
24. Dalton HJ, Reeder R, Garcia-Filion P, Holubkov R, Berg RA, Zuppa A, et al. Factors associated with bleeding and thrombosis in children receiving extracorporeal membrane oxygenation. Am J Respir Crit Care Med. 2017;196(6):762–71.
25. Braune S, Sieweke A, Brettner F, Staudinger T, Joannidis M, Verbrugge S, et al. The feasibility and safety of extracorporeal carbon dioxide removal to avoid intubation in patients with COPD unresponsive to noninvasive ventilation for acute hypercapnic respiratory failure (ECLAIR study): multicentre case–control study. Intensive Care Med. 2016;42(9):1437–44.
26. Sklar MC, Beloncle F, Katsios CM, Brochard L, Friedrich JO. Extracorporeal carbon dioxide removal in patients with chronic obstructive pulmonary disease: a systematic review. Intensive Care Med. 2015;41(10):1752–62.
27. Peperstraete H, Eloot S, Depuydt P, De Somer F, Roosens C, Hoste E. Low flow extracorporeal CO(2) removal in ARDS patients: a prospective short-term crossover pilot study. BMC Anesthesiol. 2017;17(1):155.
28. Thongprayoon C, Cheungpasitporn W, Lertjitbanjong P, Aeddula NR, Bathini T, Watthanasuntorn K, et al. Incidence and impact of acute kidney injury in patients receiving extracorporeal membrane oxygenation: a meta-analysis. J Clin Med. 2019;8(7):981.
29. Larsson M, Rayzman V, Nolte MW, Nickel KF, Björkqvist J, Jämsä A, et al. A factor XIIa inhibitory antibody provides thromboprotection in extracorporeal circulation without increasing bleeding risk. Sci Transl Med. 2014;6(222):222ra17.
30. Wachtfogel YT, Hack CE, Nuijens JH, Kettner C, Reilly TM, Knabb RM, et al. Selective kallikrein inhibitors alter human neutrophil elastase release during extracorporeal circulation. Am J Phys. 1995;268(3 Pt 2):H1352–7.
31. Plotz FB, van Oeveren W, Bartlett RH, Wildevuur CR. Blood activation during neonatal extracorporeal life support. J Thorac Cardiovasc Surg. 1993;105(5):823–32.
32. Wendel HP, Scheule AM, Eckstein FS, Ziemer G. Haemocompatibility of paediatric membrane oxygenators with heparin-coated surfaces. Perfusion. 1999;14(1):21–8.
33. Frank RD, Weber J, Dresbach H, Thelen H, Weiss C, Floege J. Role of contact system activation in hemodialyzer-induced thrombogenicity. Kidney Int. 2001;60(5):1972–81.

34. François K, Orlando C, Jochmans K, Cools W, De Meyer V, Tielemans C, et al. Hemodialysis does not induce detectable activation of the contact system of coagulation. Kidney Int Rep. 2020;5(6):831–8.

35. Cugno M, Nussberger J, Biglioli P, Giovagnoni MG, Gardinali M, Agostoni A. Cardiopulmonary bypass increases plasma bradykinin concentrations. Immunopharmacology. 1999;43(2–3):145–7.

36. Rodell TC, Naidoo Y, Bhoola KD. Role of kinins in inflammatory responses. Clin Immunotherap. 1995;3(5):352–61.

37. Marney AM, Ma J, Luther JM, Ikizler TA, Brown NJ. Endogenous bradykinin contributes to increased plasminogen activator inhibitor 1 antigen following hemodialysis. J Am Soc Nephrol. 2009;20(10):2246–52.

38. Morgan EN, Pohlman TH, Vocelka C, Farr A, Lindley G, Chandler W, et al. Nuclear factor kappaB mediates a procoagulant response in monocytes during extracorporeal circulation. J Thorac Cardiovasc Surg. 2003;125(1):165–71.

39. Szotowski B, Antoniak S, Poller W, Schultheiss HP, Rauch U. Procoagulant soluble tissue factor is released from endothelial cells in response to inflammatory cytokines. Circ Res. 2005;96(12):1233–9.

40. Ocak G, Vossen CY, Rotmans JI, Lijfering WM, Rosendaal FR, Parlevliet KJ, et al. Venous and arterial thrombosis in dialysis patients. Thromb Haemost. 2011;106(6):1046–52.

41. Oudemans-van Straaten HM. Hemostasis and thrombosis in continuous renal replacement treatment. Semin Thromb Hemost. 2015;41(1):91–8.

42. Skinner SC, Derebail VK, Poulton CJ, Bunch DC, Roy-Chaudhury P, Key NS. Hemodialysis-related complement and contact pathway activation and cardiovascular risk: a narrative review. Kidney Med. 2021;3(4):607–18.

43. Lappegård KT, Christiansen D, Pharo A, Thorgersen EB, Hellerud BC, Lindstad J, et al. Human genetic deficiencies reveal the roles of complement in the inflammatory network: lessons from nature. Proc Natl Acad Sci U S A. 2009;106(37):15861–6.

44. Moen O, Fosse E, Bråten J, Andersson C, Fagerhol MK, Venge P, et al. Roller and centrifugal pumps compared in vitro with regard to haemolysis, granulocyte and complement activation. Perfusion. 1994;9(2):109–17.

45. Graulich J, Sonntag J, Marcinkowski M, Bauer K, Kössel H, Bührer C, et al. Complement activation by in vivo neonatal and in vitro extracorporeal membrane oxygenation. Mediat Inflamm. 2002;11(2):69–73.

46. Vallhonrat H, Swinford RD, Ingelfinger JR, Williams WW, Ryan DP, Tolkoff-Rubin N, et al. Rapid activation of the alternative pathway of complement by extracorporeal membrane oxygenation. ASAIO J. 1999;45(1):113–4.

47. Poppelaars F, da Costa MG, Faria B, Berger SP, Assa S, Daha MR, et al. Intradialytic complement activation precedes the development of cardiovascular events in hemodialysis patients. Front Immunol. 2018;9:2070.

48. Lhotta K, Würzner R, Kronenberg F, Oppermann M, König P. Rapid activation of the complement system by cuprophane depends on complement component C4. Kidney Int. 1998;53(4):1044–51.

49. Inoshita H, Ohsawa I, Kusaba G, Ishii M, Onda K, Horikoshi S, et al. Complement in patients receiving maintenance hemodialysis: functional screening and quantitative analysis. BMC Nephrol. 2010;11:34.

50. Hein E, Munthe-Fog L, Thiara AS, Fiane AE, Mollnes TE, Garred P. Heparin-coated cardiopulmonary bypass circuits selectively deplete the pattern recognition molecule ficolin-2 of the lectin complement pathway in vivo. Clin Exp Immunol. 2015;179(2):294–9.

51. Burnouf T, Eber M, Kientz D, Cazenave JP, Burkhardt T. Assessment of complement activation during membrane-based plasmapheresis procedures. J Clin Apher. 2004;19(3):142–7.

52. Eskandary F, Wahrmann M, Biesenbach P, Sandurkov C, König F, Schwaiger E, et al. ABO antibody and complement depletion by immunoadsorption combined with membrane filtration—a randomized, controlled, cross-over trial. Nephrol Dial Transplant. 2014;29(3):706–14.

53. Chenoweth DE, Cheung AK, Henderson LW. Anaphylatoxin formation during hemodialysis: effects of different dialyzer membranes. Kidney Int. 1983;24(6):764–9.

54. Stasi A, Franzin R, Divella C, Sallustio F, Curci C, Picerno A, et al. PMMA-based continuous hemofiltration modulated complement activation and renal dysfunction in LPS-induced acute kidney injury. Front Immunol. 2021;12:605212.

5

55. Warren OJ, Smith AJ, Alexiou C, Rogers PL, Jawad N, Vincent C, et al. The inflammatory response to cardiopulmonary bypass: part 1—mechanisms of pathogenesis. J Cardiothorac Vasc Anesth. 2009;23(2):223–31.

56. Ki KK, Passmore MR, Chan CHH, Malfertheiner MV, Bouquet M, Cho HJ, et al. Effect of ex vivo extracorporeal membrane oxygenation flow dynamics on immune response. Perfusion. 2019;34(1_suppl):5–14.

57. Schindler R, Linnenweber S, Schulze M, Oppermann M, Dinarello CA, Shaldon S, et al. Gene expression of interleukin-1 beta during hemodialysis. Kidney Int. 1993;43(3):712–21.

58. Risnes I, Wagner K, Ueland T, Mollnes T, Aukrust P, Svennevig J. Interleukin-6 may predict survival in extracorporeal membrane oxygenation treatment. Perfusion. 2008;23(3):173–8.

59. Mildner RJ, Taub N, Vyas JR, Killer HM, Firmin RK, Field DJ, et al. Cytokine imbalance in infants receiving extracorporeal membrane oxygenation for respiratory failure. Biol Neonate. 2005;88(4):321–7.

60. Fortenberry JD, Bhardwaj V, Niemer P, Cornish JD, Wright JA, Bland L. Neutrophil and cytokine activation with neonatal extracorporeal membrane oxygenation. J Pediatr. 1996;128(5):670–8.

61. Passmore MR, Fung YL, Simonova G, Foley SR, Dunster KR, Diab SD, et al. Inflammation and lung injury in an ovine model of extracorporeal membrane oxygenation support. Am J Physiol Lung Cell Mol Physiol. 2016;311(6):L1202–12.

62. McIlwain RB, Timpa JG, Kurundkar AR, Holt DW, Kelly DR, Hartman YE, et al. Plasma concentrations of inflammatory cytokines rise rapidly during ECMO-related SIRS due to the release of preformed stores in the intestine. Lab Invest. 2010;90(1):128–39.

63. Rungatscher A, Tessari M, Stranieri C, Solani E, Linardi D, Milani E, et al. Oxygenator is the main responsible for leukocyte activation in experimental model of extracorporeal circulation: a cautionary tale. Mediat Inflamm. 2015;2015:7.

64. Caglar K, Peng Y, Pupim LB, Flakoll PJ, Levenhagen D, Hakim RM, et al. Inflammatory signals associated with hemodialysis. Kidney Int. 2002;62(4):1408–16.

65. Servillo G, Vargas M, Pastore A, Procino A, Iannuzzi M, Capuano A, et al. Immunomodulatory effect of continuous venovenous hemofiltration during sepsis: preliminary data. Biomed Res Int. 2013;2013:108951.

66. Yong K, Dogra G, Boudville N, Lim W. Increased inflammatory response in association with the initiation of hemodialysis compared with peritoneal dialysis in a prospective study of end-stage kidney disease patients. Perit Dial Int. 2018;38(1):18–23.

67. Adrian K, Skogby M, Friberg LG, Mellgren K. The effect of s-nitroso-glutathione on platelet and leukocyte function during experimental extracorporeal circulation. Artif Organs. 2003;27(6):570–5.

68. Lisowska KA, Pindel M, Pietruczuk K, Kuźmiuk-Glembin I, Storoniak H, Dębska-Ślizień A, et al. The influence of a single hemodialysis procedure on human T lymphocytes. Sci Rep. 2019;9(1):5041.

69. Borazan A, Ustün H, Ustundag Y, Aydemir S, Bayraktaroglu T, Sert M, et al. The effects of peritoneal dialysis and hemodialysis on serum tumor necrosis factor-alpha, interleukin-6, interleukin-10 and C-reactive-protein levels. Mediat Inflamm. 2004;13(3):201–4.

70. Ziemba K, Nateri J, Hanson-Huber L, Steele L, Cismowski M, West T, et al. Innate and adaptive immune function during extracorporeal membrane oxygenation. Crit Care Med. 2016;44(12):232.

71. Beshish AG, Bradley JD, McDonough KL, Halligan NLN, McHugh WM, Sturza J, et al. The functional immune response of patients on extracorporeal life support. ASAIO J. 2018;65(1):77–83.

72. Li G, Ma H, Yin Y, Wang J. CRP, IL-2 and TNF-α level in patients with uremia receiving hemodialysis. Mol Med Rep. 2018;17(2):3350–5.

73. Haase M, Bellomo R, Baldwin I, Haase-Fielitz A, Fealy N, Davenport P, et al. Hemodialysis membrane with a high-molecular-weight cutoff and cytokine levels in sepsis complicated by acute renal failure: a phase 1 randomized trial. Am J Kidney Dis. 2007;50(2):296–304.

74. Wang J, Wu Z, Wen Q, Wang X. Effects of CRRT on renal function and toxin clearance in patients with sepsis: a case–control study. J Int Med Res. 2021;49(9):3000605211042981.

75. Wang H-J, Wang P, Li N, Wan C, Jiang C-M, He J-S, et al. Effects of continuous renal replacement therapy on serum cytokines, neutrophil gelatinase-associated lipocalin, and prognosis in patients with severe acute kidney injury after cardiac surgery. Oncotarget. 2017;8(6):10628–36.

76. Yimin H, Wenkui Y, Jialiang S, Qiyi C, Juanhong S, Zhiliang L, et al. Effects of continuous renal replacement therapy on renal inflammatory cytokines during extracorporeal membrane oxygenation in a porcine model. J Cardiothorac Surg. 2013;8:113.

77. Shen J, Yu W, Chen Q, Shi J, Hu Y, Zhang J, et al. Continuous renal replacement therapy (CRRT) attenuates myocardial inflammation and mitochondrial injury induced by venovenous extracorporeal membrane oxygenation (VV ECMO) in a healthy piglet model. Inflammation. 2013;36(5):1186–93.

78. Mu TS, Palmer EG, Batts SG, Lentz-Kapua SL, Uyehara-Lock JH, Uyehara CFT. Continuous renal replacement therapy to reduce inflammation in a piglet hemorrhage–reperfusion extracorporeal membrane oxygenation model. Pediatr Res. 2012;72(3):249–55.

79. Shi J, Chen Q, Yu W, Shen J, Gong J, He C, et al. Continuous renal replacement therapy reduces the systemic and pulmonary inflammation induced by venovenous extracorporeal membrane oxygenation in a porcine model. Artif Organs. 2014;38(3):215–23.

80. McDonald CI, Fraser JF, Shekar K, Dunster KR, Thom O, Fung YL. Transfusion of packed red blood cells reduces selenium levels and increases lipid peroxidation in an in vivo ovine model. Transfus Med. 2014;24(1):50–4.

81. Rich RR, Chaplin DD. Chapter 1—The human immune response. In: Rich RR, Fleisher TA, Shearer WT, Schroeder HW, Frew AJ, Weyand CM, editors. Clinical immunology. 5th ed. London: Content Repository Only; 2019. p. 3–17.e1.

82. Wang Y, Gao H, Shi C, Erhardt PW, Pavlovsky A, Soloviev DA, et al. Leukocyte integrin Mac-1 regulates thrombosis via interaction with platelet GPIbα. Nat Commun. 2017;8:15559.

83. Laurance S, Bertin F-R, Ebrahimian T, Kassim Y, Rys RN, Lehoux S, et al. Gas6 promotes inflammatory (CCR2 hi CX3CR1 lo) monocyte recruitment in venous thrombosis. Arterioscler Thromb Vasc Biol. 2017;37(7):1315–22.

84. von Brühl M-L, Stark K, Steinhart A, Chandraratne S, Konrad I, Lorenz M, et al. Monocytes, neutrophils, and platelets cooperate to initiate and propagate venous thrombosis in mice in vivo. J Exp Med. 2012;209(4):819–35.

85. Liu X, Xue Y, Ding T, Sun J. Enhancement of proinflammatory and procoagulant responses to silica particles by monocyte-endothelial cell interactions. Part Fibre Toxicol. 2012;9(1):36.

86. Michelson AD, Barnard MR, Krueger LA, Valeri CR, Furman MI. Circulating monocyte-platelet aggregates are a more sensitive marker of in vivo platelet activation than platelet surface P-selectin: studies in baboons, human coronary intervention, and human acute myocardial infarction. Circulation. 2001;104(13):1533–7.

87. Li W, Ai X, Ni Y, Ye Z, Liang Z. The association between the neutrophil-to-lymphocyte ratio and mortality in patients with acute respiratory distress syndrome: a retrospective cohort study. Shock. 2019;51(2):161–7.

88. Peng Y, Wang J, Xiang H, Weng Y, Rong F, Xue Y, et al. Prognostic value of neutrophil-lymphocyte ratio in cardiogenic shock: a cohort study. Med Sci Mon Int Med J Exp Clin Res. 2020;26:e922167.

89. Conway Morris A, Datta D, Shankar-Hari M, Stephen J, Weir CJ, Rennie J, et al. Cell-surface signatures of immune dysfunction risk-stratify critically ill patients: INFECT study. Intensive Care Med. 2018;44(5):627–35.

90. Allen ML, Peters MJ, Goldman A, Elliott M, James I, Callard R, et al. Early postoperative monocyte deactivation predicts systemic inflammation and prolonged stay in pediatric cardiac intensive care. Crit Care Med. 2002;30(5):1140–5.

91. Pfortmueller CA, Meisel C, Fux M, Schefold JC. Assessment of immune organ dysfunction in critical illness: utility of innate immune response markers. Intensive Care Med Exp. 2017;5(1):49.

92. Conway Morris A, Anderson N, Brittan M, Wilkinson TS, McAuley DF, Antonelli J, et al. Combined dysfunctions of immune cells predict nosocomial infection in critically ill patients. Br J Anaesth. 2013;111(5):778–87.

93. Craddock PR, Fehr J, Dalmasso AP, Brighan KL, Jacob HS, Hemodialysis leukopenia. Pulmonary vascular leukostasis resulting from complement activation by dialyzer cellophane membranes. J Clin Invest. 1977;59(5):879–88.

94. Gral T, Schroth P, De Palma JR, Gordon A. Leukocyte dynamics with three types of hemodialyzers. Trans Am Soc Artif Intern Organs. 1969;15:45–9.

95. Arnaout MA, Hakim RM, Todd RF 3rd, Dana N, Colten HR. Increased expression of an adhesion-promoting surface glycoprotein in the granulocytopenia of hemodialysis. N Engl J Med. 1985;312(8):457–62.

96. Liakopoulos V, Jeron A, Shah A, Bruder D, Mertens PR, Gorny X. Hemodialysis-related changes in phenotypical features of monocytes. Sci Rep. 2018;8(1):13964.

97. Hocker JR, Wellhausen SR, Ward RA, Simpson PM, Cook LN. Effect of extracorporeal membrane oxygenation on leukocyte function in neonates. Artif Organs. 1991;15(1):23–8.

98. Zach TL, Steinhorn RH, Georgieff MK, Mills MM, Green TP. Leukopenia associated with extracorporeal membrane oxygenation in newborn infants. J Pediatr. 1990;116(3):440–4.

99. Liu CH, Kuo SW, Ko WJ, Tsai PR, Wu SW, Lai CH, et al. Early measurement of IL-10 predicts the outcomes of patients with acute respiratory distress syndrome receiving extracorporeal membrane oxygenation. Sci Rep. 2017;7(1):1021.

100. Bredthauer A, Wilm J, Philipp A, Foltan M, Mueller T, Lehle K. The oxygenator design might influence the adhesion of leukocytes and deposits of von willebrand fibers on the surface of gas exchange membranes during ECMO. Eur J Heart Fail. 2017;19(S2):36–7.

101. Nockher WA, Wiemer J, Scherberich JE. Haemodialysis monocytopenia: differential sequestration kinetics of CD14+CD16+ and CD14++ blood monocyte subsets. Clin Exp Immunol. 2001;123(1):49–55.

102. Graulich J, Walzog B, Marcinkowski M, Bauer K, Kossel H, Fuhrmann G, et al. Leukocyte and endothelial activation in a laboratory model of extracorporeal membrane oxygenation (ECMO). Pediatr Res. 2000;48(5):679–84.

103. DePuydt LE, Schuit KE, Smith SD. Effect of extracorporeal membrane oxygenation on neutrophil function in neonates. Crit Care Med. 1993;21(9):1324–7.

104. Skogby M, Mellgren K, Adrian K, Friberg LG, Chevalier JY, Mellgren G. Induced cell trauma during in vitro perfusion: a comparison between two different perfusion systems. Artif Organs. 1998;22(12):1045–51.

105. Sirolli V, Ballone E, Di Stante S, Amoroso L, Bonomini M. Cell activation and cellular-cellular interactions during hemodialysis: effect of dialyzer membrane. Int J Artif Organs. 2002;25(6):529–37.

106. Kaupke CJ, Zhang J, Cesario T, Yousefi S, Akeel N, Vaziri ND. Effect of hemodialysis on leukocyte adhesion receptor expression. Am J Kidney Dis. 1996;27(2):244–52.

107. Rudensky B, Yinnon AM, Shutin O, Broide E, Wiener-Well Y, Bitran D, et al. The cellular immunological responses of patients undergoing coronary artery bypass grafting compared with those of patients undergoing valve replacement. Eur J Cardiothorac Surg. 2010;37(5):1056–62.

108. Asimakopoulos G, Kohn A, Stefanou DC, Haskard DO, Landis RC, Taylor KM. Leukocyte integrin expression in patients undergoing cardiopulmonary bypass. Ann Thorac Surg. 2000;69(4):1192–7.

109. Shimamura S, Kimura K, Katayama M, Mashita T, Maeda K, Kobayashi S, et al. Evaluation of neutrophil function during hemodialysis treatment in healthy dogs under anesthesia with sevoflurane. J Vet Med Sci. 2014;76(11):1539–43.

110. Schnoor M, Parkos CA. Disassembly of endothelial and epithelial junctions during leukocyte transmigration. Front Biosci. 2008;13:6638–52.

111. Rao AM, Apoorva R, Anand U, Anand CV, Venu G. Effect of Hemodialysis on plasma myeloperoxidase activity in end stage renal disease patients. Indian J Clin Biochem. 2012;27(3):253–8.

112. Ono K, Ueki K, Inose K, Tsuchida A, Yano S, Nojima Y. Plasma levels of myeloperoxidase and elastase are differentially regulated by hemodialysis membranes and anticoagulants. Res Commun Mol Pathol Pharmacol. 2000;108(5–6):341–9.

113. Pham CT. Neutrophil serine proteases: specific regulators of inflammation. Nat Rev Immunol. 2006;6(7):541–50.

114. Lewis SL, Van Epps DE, Chenoweth DE. Leukocyte C5a receptor modulation during hemodialysis. Kidney Int. 1987;31(1):112–20.

115. Verma SK, Molitoris BA. Renal endothelial injury and microvascular dysfunction in acute kidney injury. Semin Nephrol. 2015;35(1):96–107.

116. Delano MJ, Ward PA. Sepsis-induced immune dysfunction: can immune therapies reduce mortality? J Clin Invest. 2016;126(1):23–31.

117. Corley A, Lye I, Lavana J, Ahuja A, Jarrett P, Anstey C, et al. Nosocomial infection rates in patients receiving extracorporeal membrane oxygenation across Australia and New Zealand: an interim analysis. Aust Crit Care. 2019;32:S12.

118. Mailloux LU, Bellucci AG, Wilkes BM, Napolitano B, Mossey RT, Lesser M, et al. Mortality in dialysis patients: analysis of the causes of death. Am J Kidney Dis. 1991;18(3):326–35.

119. Sarnak MJ, Jaber BL. Mortality caused by sepsis in patients with end-stage renal disease compared with the general population. Kidney Int. 2000;58(4):1758–64.

120. Lewis SL, Van Epps DE. Neutrophil and monocyte alterations in chronic dialysis patients. Am J Kidney Dis. 1987;9(5):381–95.

121. Kawahito K, Kobayashi E, Misawa Y, Adachi H, Fujimura A, Ino T, et al. Recovery from lymphocytopenia and prognosis after adult extracorporeal membrane oxygenation. Arch Surg. 1998;133(2):216–7.

122. Hong TH, Hu FC, Kuo SW, Ko WJ, Chow LP, Hsu LM, et al. Predicting outcome in patients under extracorporeal membrane oxygenation due to cardiogenic shock through dynamic change of lymphocytes and interleukins. IJC Metab Endocr. 2015;7:36–44.

123. DePalma L, Short BL, Meurs KV, Luban NLC. A flow cytometric analysis of lymphocyte subpopulations in neonates undergoing extracorporeal membrane oxygenation. J Pediatr. 1991;118(1):117–20.

124. Sargin M, Mete MT, Erdogan SB, Kuplay H, Bastopcu M, Akansel S, et al. Prognostic value of neutrophil lymphocyte ratio for early renal failure in ECMO patients. J Heart Lung Transplant. 2019;38(4):S175.

125. Catabay C, Obi Y, Streja E, Soohoo M, Park C, Rhee CM, et al. Lymphocyte cell ratios and mortality among incident hemodialysis patients. Am J Nephrol. 2017;46(5):408–16.

126. Zhao W-M, Tao S-M, Liu G-L. Neutrophil-to-lymphocyte ratio in relation to the risk of all-cause mortality and cardiovascular events in patients with chronic kidney disease: a systematic review and meta-analysis. Ren Fail. 2020;42(1):1059–66.

127. Lisowska KA, Dębska-Ślizień A, Jasiulewicz A, Heleniak Z, Bryl E, Witkowski JM. Hemodialysis affects phenotype and proliferation of CD4-positive T lymphocytes. J Clin Immunol. 2012;32(1):189–200.

128. Ortega SB, Pandiyan P, Windsor J, Torres VO, Selvaraj UM, Lee A, et al. A pilot study identifying brain-targeting adaptive immunity in pediatric extracorporeal membrane oxygenation patients with acquired brain injury. Crit Care Med. 2019;47(3):e206–13.

129. Byrnes J, McKamie W, Swearingen C, Prodhan P, Bhutta A, Jaquiss R, et al. Hemolysis during cardiac extracorporeal membrane oxygenation: a case-control comparison of roller pumps and centrifugal pumps in a pediatric population. ASAIO J. 2011;57(5):456–61.

130. Morgan IS, Codispoti M, Sanger K, Mankad PS. Superiority of centrifugal pump over roller pump in paediatric cardiac surgery: prospective randomised trial. Eur J Cardiothorac Surg. 1998;13(5):526–32.

131. Mlejnsky F, Klein AA, Lindner J, Maruna P, Kvasnicka J, Kvasnicka T, et al. A randomised controlled trial of roller versus centrifugal cardiopulmonary bypass pumps in patients undergoing pulmonary endarterectomy. Perfusion. 2014;30(7):520–8.

132. Perttilä J, Salo M, Peltola O. Comparison of the effects of centrifugal versus roller pump on the immune response in open-heart surgery. Perfusion. 1995;10(4):249–56.

133. Baufreton C, Intrator L, Jansen PG, te Velthuis H, Le Besnerais P, Vonk A, et al. Inflammatory response to cardiopulmonary bypass using roller or centrifugal pumps. Ann Thorac Surg. 1999;67(4):972–7.

134. Passaroni AC, Felicio ML, de Campos NLKL, de Moraes Silva MA, Yoshida WB. Hemolysis and inflammatory response to extracorporeal circulation during on-pump CABG: comparison between roller and centrifugal pump systems. Braz J Cardiovasc Surg. 2018;33(1):64–71.

135. Papadimas E, Leow L, Tan YK, Shen L, Ramanathan K, Choong AMTL, et al. Centrifugal and roller pumps in neonatal and pediatric extracorporeal membrane oxygenation: a systematic review and meta-analysis of clinical outcomes. ASAIO J. 2022;68(3):311–7.

136. Halaweish I, Cole A, Cooley E, Lynch WR, Haft JW. Roller and centrifugal pumps: a retrospective comparison of bleeding complications in extracorporeal membrane oxygenation. ASAIO J. 2015;61(5):496–501.

137. Ronco C, Clark WR. Haemodialysis membranes. Nat Rev Nephrol. 2018;14(6):394–410.

138. Falkenhagen D, Bosch T, Brown GS, Schmidt B, Holtz M, Baurmeister U, et al. A clinical study on different cellulosic dialysis membranes. Nephrol Dial Transplant. 1987;2(6):537–45.

139. Pereira BJ, King AJ, Poutsiaka DD, Strom JA, Dinarello CA. Comparison of first use and reuse of cuprophan membranes on interleukin-1 receptor antagonist and interleukin-1 beta production by blood mononuclear cells. Am J Kidney Dis. 1993;22(2):288–95.

5

140. Hernandez MR, Palomo M, Fuste B, Carbó C, Collado S, Cases A, et al. Effect of two different dialysis membranes on leukocyte adhesion and aggregation. Nephron Clin Pract. 2007;106(1):c1–8.

141. Cases A, Reverter JC, Escolar G, Sanz C, Lopez-Pedret J, Revert L, et al. Platelet activation on hemodialysis: influence of dialysis membranes. Kidney Int Suppl. 1993;41:S217–20.

142. Hakim RM, Fearon DT, Lazarus JM, Perzanowski CS. Biocompatibility of dialysis membranes: effects of chronic complement activation. Kidney Int. 1984;26(2):194–200.

143. Floris M, Marchionna N, Clementi A, Kim JC, Cruz DN, Nalesso F, et al. Evaluation of a new polysulfone hemofilter for continuous renal replacement therapy. Blood Purif. 2011;32(2):133–8.

144. Yasuda H, Sekine K, Abe T, Suzaki S, Katsumi A, Harada N, et al. Comparison of two polysulfone membranes for continuous renal replacement therapy for sepsis: a prospective cross-over study. Ren Replace Ther. 2018;4(1):6.

145. Shibata M, Miyamoto K, Kato S. Comparison of the circulatory effects of continuous renal replacement therapy using AN69ST and polysulfone membranes in septic shock patients: a retrospective observational study. Ther Apher Dial. 2020;24(5):561–7.

146. Ozturk S, Kazancioglu R, Sahin GM, Turkmen A, Gursu M, Sever MS. The effect of the type of membrane on intradialytic complications and mortality in crush syndrome. Ren Fail. 2009;31(8):655–61.

147. Stahl RF, Fisher CA, Kucich U, Weinbaum G, Warsaw DS, Stenach N, et al. Effects of simulated extracorporeal circulation on human leukocyte elastase release, superoxide generation, and procoagulant activity. J Thorac Cardiovasc Surg. 1991;101(2):230–9.

148. Bergman P, Belboul A, Friberg LG, al-Khaja N, Mellgren G, Roberts D. The effect of prolonged perfusion with a membrane oxygenator (PPMO) on white blood cells. Perfusion. 1994;9(1):35–40.

149. Wilm J, Philipp A, Muller T, Bredthauer A, Gleich O, Schmid C, et al. Leukocyte adhesion as an indicator of oxygenator thrombosis during extracorporeal membrane oxygenation therapy? ASAIO J. 2017;64(1):24–30.

150. Steiger T, Foltan M, Philipp A, Mueller T, Gruber M, Bredthauer A, et al. Accumulations of von Willebrand factor within ECMO oxygenators: potential indicator of coagulation abnormalities in critically ill patients? Artif Organs. 2019;43(11):1065–76.

151. Obstals F, Vorobii M, Riedel T, de Los Santos Pereira A, Bruns M, Singh S, et al. Improving hemocompatibility of membranes for extracorporeal membrane oxygenators by grafting nonthrombogenic polymer brushes. Macromol Biosci. 2018;18(3):1700359.

152. Kawahito S, Maeda T, Yoshikawa M, Takano T, Nonaka K, Linneweber J, et al. Blood trauma induced by clinically accepted oxygenators. ASAIO J. 2001;47(5):492–5.

153. Meyer AD, Rishmawi AR, Kamucheka R, Lafleur C, Batchinsky AI, Mackman N, et al. Effect of blood flow on platelets, leukocytes, and extracellular vesicles in thrombosis of simulated neonatal extracorporeal circulation. J Thromb Haemost. 2020;18(2):399–410.

154. Lehle K, Philipp A, Muller T, Schettler F, Bein T, Schmid C, et al. Flow dynamics of different adult ECMO systems: a clinical evaluation. Artif Organs. 2014;38(5):391–8.

155. Sezai A, Shiono M, Nakata K-I, Hata M, Iida M, Saito A, et al. Effects of pulsatile CPB on interleukin-8 and endothelin-1 levels. Artif Organs. 2005;29(9):708–13.

156. Watkins WD, Peterson MB, Kong DL, Kono K, Buckley MJ, Levine FH, et al. Thromboxane and prostacyclin changes during cardiopulmonary bypass with and without pulsatile flow. J Thorac Cardiovasc Surg. 1982;84(2):250–6.

157. Watarida S, Mori A, Onoe M, Tabata R, Shiraishi S, Sugita T, et al. A clinical study on the effects of pulsatile cardiopulmonary bypass on the blood endotoxin levels. J Thorac Cardiovasc Surg. 1994;108(4):620–5.

158. Onorati F, Santarpino G, Rubino AS, Caroleo S, Dardano A, Scalas C, et al. Body perfusion during adult cardiopulmonary bypass is improved by pulsatile flow with intra-aortic balloon pump. Int J Artif Organs. 2009;32(1):50–61.

159. Li G, Zeng J, Liu Z, Zhang Y, Fan X. The pulsatile modification improves Hemodynamics and attenuates inflammatory responses in extracorporeal membrane oxygenation. J Inflamm Res. 2021;14:1357–64.

160. Wang S, Krawiec C, Patel S, Kunselman AR, Song J, Lei F, et al. Laboratory evaluation of hemolysis and systemic inflammatory response in neonatal nonpulsatile and pulsatile extracorporeal life support systems. Artif Organs. 2015;39(9):774–81.

161. Hall MW, Knatz NL, Vetterly C, Tomarello S, Wewers MD, Volk HD, et al. Immunoparalysis and nosocomial infection in children with multiple organ dysfunction syndrome. Intensive Care Med. 2011;37(3):525–32.

162. Zheng H-Y, Zhang M, Yang C-X, Zhang N, Wang X-C, Yang X-P, et al. Elevated exhaustion levels and reduced functional diversity of T cells in peripheral blood may predict severe progression in COVID-19 patients. Cell Mol Immunol. 2020;17(5):541–3.

163. Bhat T, Teli S, Rijal J, Bhat H, Raza M, Khoueiry G, et al. Neutrophil to lymphocyte ratio and cardiovascular diseases: a review. Expert Rev Cardiovasc Ther. 2013;11(1):55–9.

164. Tauber H, Streif W, Fritz J, Ott H, Weigel G, Loacker L, et al. Predicting transfusion requirements during extracorporeal membrane oxygenation. J Cardiothorac Vasc Anesth. 2016;30(3):692–701.

165. Millar JE, Fanning JP, McDonald CI, McAuley DF, Fraser JF. The inflammatory response to extracorporeal membrane oxygenation (ECMO): a review of the pathophysiology. Crit Care. 2016;20(1):387.

166. Doyle AJ, Hunt BJ. Current understanding of how extracorporeal membrane oxygenators activate haemostasis and other blood components. Front Med. 2018;5:352.

167. Singh S. Anticoagulation during renal replacement therapy. Indian J Crit Care Med. 2020;24(Suppl 3):S112–6.

168. Guidelines for adult respiratory failure (2013).

169. Stockmann H, Keller T, Büttner S, Jörres A, Kindgen-Milles D, Kunz JV, et al. CytoResc–"CytoSorb" rescue for critically ill patients undergoing the COVID-19 cytokine storm: a structured summary of a study protocol for a randomized controlled trial. Trials. 2020;21(1):577.

170. Iwata M, Suzuki S, Asai Y, Inoue T, Takagi K. Involvement of nitric oxide in a rat model of carrageenin-induced pleurisy. Mediat Inflamm. 2010;2010:682879.

171. Dal Secco D, Paron JA, de Oliveira SHP, Ferreira SH, Silva JS, de Queiroz Cunha F. Neutrophil migration in inflammation: nitric oxide inhibits rolling, adhesion and induces apoptosis. Nitric Oxide. 2003;9(3):153–64.

172. Carreau A, Kieda C, Grillon C. Nitric oxide modulates the expression of endothelial cell adhesion molecules involved in angiogenesis and leukocyte recruitment. Exp Cell Res. 2011;317(1):29–41.

173. James C, Millar J, Horton S, Brizard C, Molesworth C, Butt W. Nitric oxide administration during paediatric cardiopulmonary bypass: a randomised controlled trial. Intensive Care Med. 2016;42(11):1744–52.

174. Checchia PA, Bronicki RA, Muenzer JT, Dixon D, Raithel S, Gandhi SK, et al. Nitric oxide delivery during cardiopulmonary bypass reduces postoperative morbidity in children—a randomized trial. J Thorac Cardiovasc Surg. 2013;146(3):530–6.

175. Millar JE, Bartnikowski N, Passmore MR, Obonyo NG, Malfertheiner MV, von Bahr V, et al. Combined mesenchymal stromal cell therapy and ECMO in ARDS: a controlled experimental study in sheep. Am J Respir Crit Care Med. 2020;202(3):383–92.

176. von Bahr V, Millar JE, Malfertheiner MV, Ki KK, Passmore MR, Bartnikowski N, et al. Mesenchymal stem cells may ameliorate inflammation in an ex vivo model of extracorporeal membrane oxygenation. Perfusion. 2019;34(1_suppl):15–21.

177. Zen K, Guo YL, Li LM, Bian Z, Zhang CY, Liu Y. Cleavage of the CD11b extracellular domain by the leukocyte serprocidins is critical for neutrophil detachment during chemotaxis. Blood. 2011;117(18):4885–94.

178. Harlan JM, Winn RK. Leukocyte-endothelial interactions: clinical trials of anti-adhesion therapy. Crit Care Med. 2002;30(5 Suppl):S214–9.

179. Scholz M, Cinatl J, Barros RT, Lisboa AC, Genevcius CF, Margraf S, et al. First efficacy and safety results with the antibody containing leukocyte inhibition module in cardiac surgery patients with neutrophil hyperactivity. ASAIO J. 2005;51(2):144–7.

180. Abdel-Rahman U, Margraf S, Aybek T, Lögters T, Bitu-Moreno J, Francischetti I, et al. Inhibition of neutrophil activity improves cardiac function after cardiopulmonary bypass. J Inflamm. 2007;4:21.

181. de Amorim CG, Malbouisson LMS, da Silva FC Jr, Fiorelli AI, Murakami CKF, Carmona MJC. Leukocyte depletion during CPB: effects on inflammation and lung function. Inflammation. 2014;37(1):196–204.

Septic Shock

Jan Bakker

Contents

© The Author(s), under exclusive license to Springer Nature Switzerland AG 2023
Z. Molnar et al. (eds.), *Management of Dysregulated Immune Response in the Critically Ill*,
Lessons from the ICU, https://doi.org/10.1007/978-3-031-17572-5_6

Learning Objectives

After reading this chapter, you will be able
- To identify markers of tissue hypoperfusion
- To create goals of resuscitation in the hypotensive patient
- To create a holistic view of the goals, means, and efficacy of early resuscitation

6.1 Introduction

A state of vasoplegia is characterized by hypotension, especially low diastolic blood pressure (DAP), in the presence or absence of a warm and well-perfused skin [1]. The decrease in blood pressure is not only the result of the arterial vasodilation but may also be related to the venous vasodilation. The latter increases the unstressed volume and thus decreases venous return and cardiac output, thereby contributing to the loss of blood pressure [2].

This chapter is focused on sepsis as this is the most frequent cause of vasodilatory shock and associated with a high mortality. The mechanisms of vasodilation, the consequences for the patient, and the focused hemodynamic treatment of this condition are discussed.

6.2 Of Infection, Mediators, and Vasodilation

Other chapters of this book discuss the immunologic response, and especially the dysregulated response, in more detail. This part is meant to place the cause and response into the clinical perspective to design optimal treatment.

The host response to infection is characterized by the production of cytokines/mediators to facilitate fighting the infection. However, in severe cases, this response may result in hemodynamic dysfunction resulting in organ damage and possible death [3–5]. Both the macrocirculation and microcirculation are affected, and the response to vasoactive drugs is impaired [6]. In case of infection, the combination of hemodynamic support and adequate antibiotics has been shown to improve survival [7]. As in clinical practice, the infection is the key element of problem; timely antibiotics and/or removal of the septic focus is mandatory. In contrast to the experimental study, no clinical studies have shown clear guidance on when to administer antibiotics. The Surviving Sepsis Guidelines recommend on the bases of (very) low quality of evidence to administer antibiotics within the first hour of diagnosis [8], where the early administration seems to benefit septic shock patients the most [9]. However, the problem of overdiagnosing is a reality [10], and the consequences of inadequate source control while rushing to antibiotics, thus requiring a much more patient-oriented approach. The time of "treat first, ask questions later" should be history [11].

Given the association between the production of cytokines/mediators and the hemodynamic consequences and organ damage, many therapies/interventions have focused on removing/blocking/mitigating the levels and effects of these. Although many studies have shown that antibodies to different mediators are safe, facilitating the immune response and removing mediators from the blood, no clear clinical use has been identified [12, 13]. In addition, where increased nitric oxide production is a major cause of the vasodilatory response in patients with sepsis, blocking its production despite improving the hemodynamics [14] may result in increased mortality [15], the latter underscoring the problems of dealing with the hemodynamics of a profound vasodilatory state in a one-size-fits-all approach.

6.3 Parameters of Tissue Perfusion in Early Resuscitation

6.3.1 Blood Pressure

One of the misconceptions in the wording frequently used is the association between sepsis and hypovolemia [16]; this makes fluid resuscitation a logical step to correct the pathophysiology. Frequently in clinical practice, the parameters used in patients with a severe loss of circulating volume (hemorrhage) are also used in patients with septic shock. In hemorrhage, restoration of circulating volume is usually associated with an increase in blood pressure and a decrease in heart rate; this is usually not found in septic shock resuscitation [2, 17].

However, blood pressure is frequently used to indicate a state of hypoperfusion and to initiate fluid administration. However, the effect of fluid resuscitation on blood pressure is much less pronounced than the effect on cardiac output (CO) in a non-hypovolemic state at baseline [2]. In the latter study, the fluid resuscitation was aimed at returning filling pressures (pulmonary artery occlusion pressure) to baseline resulting in an 82% increase in CO with only a 7% increase in MAP. Interestingly, in models using high volumes of resuscitation (40 mL/kg), the effect on cardiac output was less (increase 44%) while the increase in blood pressure was more pronounced (increase 18%) but this at the expense of decreased vasoresponsiveness and higher lactate levels [18]. Both models however underscore that the hyperdynamic state that usually characterizes clinical septic shock is the result of the initial fluid resuscitation. This is further demonstrated by the high incidence of low central venous oxygenation ($ScvO_2$) in the study by Rivers et al. [19] recruiting patients in the very early phase of sepsis in the emergency department, while the incidence after implementation of the Surviving Sepsis Guidelines (and thus aggressive early fluid resuscitation) has dropped significantly [20]. The ultimate best blood pressure for the individual patient remains a topic of debate. The current guideline to aim for a mean arterial pressure (MAP) of 65 mmHg initially is adequate when we seek the optimal pressure while resuscitating and not stopping when 65 mmHg is reached. The latter is supported by recent studies showing the variable effects of manipulating blood pressure on tissue perfusion [21–23] and the possible beneficial effects of aiming at higher blood pressure levels in some patients [24–27].

Thus, the optimal MAP may vary significantly between patients, and the use of a vasopressor test may help to find the optimal blood pressure. This concept was introduced in the ANDROMEDA-SHOCK study [28] to assess whether increasing MAP with NE was associated with improved peripheral perfusion in which case the higher blood pressure was maintained.

6.3.2 **Lactate Levels**

Increased lactate levels have shown to increase when oxygen delivery to the tissues decreases to a critical level in both clinical and experimental conditions [29, 30]. In endotoxin models, the occurrence of the rise in lactate starts at higher levels of oxygen delivery compared to control [31]. In addition, in clinical practice, oxygen supply dependency (a state where oxygen consumption increases when oxygen delivery is increased) is characterized by the presence of increased lactate levels [32, 33]. Therefore, as shock is defined as acute circulatory failure associated with inadequate oxygen utilization by the cells [34], the presence of increased lactate levels is part of the definition of septic shock [35]. A strong association between increased lactate levels, a longer duration of increased lactate levels, and the area under the time-lactate curve with increased morbidity and mortality exists, even in the prehospital phase [36–39]. In addition, a randomized study using lactate levels to guide treatment in the early hours of circulatory failure showed improved outcome compared to the standard care, also in the subgroup analysis of patients with sepsis [40]. In general, decreases in lactate levels following the start of treatment indicate improved likelihood of survival [41]. A recent study however showed that using peripheral perfusion instead of lactate levels to guide early septic shock treatment was associated with improved outcome [28, 42, 43]. In a subgroup analysis of this study, it was further shown that continued resuscitation in patients with increased lactate levels but normal peripheral perfusion was associated with increased mortality [44]. Despite the pitfalls in the interpretation [45] and the unclear efficacy of using lactate levels to guide resuscitation [46], its use together with other parameters of tissue hypoperfusion has merit in clinical practice [47, 48]. However, prolonged resuscitation aiming to normalize lactate levels in the absence of markers of tissue hypoperfusion cannot be recommended and is likely harmful [44]. A failure to decrease lactate levels following start of resuscitation measures should direct the clinician to reevaluate the diagnosis and the adequacy of treatment.

6.3.3 **Central Venous Oxygen Saturation (ScvO$_2$)**

Both the ScvO2 and the mixed venous oxygen saturation (measured in the pulmonary artery) reflect the balance between oxygen demand and oxygen supply. As CO is the major determinant of oxygen supply, both variables are related to global blood flow [49, 50]. As the use of a pulmonary artery catheter in the management of septic shock has almost disappeared, current clinical practice mainly uses ScvO$_2$. The benefit of using an abnormal ScvO$_2$ to guide treatment was most effectively shown in the study by Rivers et al. [19] and later used to guide treatment in patients with increased lactate levels [40]. Although an abnormal ScvO$_2$ should result in an appropriate assessment of the adequacy of the balance between oxygen demand

and oxygen supply, correction of a low $ScvO_2$ in the absence of other markers of tissue hypoperfusion should be weighed against the possible side effects of interventions used to increase $ScvO_2$ [51].

6.3.4 Central Venous to Arterial PCO$_2$ Difference (dPCO$_2$)

In septic shock patients, the $dPCO_2$ has been related to CO, where an increase in $dPCO_2$ resulted in a decrease in CO and the reverse, where a cutoff of 6 mmHg or more was identified as a marker of hypoperfusion [52]. Other studies have since confirmed these findings [53–55] and could associate $dPCO_2$ to the adequacy of microvascular blood flow [56]. Also, persistence of an increased $dPCO_2$ in septic shock patients has been associated with increased mortality [57]. Although the relationship between $dPCO_2$ and global blood flow is not straightforward, an increased $dPCO_2$ should be analyzed in the context of hemodynamics and lactate and peripheral perfusion and could thus be of help in optimizing tissue perfusion.

6.3.5 Peripheral Perfusion

Although Weil et al. already more than 50 years ago used markers of peripheral perfusion to indicate the severity of the circulatory dysfunction [58], it is only recently that peripheral perfusion has come to standard clinical practice. Many studies have shown the high mortality of patients with abnormal peripheral perfusion in almost any clinical context including septic shock [59, 60]. In addition, abnormal capillary refill time (CRT) may identify a very different clinical phenotype, characterized by other markers of tissue hypoperfusion, increased organ failure, more severe hypotension, and decreased vasopressor responsiveness, when compared to patients with normal CRT [61]. As abnormal peripheral perfusion is associated with decreased vital organ perfusion [62], this represents an undesirable circulatory state. When compared to lactate-guided resuscitation [40], capillary refill time (CRT)-guided early resuscitation of septic shock patients showed that organ function and ultimate survival improved [28, 42]. Even more important, the results of the latter study showed that normalization of CRT in the presence of a minimal MAP of 65 mmHg or higher could represent an adequate circulatory state in septic shock patients [44]. A study placing normalization of CRT and phenotyping of septic shock patients has recently started [63].

6.3.6 Holistic Approach

In the early resuscitation of septic shock patients, no one parameter should be used to guide resuscitation. Rather, a holistic approach using blood pressure, central venous oxygenation, lactate, $dPCO_2$, and markers of peripheral perfusion should all be used to optimize individual diagnosis and treatment [64, 65] (◘ Fig. 6.1).

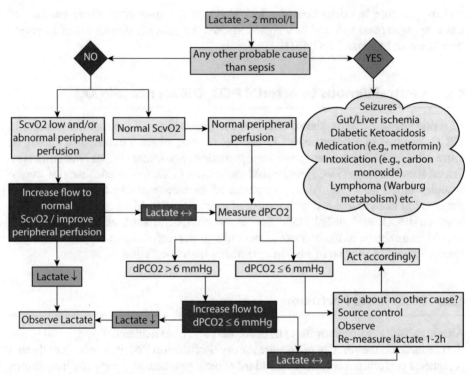

From: Hernandez et al. Intensive Care Med 2019;45(1): 82-85

🔲 **Fig. 6.1**   Flow diagram on how to address tissue perfusion in patients with increased lactate levels in a context of tissue hypoperfusion

6.4   On the Use of Fluids

Fluid resuscitation is the first choice of treatment in patients with sepsis-induced hypoperfusion or septic shock [8]. This recommendation is a one-size-fits-all approach with a volume of at least 30 mL/kg. In a worldwide study, the usual intervention consists of the infusion of 500 mL of fluids over 30 min [66]. However, an expert panel report stressed the importance of the volemic state at baseline, use of smaller volumes of infusion, and individualization of fluid resuscitation [67].

6.4.1   The Physiology

The ultimate goal of fluid resuscitation is to increase the mean systemic filling pressure in order to increase the pressure for venous return (VR) and thus, in the presence of adequate cardiac function, cardiac output [68]. Much confusion surrounds the use of right atrial pressure (RAP) or central venous pressure (CVP) in fluid resuscitation. This is caused by several publications. First is the reproduction of the Frank-Starling curve by Guyton et al. [69] where the original VR/CO (x-axis) to RAP (y-axis) graph of Frank-Starling [70] was changed into a RAP to CO graph, resulting in the interpretation that increasing RAP would result in an increase in CO, where actually RAP is the consequence of VR and cardiac function and thus passive [71]. Therefore, a rise in RAP/CVP during fluid resuscitation mandates caution and should even result in cessation of infusion when the pressure increases significantly [72] as a positive fluid balance, and increased RAP is associated with impaired microcirculatory perfusion, organ function [73, 74], and increased mortality [75]. In addition, the chances of increasing CO with fluid resuscitation are decreasing with increasing baseline RAP [76].

Frequently forgotten is the effect of fluid resuscitation on the arterial load so that initial fluid resuscitation may even decrease the baseline blood pressure [77]. The effect of fluids on the arterial pressure depends on various factors. First, not all patients that increase their cardiac output also increase their blood pressure as the increased cardiac output may decrease arterial load [78]. Second, the baseline state of the vasculature is important in that patients with lower arterial elastance are less likely to increase their blood pressure following a fluid bolus [79]. To this effect, the current ANDROMEDA-SHOCK-2 study investigates the effect of using pulse pressure and diastolic arterial pressure as markers of vasoplegia and using a vasopressor as a first-line agent to improve blood pressure and tissue perfusion rather than fluid resuscitation [63].

Where the increase in CO is the main goal of fluid resuscitation, parameters of fluid responsiveness should be used in most cases outside of clinical emergency. Fluid responsiveness can be predicted by several parameters that however require advanced hemodynamic monitoring [80, 81]. Given the risks associated with increased RAP and increased net fluid balances, fluid responsiveness should be part of standard clinical practice [74, 82, 83] and the fluid challenge should be individualized [84, 85] foregoing the reflex infusion of 30 mL/kg in sepsis patients that may harm a significant number of patients [86]. In the recent ANDROMEDA-SHOCK study [28], about 25% of the patients at study baseline were already fluid unresponsive (a pathophysiologic state) after the initial fluid resuscitation [87]. Finally, the early introduction of a vasopressor before completing a fluid resuscitation to a state of fluid unresponsiveness might further increase the chances of survival in septic shock patients [88]. This might underscore the absence of clear hypovolemia (decreased total circulating volume) but rather the presence of increased unstressed volume in patients with sepsis where norepinephrine increases VR and CO in addition to the increase in blood pressure [89, 90].

However, even when cardiac output increases regional distribution of blood flow, capillary perfusion as well as oxygen diffusion and mitochondrial function are important factors to improve oxygen metabolism and CO_2 removal [91]. In each of these processes, several parameters can be used at the bedside to evaluate the ultimate effectiveness of the fluid resuscitation (◘ Fig. 6.2).

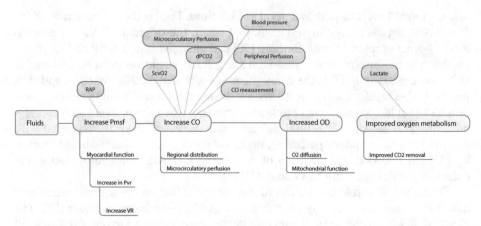

◻ Fig. 6.2 The flow of effects of fluid resuscitation to get to the goal of improved tissue oxygenation. In the red bullets, the parameters that can be used to monitor the effects of a fluid bolus. The sub-levels indicate the subsequent factors related to the main effect. (With thanks to Prof. Gustavo Ospina Tascan, Fundación Valle del Lili, Cali Columbia)

6.4.2 On the Volume of Fluids

From many studies, it is clear that positive fluid balances are associated with increased morbidity and mortality [83, 92]. Although severity of illness might confound these associations also in experimental studies, fluid resuscitation has not been shown to provide much beneficial effects [18].

The use of clear indicators of hypoperfusion, the use of fluid responsiveness parameters, and the use of small bolus fluid resuscitation seem warranted to limit the possible harm of fluid resuscitation. Repeated doses of 250 mL rather than using a fixed volume, with clear stopping rules, are in this context preferred [84, 93]. This should start immediately at the first indication of tissue hypoperfusion as restricting fluids after an initial large fluid resuscitation does not add benefit to the patient. In a recent study recruiting 1554 patients, restricting fluid resuscitation after on average a 3000 mL infusion before starting the study did not result in improved outcome [94]. Restricting the volume of infusion with a strict hypoperfusion indicator for continued fluid resuscitation is one of the main elements of the ANDROMEDA-SHOCK-2 study where the patients receive 1000 mL before start of the study and fluids are not used in patients with normal peripheral perfusion [63], a strategy shown to be safe in an earlier study [28]. Also, other studies have associated a very early start of norepinephrine to correct hypotension in septic shock patients, rather than continued fluid resuscitation, with improved outcome [88].

Continued fluid resuscitation to, ultimately, a state of fluid unresponsiveness should only be used in patients that show clear improvements in markers of tissue hypoperfusion with the ongoing fluid resuscitation as a state of fluid unresponsiveness in and of itself is a pathophysiologic state, and continuous resuscitation in patients without tissue hypoperfusion is associated with increased mortality [44].

6.5 On the Use of Vasoactive Medication

6.5.1 Vasopressors

The goal of the use of vasopressors is similar to the goal of using fluids: improving tissue hypoperfusion. However, in clinical practice, the presence of hypotension is most frequently defined as a MAP of less than 65 mmHg [95]. Hypotension in and of itself is seen as potentially harmful by most doctors and nurses in the ICU [96], thus requiring immediate treatment even in the absence of markers of tissue hypoperfusion. This follows the assumption that autoregulation of flow is lost when the MAP decreases below 60–65 mmHg [97]. However, the effect of sympathetic induced vasoconstriction may have an important role in the ultimate generation of organ blood flow [98]. Although the Surviving Sepsis Guidelines [8] specifically use a MAP of 65 mmHg as an initial goal, a minority of ICUs have a protocol in place on how to treat hypotension [96] so that this MAP is frequently maintained. The use of vasopressors in clinical practice is highly variable and seems to be more hospital associated than evidence associated [99].

Norepinephrine

The agent of choice to treat hypotension when fluid resuscitation is not successful in restoring blood pressure is norepinephrine (NE) [8]. It is sometimes suggested that norepinephrine can result in an increase in heart rate (HR), and thus a change to a non-adrenergic agent is advocated. However, in general, in septic shock patients, the use of NE is not associated with an increase in HR. When reviewing 12 early studies [100–111] on the start/increase of NE in sepsis, the HR before start/change in NE was 117 ± 12 without a significant change after the adjustment (HR: 116 ± 11). Patients with atrial fibrillation might be more susceptible to increases in HR with the use of NE. However, in a recent study, the use of a non-adrenergic agent in patients with septic shock and atrial fibrillation was associated with only a modestly lower heart rate (−4 b/min) [112]. In a study in patients with vasodilatory shock, there was a small rise in HR despite the significant lowering in the use of NE [113].

NE not only increases blood pressure by its alpha-adrenergic effect, but this effect extends to the venous circulation so that venous return increases [89] that, together with the increase in myocardial contractility, results in an increase in CO so that NE is more than just a vasopressor [114]. In addition, this combined effect on pressure and flow may result in improved microcirculatory perfusion in patients with hypoperfusion [115]. This adds to the recommendation earlier, to use a vasopressor test to find the optimal blood pressure.

As during a shortage of NE in the USA the substitution with other agents was associated with an increase in the mortality rate of septic shock [116], we can conclude that using NE as a first-line agent is safe.

Vasopressin

Vasopressin (VP) is mostly started when the NE dosage used reaches a certain level. The Surviving Sepsis Guidelines recommend its use aiming to potentiate vasoconstriction to further increase blood pressure when failed to reach a MAP of 65 mmHg with a limited dose of NE, thereby also limiting possible adrenergic side effects due to increased NE dosages [8]. Although there is a physiological rationale for the use of VP and additional increases in MAP can be achieved, adding VP to a baseline infusion of NE has not shown to be of major benefit to the patient with septic shock when compared to treatment with NE alone [117, 118]. A systematic review did not show improved day-28 mortality using vasopressin. Although there was a possibly beneficial effect on tachyarrhythmias and the requirement for renal replacement therapy this came with a higher incidence of adverse events like digital ischemia [119, 120, 121]. The use of the vasopressin analogs terlipressin and selepressin cannot be recommended. Recent studies have failed to show improved survival in the presence of a higher incidence of adverse events like digital ischemia [120, 121] when compared to NE.

Phenylephrine

As phenylephrine (PE) has no beta-adrenergic effects while exerting potent alpha-adrenergic effects, this vasopressor is frequently preferred especially in patients prone to tachyarrhythmias. However, a recent study in 1847 septic shock patients failed to show a clinically relevant difference in HR between patients treated with PE and those treated with NE [112]. The effect of PE on blood flow was studied in anesthetized patients during surgery. Although PE increased blood pressure, it did not increase CO [122]. Moreover, CO decreased in fluid-unresponsive patients without a change in fluid-responsive patients. Although these patients were not in septic shock, they were likely in a vasodilatory state given the active fluid resuscitation and persisting hypotension. Translating this to sepsis would indicate that PE might even be harmful when a completed fluid resuscitation does not restore MAP. Together with the finding of recent studies showing that the use of PE may be associated with increased mortality when used in septic shock patients [123, 124], PE should be used with caution and not be used as a first-line agent.

Other

Although angiotensin II has shown to significantly increase blood pressure while decreasing the requirement for NE and a possible positive effect on renal function, its use was not associated with improved outcome [113]. The use of angiotensin II has been associated with improved outcome in a specific subgroup of patients requiring renal replacement therapy irrespective of the effect on blood pressure [125, 126]. Although blocking the excessive production of nitric oxide in septic shock results in an increase in blood pressure and improved resolution of septic shock [14], the use of a nitric oxide synthase inhibitor has been shown to increase mortality [15]. Methylene blue also reduces increased nitric oxide production but has only been studied in small-sized patient groups, and clear mortality benefit has not been shown [127]. Despite the potential of both angiotensin II and methylene blue, the use as a standard vasopressor cannot be recommended at this point.

Vasoplegia in the Context of Decreased Vasoresponsiveness

Septic shock may be characterized by a decreased responsiveness to vasopressors that can be modified by the use of hydrocortisone [128]. Also, the response to a corticotropin test has been associated with the risk of mortality in septic shock [129], suggesting that a relative adrenal insufficiency might be relevant in clinical practice. However, the use of steroids in sepsis has not been associated with a significant improvement in mortality [130, 131]. Nevertheless, the use of hydrocortisone is suggested when patients require a high dose of vasopressors possibly indicating decreased vasoresponsiveness [8].

6.5.2 Inodilators

Dobutamine

Inadequate blood flow might result from impaired cardiac function that has been reported frequently and is related to released cytokines rather than impaired coronary perfusion [132]. This impaired myocardial function is usually present in the acute phase and thus might contribute to the hypoperfusion and limit the fluid resuscitation. A decreased CO in and of itself does not imply myocardial dysfunction as in many cases (as discussed before) fluid resuscitation will increase CO significantly. Fluid resuscitation creating strong positive fluid balances as well as increased RAP/CVP is associated with morbidity and mortality and should thus be avoided [74, 75, 133]. The therapy of choice when fluids do not increase CO and tissue perfusion to an adequate level is the use of an inotropic agent, preferably dobutamine. Dobutamine has been shown to significantly improve cardiac function and cardiac output in septic shock patients [134–136]. In addition, low-dose dobutamine also improves regional distribution of blood flow, microcirculatory perfusion, and thus oxygen delivery and oxygen consumption [134, 135, 137–141]. In general, the use of dobutamine is associated with only a modest increase in HR [142] and a significant improvement in survival [143]. A trial studying the effects of dobutamine in the context of septic cardiomyopathy and tissue hypoperfusion is underway (▶ https://clinicaltrials.gov/ct2/show/NCT04166331).

As the effects of dobutamine might also be related to the vasodilatory effects rather than to the increase in CO [141] and the individual response is difficult to predict [144], a trial of a low dose (5 mcg/kg.min) might be helpful in patients with sustained hypoperfusion following initial fluid resuscitation. This approach (similar to the vasopressor test described earlier) has been used in the ANDROMEDA-SHOCK study [28] and its follow-up study [63].

Use of Alternative Inotropes

Other drugs, like levosimendan, milrinone, and enoximone, also have inotropic and vasodilatory effects. The efficacy beyond an increase in CO has been shown in some studies where improvement in microcirculatory perfusion was shown in both experimental and clinical sepsis [145–148]. The use of milrinone/enoximone may be limited given the long half-life and its possible significant effect on blood pressure in a vasoplegic state. So, despite the possible positive effects on CO and tissue perfusion, the general use of inodilators in septic shock is still controversial as also large outcome-focused studies are missing [149].

Levosimendan, a calcium sensitizer, has shown positive hemodynamic effects in clinical and experimental studies [145, 146, 150]. However, a randomized controlled trial failed to show clear clinical benefit when adding levosimendan to standard therapy [151].

The use of these agents should thus be directed by a persisting clinical problem of hypoperfusion not responding to dobutamine or where dobutamine use has side effects or where the use of beta-blockers resulted in impaired cardiac function. Individualization in the use of these agents is thus paramount.

6.5.3 Mitigating the Adrenergic Response

Both the hyperadrenergic state of patients with septic shock and the additional use of adrenergic agents have been shown to exert negative hemodynamic and inflammatory effects [152, 153]. Several drugs (like beta-blockers and dexmedetomidine) with mitigating adrenergic effects have been studied in experimental and clinical conditions showing possible beneficial effects [154–156]. Although a few clinical studies have shown improved outcome with the use of beta-blockers [157, 158], the evidence for a favorable effect of dexmedetomidine on morbidity and mortality is missing [159]. Clinical use is still a matter of debate as possible significant side effects are present [160, 161]. The use of these agents should thus also be directed by a persisting clinical problem of an individual patient.

Similarly, extracorporeal removal of mediators through the use of various techniques [162] has not been introduced in the standard clinical practice of treating septic shock despite a possible clear rationale in patients with refractory shock where the use of hydrocortisone is not effective [12, 163, 164].

Summary

The resuscitation of septic shock patients with signs of hypoperfusion and/or hypotension is to maintain tissue oxygenation, mainly by increasing perfusion and perfusion pressure to restore tissue oxygenation [34]. This is primarily accomplished using fluids and vasoactive agents guided by indicators of fluid overload and markers of tissue hypoperfusion. The use of population-based median values as the goal of treatment may not serve the individual patient. That does not mean that protocols should not be used to treat septic shock as they can represent a starting strategy and a subsequent guide to get to an adequate circulatory state even though that may not represent normality. Many questions still remain [165]. However, a holistic approach where fluids, vasopressors, inotropes, inodilators, and immune/adrenergic modulators are used in an individual approach of the patients is most likely the optimal approach as the days of a one-size-fits-all approach have passed [166–168].

┌─ **Take-Home Messages** ─────────────────────────────────────

- Septic shock is a state in which the immune response to the infection results in inadequate tissue perfusion.
- The resuscitation of septic shock patients should not be focused on the correction of individual variables but should place these in a holistic view of the circulatory state.
- The goal of the initial treatment of septic shock is to get the patient into a state of adequate rather than normal tissue perfusion.
- Fluid resuscitation is the first line of treatment, but the volume of fluids used should be individualized aiming at the lowest volume possible as fluids may cause significant harm.
- A rise in central venous pressure during fluid resuscitation should be a warning/stop sign.
- Fluid resuscitation is best done using boluses of limited amounts of fluids with assessment of efficacy and side effects after each bolus.
- A standard infusion of 30 mL/kg as advocated by the Surviving Sepsis Campaign Guidelines is missing physiologic basis and imposes harm to a relevant number of patients.
- Early start of vasopressors before completed fluid resuscitation should be considered in every patient.
- The goal of blood pressure should be individualized as the relationship between perfusion pressure and tissue blood flow varies among patients.
- The use of a vasopressor test and/or an inodilator test may be helpful in finding the adequate state of tissue perfusion after the initial fluid resuscitation in patients.
- Norepinephrine and dobutamine are the main pillars in optimizing tissue perfusion when the initial fluid resuscitation if not successful.
- Other vasoactive drugs are available but should be used with caution and with specific goals and safety measures.

└──

References

1. Hernandez G, Messina A, Kattan E. Invasive arterial pressure monitoring: much more than mean arterial pressure! Intensive Care Med. 2022;48(10):1495–7.
2. Bakker J, Vincent JL. Effects of norepinephrine and dobutamine on oxygen transport and consumption in a dog model of endotoxic shock. Crit Care Med. 1993;21(3):425–32.
3. Taveira da Silva AM, Kaulbach HC, Chuidian FS, Lambert DR, Suffredini AF, Danner RL. Shock and multiple organ dysfunction after selfadministration of salmonella endotoxin. N Engl J Med. 1993;328:1457–60.
4. Van Deventer SJH, Buller HR, Ten Cate JW, Aarden LA, Hack CE, Sturk A. Experimental endotoxemia in humans: analysis of cytokine release and coagulation, fibrinolytic, and complement pathways. Blood. 1990;76(12):2520–6.
5. Martich GD, Danner RL, Ceska M, Suffredini AF. Detection of interleukin 8 and tumor necrosis factor in normal humans after intravenous endotoxin: the effect of antiinflammatory agents. J Exp Med. 1991;173(4):1021–4.

6. van Loon LM, Stolk RF, van der Hoeven JG, Veltink PH, Pickkers P, Lemson J, et al. Effect of vasopressors on the macro- and microcirculation during systemic inflammation in humans in vivo. Shock. 2020;53(2):171–4.

7. Natanson C, Danner RL, Reilly JM, Doerfler ML, Hoffman WD, Akin GL, et al. Antibiotics versus cardiovascular support in a canine model of human septic shock. Am J Physiol. 1990;259(5 Pt 2):H1440–7.

8. Evans L, Rhodes A, Alhazzani W, Antonelli M, Coopersmith CM, French C, et al. Surviving sepsis campaign: international guidelines for management of sepsis and septic shock 2021. Intensive Care Med. 2021;47(11):1181–247.

9. Seymour CW, Gesten F, Prescott HC, Friedrich ME, Iwashyna TJ, Phillips GS, et al. Time to treatment and mortality during mandated emergency care for sepsis. N Engl J Med. 2017;376(23):2235–44.

10. Klein Klouwenberg PM, Cremer OL, van Vught LA, Ong DS, Frencken JF, Schultz MJ, et al. Likelihood of infection in patients with presumed sepsis at the time of intensive care unit admission: a cohort study. Crit Care. 2015;19:319.

11. Klompas M, Calandra T, Singer M. Antibiotics for sepsis-finding the equilibrium. JAMA. 2018;320(14):1433–4.

12. Shankar-Hari M, Madsen MB, Turgeon AF. Immunoglobulins and sepsis. Intensive Care Med. 2018;44(11):1923–5.

13. Koutroulis I, Batabyal R, McNamara B, Ledda M, Hoptay C, Freishtat RJ. Sepsis immunometabolism: from defining sepsis to understanding how energy production affects immune response. Crit Care Explor. 2019;1(11):e0061.

14. Bakker J, Grover R, McLuckie A, Holzapfel L, Andersson J, Lodato R, et al. Administration of the nitric oxide synthase inhibitor NG-methyl-L-arginine hydrochloride (546C88) by intravenous infusion for up to 72 hours can promote the resolution of shock in patients with severe sepsis: results of a randomized, double-blind, placebo-controlled multicenter study (study no. 144-002). Crit Care Med. 2004;32(1):1–12.

15. Lopez A, Lorente JA, Steingrub J, Bakker J, McLuckie A, Willatts S, et al. Multiple-center, randomized, placebo-controlled, double-blind study of the nitric oxide synthase inhibitor 546C88: effect on survival in patients with septic shock. Crit Care Med. 2004;32(1):21–30.

16. Perner A, Cecconi M, Cronhjort M, Darmon M, Jakob SM, Pettila V, et al. Expert statement for the management of hypovolemia in sepsis. Intensive Care Med. 2018;44(6):791–8.

17. van Genderen ME, Klijn E, Lima A, de Jonge J, Visser SS, Voorbeijtel J, et al. Microvascular perfusion as a target for fluid resuscitation in experimental circulatory shock. Crit Care Med. 2014;42(2):E96–E105.

18. Byrne L, Obonyo NG, Diab SD, Dunster KR, Passmore MR, Boon AC, et al. Unintended consequences; fluid resuscitation worsens shock in an ovine model of endotoxemia. Am J Respir Crit Care Med. 2018;198(8):1043–54.

19. Rivers E, Nguyen B, Havstad S, Ressler J, Muzzin A, Knoblich B, et al. Early goal-directed therapy in the treatment of severe sepsis and septic shock. N Engl J Med. 2001;345(19):1368–77.

20. van Beest PA, Hofstra JJ, Schultz MJ, Boerma EC, Spronk PE, Kuiper MA. The incidence of low venous oxygen saturation on admission to the intensive care unit: a multi-center observational study in the Netherlands. Crit Care. 2008;12(2):R33.

21. Thooft A, Favory R, Salgado DR, Taccone FS, Donadello K, De Backer D, et al. Effects of changes in arterial pressure on organ perfusion during septic shock. Crit Care. 2011;15(5):R222.

22. Pierrakos C, Velissaris D, Scolletta S, Heenen S, De Backer D, Vincent JL. Can changes in arterial pressure be used to detect changes in cardiac index during fluid challenge in patients with septic shock? Intensive Care Med. 2012;38(3):422–8.

23. Dunser MW, Takala J, Brunauer A, Bakker J. Re-thinking resuscitation: leaving blood pressure cosmetics behind and moving forward to permissive hypotension and a tissue perfusion-based approach. Crit Care. 2013;17(5):326.

24. Asfar P, Meziani F, Hamel JF, Grelon F, Megarbane B, Anguel N, et al. High versus low blood-pressure target in patients with septic shock. N Engl J Med. 2014;370(17):1583–93.

25. Patel BM, Chittock DR, Russell JA, Walley KR. Beneficial effects of short-term vasopressin infusion during severe septic shock. Anesthesiology. 2002;96(3):576–82.

26. Fiorese Coimbra KT, de Freitas FGR, Bafi AT, Pinheiro TT, Nunes NF, de Azevedo LCP, et al. Effect of increasing blood pressure with noradrenaline on the microcirculation of patients with septic shock and previous arterial hypertension. Crit Care Med. 2019;47(8):1033–40.

27. Lamontagne F, Richards-Belle A, Thomas K, Harrison DA, Sadique MZ, Grieve RD, et al. Effect of reduced exposure to vasopressors on 90-day mortality in older critically ill patients with vasodilatory hypotension: a randomized clinical trial. JAMA. 2020;323(10):938–49.

28. Hernandez G, Ospina-Tascon GA, Damiani LP, Estenssoro E, Dubin A, Hurtado J, et al. Effect of a resuscitation strategy targeting peripheral perfusion status vs serum lactate levels on 28-day mortality among patients with septic shock: the ANDROMEDA-SHOCK randomized clinical trial. JAMA. 2019;321(7):654–64.

29. Cain SM. Appearance of excess lactate in anesthetized dogs during anemic and hypoxic hypoxia. Am J Physiol. 1965;209(3):604–10.

30. Ronco JJ, Fenwick JC, Tweeddale MG, Wiggs BR, Phang PT, Cooper DJ, et al. Identification of the critical oxygen delivery for anaerobic metabolism in critically ill septic and nonseptic humans. JAMA. 1993;270(14):1724–30.

31. Zhang H, Vincent JL. Oxygen extraction is altered by endotoxin during tamponade-induced stagnant hypoxia in the dog. Circ Shock. 1993;40(3):168–76.

32. Bakker J, Vincent J. The oxygen-supply dependency phenomenon is associated with increased blood lactate levels. J Crit Care. 1991;6(3):152–9.

33. Friedman G, De Backer D, Shahla M, Vincent JL. Oxygen supply dependency can characterize septic shock. Intensive Care Med. 1998;24(2):118–23.

34. Cecconi M, De Backer D, Antonelli M, Beale R, Bakker J, Hofer C, et al. Consensus on circulatory shock and hemodynamic monitoring. Task force of the European Society of Intensive Care Medicine. Intensive Care Med. 2014;40(12):1795–815.

35. Singer M, Deutschman CS, Seymour CW, Shankar-Hari M, Annane D, Bauer M, et al. The third international consensus definitions for sepsis and septic shock (Sepsis-3). JAMA. 2016;315(8):801–10.

36. Bakker J, Coffernils M, Leon M, Gris P, Vincent J. Blood lactate levels are superior to oxygen-derived variables in predicting outcome in human septic shock. Chest. 1991;99(4):956–62.

37. Bakker J, Gris P, Coffernils M, Kahn R, Vincent J. Serial blood lactate levels can predict the development of multiple organ failure following septic shock. Am J Surg. 1996;171(2):221–6.

38. Jansen TC, van Bommel J, Woodward R, Mulder PG, Bakker J. Association between blood lactate levels, sequential organ failure assessment subscores, and 28-day mortality during early and late intensive care unit stay: a retrospective observational study. Crit Care Med. 2009;37(8):2369–74.

39. Jouffroy R, Leguillier T, Gilbert B, Tourtier JP, Bloch-Laine E, Ecollan P, et al. Prehospital lactate clearance is associated with reduced mortality in patients with septic shock. Am J Emerg Med. 2021;46:367–73.

40. Jansen TC, van Bommel J, Schoonderbeek FJ, Visser SJS, van der Klooster JM, Lima AP, et al. Early lactate-guided therapy in intensive care unit patients a multicenter, open-label, randomized controlled trial. Am J Respir Crit Care Med. 2010;182(6):752–61.

41. Vincent JL, Quintairos ESA, Couto L Jr, Taccone FS. The value of blood lactate kinetics in critically ill patients: a systematic review. Crit Care. 2016;20(1):257.

42. Zampieri FG, Damiani LP, Bakker J, Ospina-Tascon GA, Castro R, Cavalcanti AB, et al. Effects of a resuscitation strategy targeting peripheral perfusion status vs serum lactate levels among patients with septic shock: a Bayesian reanalysis of the ANDROMEDA-SHOCK trial. Am J Respir Crit Care Med. 2020;201(4):423–9.

43. Gu WJ, Zhang Z, Bakker J. Early lactate clearance-guided therapy in patients with sepsis: a meta-analysis with trial sequential analysis of randomized controlled trials. Intensive Care Med. 2015;41(10):1862–3.

44. Kattan E, Hernandez G, Ospina-Tascon G, Valenzuela ED, Bakker J, Castro R, et al. A lactate-targeted resuscitation strategy may be associated with higher mortality in patients with septic shock and normal capillary refill time: a post hoc analysis of the ANDROMEDA-SHOCK study. Ann Intensive Care. 2020;10(1):114.

45. Hernandez G, Bellomo R, Bakker J. The ten pitfalls of lactate clearance in sepsis. Intensive Care Med. 2019;45(1):82–5.

46. Bakker J, de Backer D, Hernandez G. Lactate-guided resuscitation saves lives: we are not sure. Intensive Care Med. 2016;42(3):472–4.

47. Alegria L, Vera M, Dreyse J, Castro R, Carpio D, Henriquez C, et al. A hypoperfusion context may aid to interpret hyperlactatemia in sepsis-3 septic shock patients: a proof-of-concept study. Ann Intensive Care. 2017;7(1):29.

48. Bakker J, Nijsten MW, Jansen TC. Clinical use of lactate monitoring in critically ill patients. Ann Intensive Care. 2013;3(1):12.

49. Marx G, Reinhart K. Venous oximetry. Curr Opin Crit Care. 2006;12(3):263–8.

50. Rivers EP, Ander DS, Powell D. Central venous oxygen saturation monitoring in the critically ill patient. Curr Opin Crit Care. 2001;7(3):204–11.

51. Walley KR. Use of central venous oxygen saturation to guide therapy. Am J Respir Crit Care Med. 2011;184(5):514–20.

52. Bakker J, Vincent JL, Gris P, Leon M, Coffernils M, Kahn RJ. Veno-arterial carbon dioxide gradient in human septic shock. Chest. 1992;101(2):509–15.

53. Zhang H, Vincent JL. Arteriovenous differences in PCO2 and pH are good indicators of critical hypoperfusion. Am Rev Respir Dis. 1993;148:867–71.

54. Teboul JL, Mercat A, Lenique F, Berton C, Richard C. Value of the venous-arterial PCO2 gradient to reflect the oxygen supply to demand in humans: effects of dobutamine [see comments]. Crit Care Med. 1998;26(6):1007–10.

55. Cuschieri J, Rivers EP, Donnino MW, Katilius M, Jacobsen G, Nguyen HB, et al. Central venous-arterial carbon dioxide difference as an indicator of cardiac index. Intensive Care Med. 2005;31(6):818–22.

56. Ospina-Tascon GA, Umana M, Bermudez WF, Bautista-Rincon DF, Valencia JD, Madrinan HJ, et al. Can venous-to-arterial carbon dioxide differences reflect microcirculatory alterations in patients with septic shock? Intensive Care Med. 2016;42(2):211–21.

57. Muller G, Mercier E, Vignon P, Henry-Lagarrigue M, Kamel T, Desachy A, et al. Prognostic significance of central venous-to-arterial carbon dioxide difference during the first 24 hours of septic shock in patients with and without impaired cardiac function. Br J Anaesth. 2017;119(2):239–48.

58. Joly HR, Weil MH. Temperature of the great toe as an indication of the severity of shock. Circulation. 1969;39(1):131–8.

59. Lima A, Bakker J. Clinical assessment of peripheral circulation. Curr Opin Crit Care. 2015;21(3):226–31.

60. Ait-Oufella H, Lemoinne S, Boelle PY, Galbois A, Baudel JL, Lemant J, et al. Mottling score predicts survival in septic shock. Intensive Care Med. 2011;37(5):801–7.

61. Hernandez G, Kattan E, Ospina-Tascon G, Bakker J, Castro R, ANDROMEDA-SHOCK Study Investigators and the Latin America Intensive Care Network (LIVEN), et al. Capillary refill time status could identify different clinical phenotypes among septic shock patients fulfilling Sepsis-3 criteria: a post hoc analysis of ANDROMEDA-SHOCK trial. Intensive Care Med. 2020;46(4):816–8.

62. Brunauer A, Kokofer A, Bataar O, Gradwohl-Matis I, Dankl D, Bakker J, et al. Changes in peripheral perfusion relate to visceral organ perfusion in early septic shock: a pilot study. J Crit Care. 2016;35:105–9.

63. Kattan E, Bakker J, Estenssoro E, Ospina-Tascon G, Biasi Cavalcanti A, De Backer D, et al. Hemodynamic phenotype-based, capillary refill time-targeted resuscitation in early septic shock: the ANDROMEDA-SHOCK-2 randomized clinical trial study protocol. Rev Bras Ter Intensiva. 2022;34(1):96–106.

64. Wittayachamnankul B, Chentanakij B, Sruamsiri K, Chattipakorn N. The role of central venous oxygen saturation, blood lactate, and central venous-to-arterial carbon dioxide partial pressure difference as a goal and prognosis of sepsis treatment. J Crit Care. 2016;36:223–9.

65. Ait-Oufella H, Bakker J. Understanding clinical signs of poor tissue perfusion during septic shock. Intensive Care Med. 2016;42(12):2070–2.

66. Cecconi M, Hofer C, Teboul JL, Pettila V, Wilkman E, Molnar Z, et al. Fluid challenges in intensive care: the FENICE study : a global inception cohort study. Intensive Care Med. 2015;41(9):1529–37.

67. Cecconi M, Hernandez G, Dunser M, Antonelli M, Baker T, Bakker J, et al. Fluid administration for acute circulatory dysfunction using basic monitoring: narrative review and expert panel recommendations from an ESICM task force. Intensive Care Med. 2019;45(1):21–32.

68. Berlin DA, Bakker J. Understanding venous return. Intensive Care Med. 2014;40(10):1564–6.
69. Guyton AC, Jones CE, Coleman TG. Circulatory physiology; cardiac output and its regulation. 2nd ed. Saunders; 1973.
70. Patterson SW, Starling EH. On the mechanical factors which determine the output of the ventricles. J Physiol. 1914;48(5):357–79.
71. Berlin DA, Bakker J. Starling curves and central venous pressure. Crit Care. 2015;19(1):55.
72. Vincent JL, Weil MH. Fluid challenge revisited. Crit Care Med. 2006;34(5):1333–7.
73. Vellinga NA, Ince C, Boerma EC. Elevated central venous pressure is associated with impairment of microcirculatory blood flow in sepsis: a hypothesis generating post hoc analysis. BMC Anesthesiol. 2013;13:17.
74. Legrand M, Dupuis C, Simon C, Gayat E, Mateo J, Lukaszewicz AC, et al. Association between systemic hemodynamics and septic acute kidney injury in critically ill patients: a retrospective observational study. Crit Care. 2013;17(6):R278.
75. Boyd JH, Forbes J, Nakada TA, Walley KR, Russell JA. Fluid resuscitation in septic shock: a positive fluid balance and elevated central venous pressure are associated with increased mortality. Crit Care Med. 2011;39(2):259–65.
76. Magder S, Bafaqeeh F. The clinical role of central venous pressure measurements. J Intensive Care Med. 2007;22(1):44–51.
77. Magder S, Vanelli G. Circuit factors in the high cardiac output of sepsis. J Crit Care. 1996;11(4):155–66.
78. Monge Garcia MI, Guijo Gonzalez P, Gracia Romero M, Gil Cano A, Oscier C, Rhodes A, et al. Effects of fluid administration on arterial load in septic shock patients. Intensive Care Med. 2015;41(7):1247–55.
79. Garcia MI, Romero MG, Cano AG, Aya HD, Rhodes A, Grounds RM, et al. Dynamic arterial elastance as a predictor of arterial pressure response to fluid administration: a validation study. Crit Care. 2014;18(6):626.
80. Pinsky MR. Understanding preload reserve using functional hemodynamic monitoring. Intensive Care Med. 2015;41(8):1480–2.
81. Monnet X, Shi R, Teboul JL. Prediction of fluid responsiveness. What's new? Ann Intensive Care. 2022;12(1):46.
82. van den Akker JPC, Bakker J, Groeneveld ABJ, den Uil CA. Risk indicators for acute kidney injury in cardiogenic shock. J Crit Care. 2019;50:11–6.
83. Malbrain MLNG, Van Regenmortel N, Saugel B, De Tavernier B, Van Gaal PJ, Joannes-Boyau O, et al. Principles of fluid management and stewardship in septic shock: it is time to consider the four D's and the four phases of fluid therapy. Ann Intensive Care. 2018;8(1):66.
84. Vincent JL, Cecconi M, De Backer D. The fluid challenge. Crit Care. 2020;24(1):703.
85. Guarracino F, Bertini P, Pinsky MR. Heterogeneity of cardiovascular response to standardized sepsis resuscitation. Crit Care. 2020;24(1):99.
86. Douglas IS, Alapat PM, Corl KA, Exline MC, Forni LG, Holder AL, et al. Fluid response evaluation in sepsis hypotension and shock: a randomized clinical trial. Chest. 2020;158(4):1431–45.
87. Kattan E, Ospina-Tascon GA, Teboul JL, Castro R, Cecconi M, Ferri G, et al. Systematic assessment of fluid responsiveness during early septic shock resuscitation: secondary analysis of the ANDROMEDA-SHOCK trial. Crit Care. 2020;24(1):23.
88. Ospina-Tascon GA, Hernandez G, Alvarez I, Calderon-Tapia LE, Manzano-Nunez R, Sanchez-Ortiz AI, et al. Effects of very early start of norepinephrine in patients with septic shock: a propensity score-based analysis. Crit Care. 2020;24(1):52.
89. Persichini R, Silva S, Teboul JL, Jozwiak M, Chemla D, Richard C, et al. Effects of norepinephrine on mean systemic pressure and venous return in human septic shock. Crit Care Med. 2012;40(12):3146–53.
90. Hamzaoui O, Georger JF, Monnet X, Ksouri H, Maizel J, Richard C, et al. Early administration of norepinephrine increases cardiac preload and cardiac output in septic patients with life-threatening hypotension. Crit Care. 2010;14(4):R142.
91. Bennett VA, Vidouris A, Cecconi M. Effects of fluids on the macro- and microcirculations. Crit Care. 2018;22(1):74.
92. Acheampong A, Vincent JL. A positive fluid balance is an independent prognostic factor in patients with sepsis. Crit Care. 2015;19:251.

93. Barthelemy R, Kindermans M, Delval P, Collet M, Gaugain S, Cecconi M, et al. Accuracy of cumulative volumes of fluid challenge to assess fluid responsiveness in critically ill patients with acute circulatory failure: a pharmacodynamic approach. Br J Anaesth. 2022;128(2):236–43.

94. Meyhoff TS, Hjortrup PB, Wetterslev J, Sivapalan P, Laake JH, Cronhjort M, et al. Restriction of intravenous fluid in ICU patients with septic shock. N Engl J Med. 2022;386(26):2459–70.

95. Schenk J, van der Ven WH, Schuurmans J, Roerhorst S, Cherpanath TGV, Lagrand WK, et al. Definition and incidence of hypotension in intensive care unit patients, an international survey of the European Society of Intensive Care Medicine. J Crit Care. 2021;65:142–8.

96. van der Ven WH, Schuurmans J, Schenk J, Roerhorst S, Cherpanath TGV, Lagrand WK, et al. Monitoring, management, and outcome of hypotension in intensive care unit patients, an international survey of the European Society of Intensive Care Medicine. J Crit Care. 2022;67:118–25.

97. Leone M, Asfar P, Radermacher P, Vincent JL, Martin C. Optimizing mean arterial pressure in septic shock: a critical reappraisal of the literature. Crit Care. 2015;19(1):794.

98. Kato R, Pinsky MR. Personalizing blood pressure management in septic shock. Ann Intensive Care. 2015;5(1):41.

99. Bosch NA, Teja B, Wunsch H, Walkey AJ. Practice patterns in the initiation of secondary vasopressors and adjunctive corticosteroids during septic shock in the United States. Ann Am Thorac Soc. 2021;18(12):2049–57.

100. Martin C, Saux P, Eon B, Aknin P, Gouin F. Septic shock: a goal-directed therapy using volume loading, dobutamine and/or norepinephrine. Acta Anaesthesiol Scand. 1990;34(5):413–7.

101. Martin C, Papazian L, Perrin G, Saux P, Gouin F. Norepinephrine or dopamine for the treatment of hyperdynamic septic shock? Chest. 1993;103(6):1826–31.

102. Schreuder WO, Schneider AJ, Groeneveld ABJ, Thijs LG. Effect of dopamine vs norepinephrine on hemodynamics in septic shock. Emphasis on right ventricular performance. Chest. 1989;95(6):1282–8.

103. Martin C, Eon B, Saux P, Aknin P, Gouin F. Renal effects of norepinephrine used to treat septic shock patients. Crit Care Med. 1990;18(3):282–5.

104. Meadows D, Edwards JD, Wilkins RG, Nightingale P. Reversal of intractable septic shock with norepinephrine therapy. Crit Care Med. 1988;16(7):663–6.

105. Desjars P, Pinaud M, Potel G, Tasseau F, Touze MD. A reappraisal of norepinephrine therapy in human septic shock. Crit Care Med. 1987;15(2):134–7.

106. Fukuoka T, Nishimura M, Imanaka H, Taenaka N, Yoshiya I, Takezawa J. Effects of norepinephrine on renal function in septic patients with normal and elevated serum lactate levels. Crit Care Med. 1989;17(11):1104–7.

107. Hesselvik JF, Brodin B. Low dose norepinephrine in patients with septic shock and oliguria: effects on afterload, urine flow and oxygen transport. Crit Care Med. 1989;17:179–80.

108. Martin C, Viviand X, Arnaud S, Vialet R, Rougnon T. Effects of norepinephrine plus dobutamine or norepinephrine alone on left ventricular performance of septic shock patients. Crit Care Med. 1999;27(9):1708–13.

109. Martin C, Perrin G, Saux P, Papazian L, Gouin F. Effects of norepinephrine on right ventricular function in septic shock patients. Intensive Care Med. 1994;20(6):444–7.

110. Redl-Wenzl EM, Armbruster C, Edelmann G, Fischl E, Kolacny M, Wechsler-Fördôs A, et al. The effects of norepinephrine on hemodynamics and renal function in severe septic shock states. Intensive Care Med. 1993;19(3):151–4.

111. Marik PE, Mohedin M. The contrasting effects of dopamine and norepinephrine on systemic and splanchnic oxygen utilization in hyperdynamic sepsis. JAMA. 1994;272:1354–7.

112. Law AC, Bosch NA, Peterson D, Walkey AJ. Comparison of heart rate after phenylephrine versus norepinephrine initiation in patients with septic shock and atrial fibrillation. Chest. 2022;162(4):796–803.

113. Khanna A, English SW, Wang XS, Ham K, Tumlin J, Szerlip H, et al. Angiotensin II for the treatment of vasodilatory shock. N Engl J Med. 2017;377(5):419–30.

114. Espinoza EDV, Hernandez G, Bakker J. Norepinephrine, more than a vasopressor. Ann Transl Med. 2019;7(S1):S25.

115. Dubin A, Pozo MO, Casabella CA, Palizas F Jr, Murias G, Moseinco MC, et al. Increasing arterial blood pressure with norepinephrine does not improve microcirculatory blood flow: a prospective study. Crit Care. 2009;13(3):R92.

116. Vail E, Gershengorn HB, Hua M, Walkey AJ, Rubenfeld G, Wunsch H. Association between US norepinephrine shortage and mortality among patients with septic shock. JAMA. 2017;317(14):1433–42.

117. Gordon AC, Mason AJ, Thirunavukkarasu N, Perkins GD, Cecconi M, Cepkova M, et al. Effect of early vasopressin vs norepinephrine on kidney failure in patients with septic shock: the VANISH randomized clinical trial. JAMA. 2016;316(5):509–18.

118. Russell JA, Walley KR, Singer J, Gordon AC, Hebert PC, Cooper DJ, et al. Vasopressin versus norepinephrine infusion in patients with septic shock. N Engl J Med. 2008;358(9):877–87.

119. Nagendran M, Russell JA, Walley KR, Brett SJ, Perkins GD, Hajjar L, et al. Vasopressin in septic shock: an individual patient data meta-analysis of randomised controlled trials. Intensive Care Med. 2019;45(6):844–55.

120. Liu ZM, Chen J, Kou Q, Lin Q, Huang X, Tang Z, et al. Terlipressin versus norepinephrine as infusion in patients with septic shock: a multicentre, randomised, double-blinded trial. Intensive Care Med. 2018;44(11):1816–25.

121. Laterre PF, Berry SM, Blemings A, Carlsen JE, Francois B, Graves T, et al. Effect of selepressin vs placebo on ventilator- and vasopressor-free days in patients with septic shock: the SEPSIS-ACT randomized clinical trial. JAMA. 2019;322(15):1476–85.

122. Rebet O, Andremont O, Gerard JL, Fellahi JL, Hanouz JL, Fischer MO. Preload dependency determines the effects of phenylephrine on cardiac output in anaesthetised patients: a prospective observational study. Eur J Anaesthesiol. 2016;33(9):638–44.

123. Patel VV, Sullivan JB, Cavanaugh J. Analysis of mortality in patients treated with phenylephrine in septic shock. J Pharm Pract. 2021:8971900211000218.

124. Hawn JM, Bauer SR, Yerke J, Li M, Wang X, Reddy AJ, et al. Effect of phenylephrine push before continuous infusion norepinephrine in patients with septic shock. Chest. 2021;159(5):1875–83.

125. Bellomo R, Forni LG, Busse LW, McCurdy MT, Ham KR, Boldt DW, et al. Renin and survival in patients given angiotensin II for catecholamine-resistant vasodilatory shock. A clinical trial. Am J Respir Crit Care Med. 2020;202(9):1253–61.

126. Tumlin JA, Murugan R, Deane AM, Ostermann M, Busse LW, Ham KR, et al. Outcomes in patients with vasodilatory shock and renal replacement therapy treated with intravenous angiotensin II. Crit Care Med. 2018;46(6):949–57.

127. Hosseinian L, Weiner M, Levin MA, Fischer GW. Methylene blue: magic bullet for vasoplegia? Anesth Analg. 2016;122(1):194–201.

128. Bellissant E, Annane D. Effect of hydrocortisone on phenylephrine—mean arterial pressure dose- response relationship in septic shock. Clin Pharmacol Ther. 2000;68(3):293–303.

129. Annane D, Sebille V, Troche G, Raphael JC, Gajdos P, Bellissant E. A 3-level prognostic classification in septic shock based on cortisol levels and cortisol response to corticotropin. JAMA. 2000;283(8):1038–45.

130. Rochwerg B, Oczkowski SJ, Siemieniuk RAC, Agoritsas T, Belley-Cote E, D'Aragon F, et al. Corticosteroids in sepsis: an updated systematic review and meta-analysis. Crit Care Med. 2018;46(9):1411–20.

131. Volbeda M, Wetterslev J, Gluud C, Zijlstra JG, van der Horst IC, Keus F. Glucocorticosteroids for sepsis: systematic review with meta-analysis and trial sequential analysis. Intensive Care Med. 2015;41(7):1220–34.

132. Vieillard-Baron A. Septic cardiomyopathy. Ann Intensive Care. 2011;1(1):6.

133. Vincent JL, Sakr Y, Sprung CL, Ranieri VM, Reinhart K, Gerlach H, et al. Sepsis in European intensive care units: results of the SOAP study. Crit Care Med. 2006;34(2):344–53.

134. Vincent JL, Roman A, De Backer D, Kahn RJ. Oxygen uptake/supply dependency. Effects of short-term dobutamine infusion. Am J Respir Crit Care Med. 1990;142(1):2–7.

135. De Backer D, Moraine JJ, Berre J, Kahn RJ, Vincent JL. Effects of dobutamine on oxygen consumption in septic patients. Direct versus indirect determinations. Am J Respir Crit Care Med. 1994;150(1):95–100.

136. Geri G, Vignon P, Aubry A, Fedou AL, Charron C, Silva S, et al. Cardiovascular clusters in septic shock combining clinical and echocardiographic parameters: a post hoc analysis. Intensive Care Med. 2019;45(5):657–67.

137. Joly LM, Monchi M, Cariou A, Chiche JD, Bellenfant F, Brunet F, et al. Effects of dobutamine on gastric mucosal perfusion and hepatic metabolism in patients with septic shock. Am J Respir Crit Care Med. 1999;160:1983–6.

138. Price K, Clark C, Gutierrez G. Intravenous dobutamine improves gastric intramucosal pH in septic patients. Am Rev Respir Dis. 1992;145:A316.

139. Reinelt H, Radermacher P, Fischer G, Geisser W, Wachter U, Wiedeck H, et al. Effects of a dobutamine-induced increase in splanchnic blood flow on hepatic metabolic activity in patients with septic shock. Anesthesiology. 1997;86(4):818–24.

140. Hernandez G, Bruhn A, Luengo C, Regueira T, Kattan E, Fuentealba A, et al. Effects of dobutamine on systemic, regional and microcirculatory perfusion parameters in septic shock: a randomized, placebo-controlled, double-blind, crossover study. Intensive Care Med. 2013;39(8):1435–43.

141. De Backer D, Creteur J, Dubois MJ, Sakr Y, Koch M, Verdant C, et al. The effects of dobutamine on microcirculatory alterations in patients with septic shock are independent of its systemic effects. Crit Care Med. 2006;34(2):403–8.

142. Vieillard-Baron A, Caille V, Charron C, Belliard G, Page B, Jardin F. Actual incidence of global left ventricular hypokinesia in adult septic shock. Crit Care Med. 2008;36(6):1701–6.

143. Belletti A, Benedetto U, Biondi-Zoccai G, Leggieri C, Silvani P, Angelini GD, et al. The effect of vasoactive drugs on mortality in patients with severe sepsis and septic shock. A network meta-analysis of randomized trials. J Crit Care. 2017;37:91–8.

144. Potter EK, Hodgson L, Creagh-Brown B, Forni LG. Manipulating the microcirculation in sepsis - the impact of vasoactive medications on microcirculatory blood flow: a systematic review. Shock. 2019;52(1):5–12.

145. Fries M, Ince C, Rossaint R, Bleilevens C, Bickenbach J, Rex S, et al. Levosimendan but not norepinephrine improves microvascular oxygenation during experimental septic shock. Crit Care Med. 2008;36(6):1886–91.

146. Morelli A, Donati A, Ertmer C, Rehberg S, Lange M, Orecchioni A, et al. Levosimendan for resuscitating the microcirculation in patients with septic shock: a randomized controlled study. Crit Care. 2010;14(6):R232.

147. Schmidt W, Tinelli M, Secchi A, Gebhard MM, Martin E, Schmidt H. Milrinone improves intestinal villus blood flow during endotoxemia. Can J Anaesth. 2000;47(7):673–9.

148. de Miranda ML, Pereira SJ, Santos AO, Villela NR, Kraemer-Aguiar LG, Bouskela E. Milrinone attenuates arteriolar vasoconstriction and capillary perfusion deficits on endotoxemic hamsters. PLoS One. 2015;10(2):e0117004.

149. Ospina-Tascon GA, Calderon-Tapia LE. Inodilators in septic shock: should these be used? Ann Transl Med. 2020;8(12):796.

150. Rehberg S, Ertmer C, Vincent JL, Spiegel HU, Kohler G, Erren M, et al. Effects of combined arginine vasopressin and levosimendan on organ function in ovine septic shock. Crit Care Med. 2010;38(10):2016–23.

151. Gordon AC, Perkins GD, Singer M, McAuley DF, Orme RM, Santhakumaran S, et al. Levosimendan for the prevention of acute organ dysfunction in sepsis. N Engl J Med. 2016;375(17):1638–48.

152. Stolk RF, van der Pasch E, Naumann F, Schouwstra J, Bressers S, van Herwaarden AE, et al. Norepinephrine dysregulates the immune response and compromises host defense during sepsis. Am J Respir Crit Care Med. 2020;202(6):830–42.

153. Stolk RF, van der Poll T, Angus DC, van der Hoeven JG, Pickkers P, Kox M. Potentially inadvertent immunomodulation: norepinephrine use in sepsis. Am J Respir Crit Care Med. 2016;194(5):550–8.

154. Cioccari L, Luethi N, Bailey M, Shehabi Y, Howe B, Messmer AS, et al. The effect of dexmedetomidine on vasopressor requirements in patients with septic shock: a subgroup analysis of the sedation practice in intensive care evaluation [SPICE III] trial. Crit Care. 2020;24(1):441.

155. Hernandez G, Tapia P, Alegria L, Soto D, Luengo C, Gomez J, et al. Effects of dexmedetomidine and esmolol on systemic hemodynamics and exogenous lactate clearance in early experimental septic shock. Crit Care. 2016;20(1):234.

156. Miyamoto K, Nakashima T, Shima N, Kato S, Ueda K, Kawazoe Y, et al. Effect of dexmedetomidine on lactate clearance in patients with septic shock: a subanalysis of a Multicenter randomized controlled trial. Shock. 2018;50(2):162–6.

157. Orbegozo Cortes D, Njimi H, Dell'Anna AM, Taccone FS. Esmolol for septic shock: more than just heart rate control? Minerva Anestesiol. 2014;80(2):254–8.

158. Morelli A, Ertmer C, Westphal M, Rehberg S, Kampmeier T, Ligges S, et al. Effect of heart rate control with esmolol on hemodynamic and clinical outcomes in patients with septic shock: a randomized clinical trial. JAMA. 2013;310(16):1683–91.

159. Kawazoe Y, Miyamoto K, Morimoto T, Yamamoto T, Fuke A, Hashimoto A, et al. Effect of dexmedetomidine on mortality and ventilator-free days in patients requiring mechanical ventilation with sepsis: a randomized clinical trial. JAMA. 2017;317(13):1321–8.

160. Levy B, Fritz C, Piona C, Duarte K, Morelli A, Guerci P, et al. Hemodynamic and anti-inflammatory effects of early esmolol use in hyperkinetic septic shock: a pilot study. Crit Care. 2021;25(1):21.

161. Jacquet-Lagreze M, Allaouchiche B, Restagno D, Paquet C, Ayoub JY, Etienne J, et al. Gut and sublingual microvascular effect of esmolol during septic shock in a porcine model. Crit Care. 2015;19:241.

162. Venkataraman R, Subramanian S, Kellum JA. Clinical review: extracorporeal blood purification in severe sepsis. Crit Care. 2003;7(2):139–45.

163. Stahl K, Wendel-Garcia PD, Bode C, David S. Unraveling the secret of re-balancing homeostasis in sepsis: a critical view on extracorporeal blood purification modalities. Intensive Care Med. 2022;48(1):130–2.

164. Pickkers P, Payen D. What's new in the extracorporeal treatment of sepsis? Intensive Care Med. 2017;43(10):1498–500.

165. Bakker J, Kattan E, Annane D, Castro R, Cecconi M, De Backer D, et al. Current practice and evolving concepts in septic shock resuscitation. Intensive Care Med. 2022;48(2):148–63.

166. Einav S, Helviz Y, Ippolito M, Cortegiani A. Vasopressor and inotrope treatment for septic shock: an umbrella review of reviews. J Crit Care. 2021;65:65–71.

167. Vincent JL, Singer M, Einav S, Moreno R, Wendon J, Teboul JL, et al. Equilibrating SSC guidelines with individualized care. Crit Care. 2021;25:397.

168. Scheeren TWL, Bakker J, Kaufmann T, Annane D, Asfar P, Boerma EC, et al. Current use of inotropes in circulatory shock. Ann Intensive Care. 2021;11(1):21.

Assessing Dysregulated Immune Response at the Bedside

Contents

Pro- and Anti-inflammatory Biomarkers

Jean-Louis Vincent

Contents

⊛ Learning Objectives
- To understand what a biomarker of sepsis is, and list some of the most widely studied and used
- To explain the four key uses of biomarkers (diagnosis, prognostication, therapeutic response, therapeutic choice)
- To appreciate why separating biomarkers into pro- or anti-inflammatory groups is not useful
- To realize how biomarkers could be used in combination with other factors to define the endotypes of patients with sepsis

7.1 Introduction

Characterization of the host response to conditions such as sepsis is essential to better understand the nature of the response in a patient and the extent of the alterations, and thereby to potentially guide the most appropriate therapeutic choices. This characterization can be achieved by the use of biological markers (biomarkers) and objective quantifiable variables that indicate an ongoing normal or pathological biological process [1, 2]. Biomarkers can range from clinical signs, such as heart rate and blood pressure, to common and more complex laboratory-measured compounds, through to data measured by digital devices ("digital biomarkers") [3].

Our discussions in this chapter focus on biomarkers of inflammation present in the blood compartment, although biomarkers can also be measured in other body fluids, such as bronchoalveolar lavage, cerebrospinal fluid, or drainage fluids. Many—more than 200 [4]—biomarkers that can be measured in humans have been proposed for use in sepsis, and more continue to be identified and evaluated. It is not possible or meaningful to discuss them all, so we will restrict our discussion to general principles and to the markers that have been most widely studied. We will not discuss blood lactate levels in this review, because they reflect oxygen metabolism more than altered inflammation. Blood lactate levels are elevated in all forms of shock, including those primarily due to a critical decrease in blood flow in the absence of any major inflammatory reaction in hypovolemic, cardiogenic, or obstructive types of shock [5].

7.2 Pro- and Anti-inflammatory Biomarkers

The immune response to sepsis comprises pro- and anti-inflammatory elements that are present simultaneously and in different degrees according to individual patient factors and evolution of the disease [6]. Cytokines play a central role in mediating and regulating the immune response to sepsis, and excessive, dysregulated activity can result in organ failure. Many cytokines have therefore been proposed as biomarkers of sepsis. As the pathophysiology of sepsis began to be unraveled and different mediators were discovered, it was popular to categorize them according to their known main pro- or anti-inflammatory role. It may therefore seem logical to separate biomarkers, many of which are cytokines, into pro- and anti-inflammatory markers.

If one had to name a cytokine that was "typically" pro-inflammatory, one would probably cite tumor necrosis factor (TNF) or interleukin (IL)-1. However, these cytokines act locally and do not circulate much in the blood, making them of little use as biomarkers of sepsis in this context. But they stimulate the production of IL-6, which circulates more and has been widely studied as a biomarker in sepsis. In healthy individuals, serum concentrations of IL-6 are low, around 1–5 pg/mL, which is close to the limit of detection [7]. In patients with sepsis, IL-6 concentrations are often raised, but a single IL-6 value is not a very reliable diagnostic indicator of sepsis [8, 9]. IL-6 must circulate in the blood to reach the liver where it induces the production of acute-phase reactant C-reactive protein (CRP) via the membrane-bound IL-6 receptor (IL-6R). CRP and procalcitonin (PCT), another acute-phase reactant, are therefore conveniently used as "pro-inflammatory" markers that can reflect the presence of an infection, especially when changes in concentration over time are considered [10, 11].

If one had to name a cytokine that had "typical" anti-inflammatory effects, one would probably cite IL-10, which inhibits the effects of TNF and other strong pro-inflammatory mediators. IL-10 has also been widely studied as a biomarker of sepsis. We were the first to show that IL-10 is released very early in sepsis [12, 13]. The higher the IL-10 levels are, the higher the mortality rate [14, 15]. Other "anti-inflammatory" cytokines include type I interferons [16], and other anti-inflammatory biomarkers include alpha-1 antitrypsin (AAT) [17].

7.3 Separating Pro- and Anti-inflammatory Biomarkers?

Although it could be considered potentially beneficial to be able to identify whether a patient with sepsis has a predominantly pro- or anti-inflammatory response in order to personalize immunomodulatory therapies, separating individual biomarkers into pro- or anti-inflammatory actually makes little sense. Indeed, many (if not most) biomarkers could be considered to fall somewhere between the extremes of the anti- and pro-inflammatory spectrum. Some of the best studied are heparin-binding protein (HBP) [18], presepsin (sCD14) [19], soluble triggering receptor expressed on myeloid cells 1 (sTREM-1) [20], monocyte chemoattractant protein (MCP) 1, and soluble urokinase-type plasminogen-activator receptor (suPAR) [21]. One could also cite high-affinity immunoglobulin receptor CD64 [22] or changes in white blood cell morphology [23].

It is impossible to list sepsis mediators in order from the most pro-inflammatory to the most anti-inflammatory, as it is now well established that their function is highly complex, affected by their location, environment, and presence of other cytokines. This realization supports the use of purification techniques, which could eliminate different mediators that are released in excessive amounts, regardless of their predominantly pro- or anti-inflammatory profile.

7.4 Combining Cytokine Levels?

One could consider that using the ratio between IL-6 levels (taken as a surrogate for TNF and IL-1 activation, i.e., a pro-inflammatory biomarker) and IL-10 levels (an anti-inflammatory biomarker) [24] may make sense to appropriately orient the therapeutic strategy, but this approach has not been adopted. In patients with coronavirus disease 2019 (COVID-19), higher IL-6/IL-10 ratios were associated with worse outcomes [25] and the IL-6:AAT ratio was markedly higher in patients requiring ICU admission than in less severe cases [26].

A combination biomarker "panel" of cytokines and other mediators without particular reference to their pro- or anti-inflammatory profile may be more useful to identify and monitor sepsis. Such systems include SeptiCyte (Immunexpress, Seattle), but there are many others [27].

7.5 Clinical Applications of Biomarkers

In general, biomarkers could help in the assessment of four important clinical questions (◘ Table 7.1):
1. Is the patient infected? The implications of this purpose on guiding antibiotic therapy are evident, not only for decisions about when to start treatment but also about withholding it if the probability of an infection is quite low, and thus avoiding adverse effects associated with antibiotic use and unnecessary costs. A positive biomarker result could also help to determine whether additional tests or procedures are warranted, for example, X-ray or CT scan and blood cultures. Biomarkers considered as typically pro-inflammatory, such as IL-6, CRP, or PCT, are usually used in this context.
2. Is the patient severely ill? Most biomarker levels are higher (a few are lower) in more severely ill patients, usually characterized as patients with sepsis with or without shock or survivors vs. non-survivors (◘ Fig. 7.1). This important feature can help the clinician to evaluate whether or not a patient needs to be admitted or could be discharged home from the emergency room, to assess whether a patient should be admitted or transferred to the ICU, or to suggest the need for an expert opinion (surgeon, infectious disease specialist …). A number of mediators could be considered for this purpose, such as heparin-binding protein [28].
3. Is the patient responding to therapy? Or should we consider surgical (re)exploration or a change in antibiotic? A change in antibiotic therapy could include esca-

◘ **Table 7.1** Potential applications of biomarkers

Use *Question asked*	Implication
– **Identification of an infection** *Is the patient infected or not?*	– Antibiotics? (add or withhold) – Look for a source (X-ray, CT) (do or don't)
– **Severity assessment** *Is the patient very ill/at risk of complications?*	– Send the patient home? – Admit to ICU? – Ask for expert opinion?
– **Monitoring of the patient's response** *Is the patient responding to therapy?*	– Consider surgical (re)exploration? – Change or stop antibiotic therapy?
– **Individualized selection of relevant therapies** *Does the patient qualify for this treatment?*	– Consider adding a new drug/intervention?

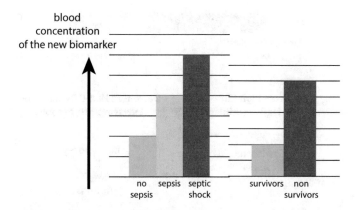

Fig. 7.1 A summary matrix of most figures that show data on a new sepsis biomarker, showing higher levels in patients with sepsis and septic shock and in non-survivors

lation with addition of another antibiotic or de-escalation with discontinuation of all or some of the antibiotics. Decisions to repeat imaging studies (like a CT scan) could also potentially be influenced by these data. Pro-inflammatory markers like PCT [29] and CRP [30, 31] have havebeen used for this purpose. Following the time course of CRP [32] or PCT [33] could help indicate the response to treatment, with decreasing values suggesting a good response. Conversely, no decrease in levels over time should suggest the need for the therapeutic strategy to be reevaluated. A change in antibiotic therapy could include escalation with addition of another antibiotic or de-escalation with discontinuation of all or some of the antibiotics. These aspects are discussed in more detail in another chapter.

4. Is this patient eligible for a particular therapeutic intervention? Randomized clinical trials targeting a single mediator in heterogeneous patient populations have not resulted in a clear benefit. Nevertheless, high IL-6 levels and/or ferritin levels may help to identify patients who could benefit from immunomodulating therapies in sepsis, including in COVID-19 [34]. Likewise, SuPAR levels have been used to identify COVID-19 patients likely to benefit from IL-1ra administration [35].

At the other end of the spectrum, immune stimulatory cytokines, like IL-7, IL-15, or interferon (IFN)γ, and antibodies against checkpoint protein ligation may also have a place in the treatment of sepsis [36]. However, as for pro-inflammatory strategies, these agents may not be effective in heterogeneous patient populations but could potentially be applied in selected patients with a clear immunosuppressed profile (■ Fig. 7.2). As an example, we successfully treated a patient with severe and resistant mucormycosis following trauma with combined anti-PD-L1 and IFNγ [37]. New methods are available to rapidly identify patients who have a profound anti-inflammatory profile and may benefit from immunostimulating strategies. Functional testing is also very attractive [38, 39], rather than applying new strategies in heterogeneous patient populations such as simply with "sepsis" or "ARDS." As endotoxin levels may guide the application of anti-endotoxin strategies, one can consider specific therapeutic interventions guided by biomarkers. As an example, a retrospective subgroup analysis suggested that stratification by baseline plasma IL-1ra concentrations resulted in more convincing results, as those with high plasma IL-1ra concentrations appeared to benefit

Pro-inflammatory state	Acquired Immunosuppression
Diagnosis	
Very high CRP	**Decreased HLA-DR expression**
High ferritin	**Low lymphocyte count**
Some therapeutic options	
Corticosteroids	**Interferon-γ**
Anti-TNF	**IL-7**
IL-1ra	**GM-CSF**
	Anti-PD1

▢ **Fig. 7.2** Schematic showing some suggested biomarkers and therapeutic options for patients with a pro-inflammatory state and those with acquired immunosuppression. *TNF* tumor necrosis factor, *IL-1ra* interleukin-1 receptor antagonist, *GM-CSF* granulocyte-macrophage colony-stimulating factor, *PD1* programmed cell death protein 1

7

from recombinant IL-1ra therapy [40]. Pickkers and colleagues are currently investigating the potential value of adrecizumab, a humanized monoclonal adrenomedullin antibody, in septic shock patients with high adrenomedullin levels [41]. Biomarker levels could help to define endotypes (biological subtypes characterized by distinct pathophysiological mechanisms) of patients more likely to respond to certain therapies [42].

Summary
Even though some mediators, like TNF, IL-1, or AAT, can be considered as typically pro-inflammatory and IL-10 typically anti-inflammatory, most mediators have both properties and cannot be easily confined into one or other category. The attempt to develop therapies to control the effects of a single pro- or anti-inflammatory mediator has been abandoned. Assessment of a combination of biomarkers could be helpful to identify a profile that may benefit from a particular therapeutic intervention.

Take-Home Messages

- Sepsis is associated with the release of many pro- and anti-inflammatory substances, and it is difficult to place them all in separate pro-inflammatory or anti-inflammatory baskets.
- Sepsis is a heterogeneous syndrome that should be further characterized into subtypes.
- Treatment should be guided by different features, including the presence of toxic molecules (e.g., endotoxin), immunologic tests (e.g., HLA-DR or lymphocyte counts), endogenous response (e.g., coagulopathy), or endogenous molecules that could be targeted (e.g., adrecizumab).

Conflict of Interest   No conflicts of interest to declare related to this chapter.

References

1. Strimbu K, Tavel JA. What are biomarkers? Curr Opin HIV AIDS. 2010;5(6):463–6.
2. Barichello T, Generoso JS, Singer M, Dal-Pizzol F. Biomarkers for sepsis: more than just fever and leukocytosis-a narrative review. Crit Care. 2022;26(1):14.
3. Egli A, Battegay M, Buchler AC, Buhlmann P, Calandra T, Eckert P, et al. SPHN/PHRT: forming a Swiss-wide infrastructure for data-driven sepsis research. Stud Health Technol Inform. 2020;270:1163–7.
4. Pierrakos C, Velissaris D, Bisdorff M, Marshall JC, Vincent JL. Biomarkers of sepsis: time for a reappraisal. Crit Care. 2020;24(1):287.
5. Vincent JL, De Backer D. Circulatory shock. N Engl J Med. 2013;369(18):1726–34.
6. Hotchkiss RS, Moldawer LL, Opal SM, Reinhart K, Turnbull IR, Vincent JL. Sepsis and septic shock. Nat Rev Dis Primers. 2016;2:16045.
7. McElvaney OJ, Curley GF, Rose-John S, McElvaney NG. Interleukin-6: obstacles to targeting a complex cytokine in critical illness. Lancet Respir Med. 2021;9(6):643–54.
8. Badea IM, Timar AE, Coman O, Negrea V. Establishing the diagnostic and prognostic value of serum interleukin 6 levels in sepsis. Acta Marisiensis Seria Med. 2020;66:83–7.
9. Molano FD, Arevalo-Rodriguez I, Roque IF, Montero Oleas NG, Nuvials X, Zamora J. Plasma interleukin-6 concentration for the diagnosis of sepsis in critically ill adults. Cochrane Database Syst Rev. 2019;4:CD011811.
10. Vincent JL, Donadello K, Schmit X. Biomarkers in the critically ill patient: C-reactive protein. Crit Care Clin. 2011;27(2):241–51.
11. Vincent JL, Van Nuffelen M, Lelubre C. Host response biomarkers in sepsis: the role of procalcitonin. Methods Mol Biol. 2015;1237:213–24.
12. Marchant A, Alegre ML, Hakim A, Pierard G, Marecaux G, Friedman G, et al. Clinical and biological significance of interleukin-10 plasma levels in patients with septic shock. J Clin Immunol. 1995;15(5):266–73.
13. Marchant A, Deviere J, Byl B, De GD, Vincent JL, Goldman M. Interleukin-10 production during septicaemia. Lancet. 1994;343(8899):707–8.
14. Friedman G, Jankowski S, Marchant A, Goldman M, Kahn RJ, Vincent JL. Blood interleukin 10 levels parallel the severity of septic shock. J Crit Care. 1997;12(4):183–7.
15. Kellum JA, Kong L, Fink MP, Weissfeld LA, Yealy DM, Pinsky MR, et al. Understanding the inflammatory cytokine response in pneumonia and sepsis: results of the genetic and inflammatory markers of sepsis (GenIMS) study. Arch Intern Med. 2007;167(15):1655–63.
16. Benveniste EN, Qin H. Type I interferons as anti-inflammatory mediators. Sci STKE. 2007;2007(416):e70.
17. Stockley RA. The multiple facets of alpha-1-antitrypsin. Ann Transl Med. 2015;3(10):130.
18. Wu YL, Yo CH, Hsu WT, Qian F, Wu BS, Dou QL, et al. Accuracy of heparin-binding protein in diagnosing sepsis: a systematic review and meta-analysis. Crit Care Med. 2021;49(1):e80–90.
19. Yang HS, Hur M, Yi A, Kim H, Lee S, Kim SN. Prognostic value of presepsin in adult patients with sepsis: systematic review and meta-analysis. PLoS One. 2018;13(1):e0191486.
20. Wu Y, Wang F, Fan X, Bao R, Bo L, Li J, et al. Accuracy of plasma sTREM-1 for sepsis diagnosis in systemic inflammatory patients: a systematic review and meta-analysis. Crit Care. 2012;16(6):R229.
21. Donadello K, Scolletta S, Covajes C, Vincent JL. suPAR as a prognostic biomarker in sepsis. BMC Med. 2012;10:2.
22. Wang X, Li ZY, Zeng L, Zhang AQ, Pan W, Gu W, et al. Neutrophil CD64 expression as a diagnostic marker for sepsis in adult patients: a meta-analysis. Crit Care. 2015;19:245.
23. Hausfater P, Robert BN, Morales IC, Cancella de Abreu M, Marin AM, Pernet J, et al. Monocyte distribution width (MDW) performance as an early sepsis indicator in the emergency department: comparison with CRP and procalcitonin in a multicenter international European prospective study. Crit Care. 2021;25(1):227.
24. Taniguchi T, Koido Y, Aiboshi J, Yamashita T, Suzaki S, Kurokawa A. Change in the ratio of interleukin-6 to interleukin-10 predicts a poor outcome in patients with systemic inflammatory response syndrome. Crit Care Med. 1999;27(7):1262–4.

25. McElvaney OJ, Hobbs BD, Qiao D, McElvaney OF, Moll M, McEvoy NL, et al. A linear prognostic score based on the ratio of interleukin-6 to interleukin-10 predicts outcomes in COVID-19. EBioMedicine. 2020;61:103026.

26. McElvaney OJ, McEvoy NL, McElvaney OF, Carroll TP, Murphy MP, Dunlea DM, et al. Characterization of the inflammatory response to severe COVID-19 illness. Am J Respir Crit Care Med. 2020;202(6):812–21.

27. Reddy B Jr, Hassan U, Seymour C, Angus DC, Isbell TS, White K, et al. Point-of-care sensors for the management of sepsis. Nat Biomed Eng. 2018;2(9):640–8.

28. Katsaros K, Renieris G, Safarika A, Adami EM, Gkavogianni T, Giannikopoulos G, et al. Heparin binding protein for the early diagnosis and prognosis of sepsis in the emergency department: the prompt multicenter study. Shock. 2022;57(4):518–25.

29. Schuetz P, Wirz Y, Sager R, Christ-Crain M, Stolz D, Tamm M, et al. Effect of procalcitonin-guided antibiotic treatment on mortality in acute respiratory infections: a patient level meta-analysis. Lancet Infect Dis. 2018;18(1):95–107.

30. Borges I, Carneiro R, Bergo R, Martins L, Colosimo E, Oliveira C, et al. Duration of antibiotic therapy in critically ill patients: a randomized controlled trial of a clinical and C-reactive protein-based protocol versus an evidence-based best practice strategy without biomarkers. Crit Care. 2020;24(1):281.

31. von Dach E, Albrich WC, Brunel AS, Prendki V, Cuvelier C, Flury D, et al. Effect of C-reactive protein-guided antibiotic treatment duration, 7-day treatment, or 14-day treatment on 30-day clinical failure rate in patients with uncomplicated Gram-negative bacteremia: a randomized clinical trial. JAMA. 2020;323(21):2160–9.

32. Schmit X, Vincent JL. The time course of blood C-reactive protein concentrations in relation to the response to initial antimicrobial therapy in patients with sepsis. Infection. 2008;36(3):213–9.

33. Schuetz P, Birkhahn R, Sherwin R, Jones AE, Singer A, Kline JA, et al. Serial procalcitonin predicts mortality in severe sepsis patients: results from the multicenter procalcitonin MOnitoring SEpsis (MOSES) study. Crit Care Med. 2017;45(5):781–9.

34. Ascierto PA, Fu B, Wei H. IL-6 modulation for COVID-19: the right patients at the right time? J Immunother Cancer. 2021;9(4):e002285.

35. Kyriazopoulou E, Poulakou G, Milionis H, Metallidis S, Adamis G, Tsiakos K, et al. Early treatment of COVID-19 with anakinra guided by soluble urokinase plasminogen receptor plasma levels: a double-blind, randomized controlled phase 3 trial. Nat Med. 2021;27(10):1752–60.

36. Francois B, Jeannet R, Daix T, Walton AH, Shotwell MS, Unsinger J, et al. Interleukin-7 restores lymphocytes in septic shock: the IRIS-7 randomized clinical trial. JCI Insight. 2018;3(5):e98960.

37. Grimaldi D, Pradier O, Hotchkiss RS, Vincent JL. Nivolumab plus interferon-gamma in the treatment of intractable mucormycosis. Lancet Infect Dis. 2017;17(1):18.

38. Monneret G, Demaret J, Gossez M, Reverdiau E, Malergue F, Rimmele T, et al. Novel approach in monocyte intracellular TNF measurement: application to sepsis-induced immune alterations. Shock. 2017;47(3):318–22.

39. Mazer MB, Caldwell C, Hanson J, Mannion D, Turnbull IR, Drewry A, et al. A whole blood enzyme-linked immunospot assay for functional immune endotyping of septic patients. J Immunol. 2021;206(1):23–36.

40. Meyer NJ, Reilly JP, Anderson BJ, Palakshappa JA, Jones TK, Dunn TG, et al. Mortality benefit of recombinant human interleukin-1 receptor antagonist for sepsis varies by initial interleukin-1 receptor antagonist plasma concentration. Crit Care Med. 2018;46(1):21–8.

41. Laterre PF, Pickkers P, Marx G, Wittebole X, Meziani F, Dugernier T, et al. Safety and tolerability of non-neutralizing adrenomedullin antibody adrecizumab (HAM8101) in septic shock patients: the AdrenOSS-2 phase 2a biomarker-guided trial. Intensive Care Med. 2021;47(11):1284–94.

42. Leligdowicz A, Matthay MA. Heterogeneity in sepsis: new biological evidence with clinical applications. Crit Care. 2019;23(1):80.

7

How to Interpret Procalcitonin?

Philipp Schuetz

Contents

© The Author(s), under exclusive license to Springer Nature Switzerland AG 2023
Z. Molnar et al. (eds.), *Management of Dysregulated Immune Response in the Critically Ill,*
Lessons from the ICU, https://doi.org/10.1007/978-3-031-17572-5_8

🎓 **Learning Objectives**

- Understanding the regulation and kinetic of procalcitonin during infections
- Understanding strength and limitations of traditional parameters and novel markers such as procalcitonin in the diagnostic workup of patients with suspicion of infection
- Understanding the importance of early recognition of sepsis and early and adequate treatment
- Understanding how procalcitonin can be used for monitoring of patients in and outside the ICU
- Understanding the concept of procalcitonin-guided antibiotic stewardship in sepsis in the ICU and respiratory tract infections in the emergency department and medical wards

8.1 Introduction

Acute respiratory tract infections and suspected sepsis often prompt initiation of empiric antibiotic treatment. Yet, in many cases, a bacterial pathogen cannot be detected and viruses may indeed account for a large proportion of respiratory illnesses [1, 2]. The same is true in patients presenting with clinical signs and symptoms of possible sepsis, where other inflammatory or viral illnesses may account for a significant proportion of cases. Despite the wider availability of rapid molecular diagnostics [3], antibiotics are often overprescribed due to concerns about bacterial coinfections and safety of withholding antibiotics. In addition, once started, physicians frequently use prolonged antibiotic courses due to the lack of well-validated clinical parameters providing proof that the infection has resolved and when antibiotics no longer provide benefit. Individualizing antibiotic treatment with the help of blood biomarkers has the potential to improve antibiotic stewardship efforts and mitigate the emergence of multidrug-resistant pathogens [4].

Integration of host response markers which correlate with bacterial infection into the clinical care of patients with acute respiratory illnesses and sepsis has high potential to improve individual antibiotic decisions in patients. Among such host-response markers, procalcitonin (PCT) has generated much interest as it more specifically correlates with bacterial infection compared to traditional markers such as C-reactive protein (CRP) or white blood cell count (WBC) and shows a more favorable kinetic profile allowing its use for assessing response to treatment [5–7]. However, understanding strengths and limitations of PCT is key for its safe and efficient use in clinical practice.

8.2 Evidence Regarding PCT-Guided Antibiotic Stewardship

In addition to a large body of preclinical and observational data [8], several interventional trials have tested the effects of integrating PCT into antibiotic stewardship protocols with a control group and assessed the impact on antibiotic use and clinical outcomes [9–11]. Most trials focused on patients with respiratory infection and sepsis patients. Protocols used in trials were somewhat similar and defined PCT cutoff values in low-risk patients for which bacterial infection was unlikely and antibiotic treatment could be stopped, or not initiated [12]. In clinical scenarios where the probability for bacterial infection was high, the protocol focused on PCT kinetics and cessation of antibiotics when PCT levels dropped into normal ranges or by at least 80–90%. The PCT protocols had different cutoffs for emergency department and medical ward patients (i.e., PCT <0.25 µg/L was used to recommend against antibiotic use) and intensive care patients (i.e., PCT <0.5 µg/L was used to recommend discontinuation of antibiotics). Based on the results of a recent meta-analysis [10], PCT guidance was associated with a 2.4-day reduction in antibiotic exposure (5.7 vs. 8.1 days) due to decreased rate of antibiotic initiation in patients with bronchitis and COPD and in primary care settings and shorter treatment courses in patients with pneumonia of varying clinical severity. In addition, PCT guidance resulted in a reduction in antibiotic-related side effects (16% vs. 22%) and in decreased mortality (286 [9%] deaths in 3336 procalcitonin-guided patients vs. 336 [10%] in 3372 controls [$p = 0.037$]). Another 2018 meta-analysis investigating the effects of PCT use in patients with sepsis [9] reported that PCT use was associated with earlier discontinuation of antibiotics and a significant reduction in mean treatment duration from 10.4 to 9.3 days. Again, mortality in PCT-guided patients was significantly lower compared with control group patients (21.1% vs. 23.7%, $p = 0.03$). Similar effects were also noted for a subgroup of patients who meet the definition of severe sepsis by Sequential Organ Failure Assessment (SOFA) score, the presence of septic shock or renal failure, and the need for vasopressor or ventilator support.

Importantly, the role of PCT kinetics (i.e., changes over the first 12–24 h) has been suggested to further improve individualization of AB management [13, 14], a concept similar to the use of troponin in patients with acute chest pain. Such an approach may help to diagnose new-onset infection in the ICU early for starting of antibiotics [13] and also help to assess antibiotic appropriateness early [14].

8.3 Practical Considerations for Use of PCT

Decisions regarding antibiotic use in an individual patient are complex and should be based on several considerations including the pretest probability for bacterial infection, which is based on the clinical examination and results from microbiological tests, severity of presentation, and PCT results [15]. ◻ Figures 8.1 and 8.2 provide practical guides for a rational use of PCT in low-risk settings and high-risk

Initial clinical assessment (including microbiology)	PCT (µg/L)	Probability of bacterial Infection based on PCT level	PCT Interpretation	Antibiotic management	PCT Monitoring
Bacterial infection uncertain	< 0.25	Low probability	Bacterial infection unlikely	Withhold antibiotics in low risk patients and consider other diagnostic tests	consider repeat PCT test in 6-24h before sending home
	≥ 0.25	High probability	Bacterial infection likely	Initiate appropriate empiric antibiotics	Repeat PCT every 24-48h and discontinue antibiotics when PCT <0.25 ug/L or decreases by 80%
Bacterial infection suspected	< 0.25	Low probability	Bacterial infection possible	Initiate appropriate empiric antibiotic consider other diagnostic tests	Repeat PCT test within 24-48h and stop antibiotics if PCT still <0.25 ug/L
	≥ 0.25	High probability	Bacterial infection highly likely	Initiate appropriate empiric or targeted antibiotic regimen	Repeat PCT every 24-48h and discontinue antibiotics when PCT <0.25 ug/L or decreases by 80%

◻ **Fig. 8.1** Suggested PCT protocol in primary care and emergency department/medical ward

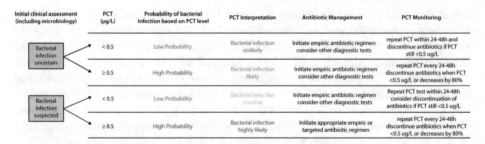

Initial clinical assessment (including microbiology)	PCT (µg/L)	Probability of bacterial Infection based on PCT level	PCT Interpretation	Antibiotic Management	PCT Monitoring
Bacterial infection uncertain	< 0.5	Low Probability	Bacterial infection unlikely	Initiate empiric antibiotic regimen consider other diagnostic tests	repeat PCT within 24-48h and discontinue antibiotics if PCT still <0.5 ug/L
	≥ 0.5	High Probability	Bacterial infection likely	Initiate empiric antibiotic regimen consider other diagnostic tests	repeat PCT every 24-48h discontinue antibiotics when PCT <0.5 ug/L or decreases by 80%
Bacterial infection suspected	< 0.5	Low Probability	Bacterial infection possible	Initiate empiric antibiotic regimen consider other diagnostic tests	Repeat PCT test within 24-48h consider discontinuation of antibiotics if PCT still <0.5 ug/L
	≥ 0.5	High Probability	Bacterial infection highly likely	Initiate appropriate empiric or targeted antibiotic regimen	repeat PCT every 24-48h discontinue antibiotics when PCT <0.5 ug/L or decreases by 80%

Fig. 8.2 Suggested PCT protocol in the intensive care unit

settings, respectively, in conjunction with the clinical assessment including interpretation of PCT and recommendations for antibiotic use [12, 16].

In the context of a low-risk situation (e.g., patient in primary care or the medical ward) and a low pretest probability for bacterial infections (e.g., a patient presenting with bronchitis), a low PCT level < 0.25 µg/L aids in ruling out bacterial infection, and empiric antibiotic therapy should be avoided (■ Fig. 8.1). If the patient does not improve clinically, PCT should be retested. If PCT is increased or the initial clinical assessment shows a high suspicion for bacterial infection, antibiotics should be considered and PCT testing every 24–48 h can be used to stop antibiotics in case PCT drops to levels ≤0.25 µg/L or if it decreases by 80% or more from its peak.

In the context of a high-risk patient with sepsis, initial antibiotics should be used irrespective of PCT results, but a low PCT value may prompt additional diagnostic measures to rule out other nonbacterial causes of illness. In these situations, monitoring of PCT over time helps to track resolution of infection and decisions regarding early stop of antibiotic treatment (■ Fig. 8.2).

8.4 Limitations of Procalcitonin

Most PCT studies were done in patients with respiratory infections or sepsis, and there is only limited data in immunosuppressed patients including those with HIV and patients with cystic fibrosis, pancreatitis, trauma, pregnancy, and high-volume transfusion. Additionally, some noninfectious conditions such as C-cell carcinoma or trauma can increase PCT levels limiting its specificity. Also, PCT-guided stewardship should also not be applied to patients with chronic infections such as osteomyelitis or endocarditis as observational studies have not shown positive results and interventional research is largely lacking [17]. Finally, there is a plentitude of novel sepsis markers and genetic tests, which may further improve the assessment of patients regarding antibiotic use when used in combination with PCT [18].

Summary
There is a strong interest in the medical community in reducing unnecessary antibiotic exposure in patients with acute respiratory illness who are at low risk for bacterial infection and reducing treatment courses in patients with known bacterial infections, thereby moving from fixed antibiotic doses to individual treatment courses. As a marker of host defense, PCT has shown promising results for respiratory infections and sepsis. PCT should not be used as a substitute for good clinical practice, but rather be part of the overall assessment of a patient. Decisions pertaining to the initiation and cessation of antibiotic treatment remain strongly dependent on an assessment of all available clinical and diagnostic parameters including a thorough patient assessment and the severity of the illness. Furthermore, the use of PCT should not delay or impede the initiation of empirical treatment in high-risk situations. However, host response markers like PCT remain the best line of defense against diagnostic uncertainty and antibiotic overuse, and further research is needed to explore the optimal use of biomarkers in combination with pathogen-directed tests.

Take-Home Messages

- The limitations of clinical signs and microbial techniques for the diagnosis of bacterial infections are eminent.
- The use of procalcitonin provides a promising approach to better diagnose infection and for individualized antibiotic stewardship.
- Interpretation of procalcitonin levels must always comprise the clinical setting and the assay characteristics, particularly the setting-specific cutoff ranges and functional assay sensitivities.
- The higher the risk of a patient, the more cautious physicians must be, and empirical antibiotic therapies must be considered despite low biomarker levels.
- Measurement of highly sensitive PCT embedded in a clearly defined setting and prospectively validated with clinical algorithms can significantly improve the diagnostic certainty and safety of patients, and still reduce the (over)utilization of antimicrobial therapy.
- This concept has been proven mostly for respiratory infections and for sepsis in the intensive care unit. For other infections, disease and setting-specific cutoff ranges must be validated and proposed and intervention studies conducted in the future.

Financial Disclosures   Drs. Schuetz reports grants from bioMerieux, Thermo Fisher, and Roche Diagnostics (paid to the institution).

References

1. Musher DM, Thorner AR. Community-acquired pneumonia. N Engl J Med. 2014;371(17):1619–28.
2. Jain S, Self WH, Wunderink RG, Fakhran S, Balk R, Bramley AM, et al. Community-acquired pneumonia requiring hospitalization among U.S. adults. N Engl J Med. 2015;373(5):415–27.
3. Mitsuma SF, Mansour MK, Dekker JP, Kim J, Rahman MZ, Tweed-Kent A, et al. Promising new assays and technologies for the diagnosis and management of infectious diseases. Clin Infect Dis. 2013;56(7):996–1002.
4. Jee Y, Carlson J, Rafai E, Musonda K, Huong TTG, Daza P, et al. Antimicrobial resistance: a threat to global health. Lancet Infect Dis. 2018;18(9):939–40.
5. Zhydkov A, Christ-Crain M, Thomann R, Hoess C, Henzen C, Werner Z, et al. Utility of procalcitonin, C-reactive protein and white blood cells alone and in combination for the prediction of clinical outcomes in community-acquired pneumonia. Clin Chem Lab Med. 2015;53(4):559–66.
6. Schuetz P, Birkhahn R, Sherwin R, Jones AE, Singer A, Kline JA, et al. Serial procalcitonin predicts mortality in severe sepsis patients: results from the Multicenter procalcitonin MOnitoring SEpsis (MOSES) study. Crit Care Med. 2017;45(5):781–9.
7. Sager R, Kutz A, Mueller B, Schuetz P. Procalcitonin-guided diagnosis and antibiotic stewardship revisited. BMC Med. 2017;15(1):15.
8. Schuetz P, Aujesky D, Muller C, Muller B. Biomarker-guided personalised emergency medicine for all—hope for another hype? Swiss Med Wkly. 2015;145:w14079.
9. Wirz Y, Meier MA, Bouadma L, Luyt CE, Wolff M, Chastre J, et al. Effect of procalcitonin-guided antibiotic treatment on clinical outcomes in intensive care unit patients with infection and sepsis patients: a patient-level meta-analysis of randomized trials. Crit Care. 2018;22(1):191.
10. Schuetz P, Wirz Y, Sager R, Christ-Crain M, Stolz D, Tamm M, et al. Effect of procalcitonin-guided antibiotic treatment on mortality in acute respiratory infections: a patient level meta-analysis. Lancet Infect Dis. 2018;18(1):95–107.
11. Schuetz P, Raad I, Amin DN. Using procalcitonin-guided algorithms to improve antimicrobial therapy in ICU patients with respiratory infections and sepsis. Curr Opin Crit Care. 2013;19(5):453–60.
12. Schuetz P, Bolliger R, Merker M, Christ-Crain M, Stolz D, Tamm M, et al. Procalcitonin-guided antibiotic therapy algorithms for different types of acute respiratory infections based on previous trials. Expert Rev Anti Infect Ther. 2018;16(7):555–64.
13. Trasy D, Tanczos K, Nemeth M, Hankovszky P, Lovas A, Mikor A, et al. Delta procalcitonin is a better indicator of infection than absolute procalcitonin values in critically ill patients: a prospective observational study. J Immunol Res. 2016;2016:3530752.
14. Trasy D, Tanczos K, Nemeth M, Hankovszky P, Lovas A, Mikor A, et al. Early procalcitonin kinetics and appropriateness of empirical antimicrobial therapy in critically ill patients: a prospective observational study. J Crit Care. 2016;34:50–5.
15. Neeser O, Branche A, Mueller B, Schuetz P. How to: implement procalcitonin testing in my practice. Clin Microbiol Infect. 2019;25(10):1226–30.
16. Schuetz P, Beishuizen A, Broyles M, Ferrer R, Gavazzi G, Gluck EH, et al. Procalcitonin (PCT)-guided antibiotic stewardship: an international experts consensus on optimized clinical use. Clin Chem Lab Med. 2019;57(9):1308–18.
17. Wolfisberg S, Gregoriano C, Schuetz P. Procalcitonin for individualizing antibiotic treatment: an update with a focus on COVID-19. Crit Rev Clin Lab Sci. 2022;59(1):54–65.
18. Schuetz P, Hausfater P, Amin D, Amin A, Haubitz S, Faessler L, et al. Biomarkers from distinct biological pathways improve early risk stratification in medical emergency patients: the multinational, prospective, observational TRIAGE study. Crit Care. 2015;19:377.

8

Assessment of the Macro- and Microcirculation

Antonio Messina, Daniel De Backer, and Maurizio Cecconi

Contents

☺ Learning Objectives
  − To couple macro- and microcirculation assessment to titrate fluid and vasopressor infusion during a septic shock in critically ill patients.
  − To deal with clinical parameters assessing macro- and microcirculation.
  − To learn about investigation of the microcirculation, which has long been difficult due to the lack of adequate tools. In fact, with the development of small handheld microscopes, the investigation of the microcirculation at bedside was made feasible.

9.1 Introduction

Sepsis is a life-threatening condition and a medical human health emergency worldwide, which has been recognized by the World Health Organization (WHO) as a Global Health Priority [1]. In fact, despite a huge scientific interest on this topic and the dissemination and the compliance with the Surviving Sepsis Campaign guidelines [2], mortality rates remain overall unbearably high, despite some differences depending on the country (i.e., 25–30% for sepsis, and up to 40–50% in cases of sepsis-related shock) [3, 4]. This syndrome is generally viewed as a dysregulated host response to infection, potentially leading to multiple-organ failure and shock, being the primary source of hemodynamic instability for patients admitted to the intensive care unit (ICU) [2, 5].

The pathophysiology of septic shock is thought to involve complex interactions between pathogens and a host immune system, and the dysregulation includes not only a variable excess of inflammation, but also immunosuppression and immunoparalysis which can exist concomitantly, and the degree of each component varies markedly. In this perspective, a previous schematic and biphasic concept that a hyperinflammatory early phase is followed by an immunosuppressive late phase is now considered outdated [6]. Interestingly, many experimental therapeutic treatments for immunomodulation during sepsis have been successful in animal sepsis models [7], which have never been proven to be effective in clinical trials. This concept is not novel and still very frustrating. However, combining an unpredictable immune response to the pathophysiology of sepsis in the heterogenous patient populations enrolled in the trials, not specifically selected on genetic backgrounds but mostly using individual medical histories, the trigger of the infection and early/late clinical pathways would inevitably bias the results of all the clinical investigations.

From a cellular perspective, the final effect of deregulated inflammation is inevitably accompanied by tissue hypoxia or dysoxia, which may be described, according to Connett et al. [8], using three theoretical thresholds. The first is crossed when cellular oxygen availability is reduced; however, ATP production is still sufficiently preserved by metabolic pathways of adaptation (i.e., alteration of phosphorylation states, increased glycolysis redox recruitment). The second occurs when ATP can be maintained only by the production of ATP from the low effective anaerobic glycolysis, and highly metabolic syndrome may rapidly develop ATP depletion and, below this threshold, dysoxia. The third threshold is crossed when glycolysis becomes insufficient to produce enough ATP to maintain cell function and structural integrity, leading to cellular damage and death. Monitoring microcirculation is basically the use of different techniques, more or less invasive, to quantify the degree of tissue dysoxia and, potentially, restore ATP production.

The hemodynamic alterations in septic shock are characterized by a combination in variable severity of a decrease in vascular tone, affecting both arterioles and venules, an initial component of hypovolemia, myocardial depression, and alteration in regional blood flow distribution. In addition, microvascular alterations occur, which include a decrease in microvascular perfusion and an increase in vascular permeability. Clinical targets and interventions should, in principle, restore the (micro) damages of the immune system dysregulation by treating (macro) hemodynamic variables, such as mean system pressure (MAP) or cardiac output (CO). This necessarily implies a continuous assessment of macro- and microcirculation. In fact, acute circulatory dysfunction due to septic shock is often a challenging clinical scenario, which should be promptly treated to avoid multiorgan dysfunction (i.e., the final macro effect of the sum of thousands of microcellular injuries).

Septic shock is initially approached, from the hemodynamic point of view, by using fluid resuscitation and vasopressors [2, 9, 10]. The physiological purpose of these combined strategies is to optimize the CO to improve the oxygen delivery (DO_2) to cells. However, as said, a single physiological or biochemical parameter defining and tracking the balance between the changes in CO and in DO_2 (i.e., coupling "macro" and "micro" circulation) is still not available.

Since at the bedside the ability of ICU physicians in estimating the exact CO value is rather low [11], the diagnosis of an acute circulatory dysfunction is primarily clinical. In fact, a very low CO, since it is a primary determinant of peripheral oxygen supply, could be harmful, but, however, there is not a mathematical correlation between the CO measurement and the adequacy of peripheral blood flow. In other words, normal or even high values or CO could be insufficient, if metabolic demand is not adequately supplied.

For all these reasons, the basic monitoring of an acute circulatory dysfunction should be focused on those parameters coupling the "macro" and "micro" response to shock and tracking the changes of the two systems in response to the therapy (◻ Table 9.1).

Table 9.1 Pros/Cons and clinical utility of the parameters coupling "macro" and "micro" response to an acute circulatory dysfunction

	Advantages	Drawbacks	Clinical utility
Skin mottling	Costless, noninvasive, easily obtainable, repeatable, does not require tools for its assessment	Observer dependent Not useful in patients with dark skin Affected by the ambient and skin temperatures	Should be part of the bedside standard clinical examination of all the ICU patients Consider a score ranging from 0 (indicating no mottling) to 5 (an extremely severe mottling area that goes beyond the fold of the groin) [46]. Scores 4–5 relate with the lowest chances of survival
CRT	Costless, noninvasive, easily obtainable, repeatable, does not require tools for its assessment	Observer dependent Depends on pressure applied, ambient and skin temperatures	Should be part of the bedside standard clinical examination of all ICU patients CRT of 2 s or less should be considered normal, CRT >4.5 is related with higher morbidity and mortality Pressure applied should be just enough to remove the blood at the tip of the physician's nail, illustrated by the appearance of a thin white distal crescent (blanching) under the nail, for 15 s [32]
Lactate	Quickly available Target of optimization May trigger further evaluation in subclinical (cryptic) shock. Prognostic value	Not a direct measure of tissue perfusion. Influenced by lactate clearance. Normal values are common in septic shock	Different prognostic implications depending on the initial values: lactate normalization is indicative of successful resuscitation, while persistence of severe hyperlactatemia (>10 mmol/L for >24 h) is associated with ominous prognosis A patient with lactate level >2 mmol/L should be carefully monitored A patient with persistent lactate level >4 mmol/L should be considered for ICU admission, unless not indicated
Body temperature gradient	Validated method for estimating microcirculatory skin perfusion	Observer dependent when measured with the dorsal face of hands. Does not reflect peripheral perfusion variations in real time. Affected by hypothermia and room temperature	Toe-to-room temperature gradient reflects tissue perfusion and correlates with prognosis in ICU patients with severe infections. Central-to-toe >7 °C related with higher morbidity and mortality Forearm-to-finger >4 °C related with higher morbidity and mortality

9

□ Table 9.1 (continued)

	Advantages	Drawbacks	Clinical utility
$ScVO_2$	Quickly available. Can detect early hemodynamic deterioration Target of optimization in the early phase of shock (when low at presentation) Surrogate of mixed venous oxygen saturation	Invasive: needs a CVC in the superior vena cava No therapy for high values of $ScVO_2$ Normal to high values common in septic shock	The optimization of low $ScVO_2$ (<70%) has been successfully used in a protocolized approach to septic shock Normal or high values are less indicative of the degree of shock
Peripheral perfusion index	Noninvasive, continuous, easy-to-obtain equipment (pulse oximeter) always available in any setting, does not depend on oxygen saturation	Not accurate during patient motion	A value of PPI <1.4% is related with higher morbidity and mortality
Near-infrared spectroscopy/ StO_2	Low cost, noninvasive. Allows for determination and continuous monitoring of tissue oxygenation. Does not require pulsatile blood flow. Provides quantitative information on microvascular function within minutes	Requires NIRS equipment and electrodes. Available data are reported with different devices. VOT is not standardized Needs special device and expertise. Response of the microcirculation to treatment is variable and cannot be predicted	More studies that explore the relationship between $ScvO_2$ and StO_2 and the use of VOT-derived parameters may be warranted before recommending its routine use in the critical care setting
Microcirculatory assessment	Detection of microcirculatory dysfunction may aid diagnosis and risk stratification in patients with sepsis. Restoration of the function of the microcirculation may be a useful therapeutic target for resuscitation	Needs special device and expertise. Response of the microcirculation to treatment is variable and cannot be predicted	The severity of microvascular alterations is associated with organ dysfunction and mortality

CRT capillary refill time, *ICU* intensive care unit, *PPI* peripheral perfusion index, *StO_2* tissue oxygen saturation, *NIRS* near-infrared spectroscopy, *VOT* vascular occlusion test

9.2   Coupling Macro- and Microcirculation: Monitoring Peripheral Perfusion in Critically Ill Patients

Septic shock resuscitation represents a fundamental challenge in the ICU because of the extreme complexity of sepsis-related circulatory disfunction and impaired tissue perfusion. Over the last decades, many parameters (macrohemodynamic, metabolic, microcirculatory) have been adopted to monitor perfusion status and resuscitation success, but none of these have earned universal consensus to be considered as the hallmark to guide resuscitation, probably because of the lack of an integrative and comprehensive protocol in which these targets are tested with a holistic approach [12].

In a shock state, blood flow is diverted from less important tissues to vital organs to maintain vital organ perfusion by reducing peripheral circulation. According to that, the rationale of peripheral perfusion monitoring is that the skin is easily accessible, hoping that triggering resuscitation based on skin circulation would improve perfusion to other tissues [13]. Impaired peripheral circulation abnormalities can be determined using several different levels of invasiveness (i.e., skin temperature measurements and optical monitoring devices). The assessment of peripheral perfusion in the context of hyperlactatemia may provide additional physiological information. An abnormal peripheral perfusion may be caused by either a low cardiac output or a hypovolemia, and thus a complementary evaluation of cardiac function and a reassessment of preload status are mandatory. Furthermore, microcirculation impairment can be present in patients with adequate perfusion and normal ScvO2 values. This means that a multimodal assessment is desirable for a more comprehensive understanding of persistent tissue hypoperfusion, especially in the context of discrepant signals from other classic parameters [12].

9.2.1   Role of Blood Lactate

Since the early studies by Weil and others, blood lactate levels have been routinely adopted in clinical practice as a marker of impaired tissue perfusion in critically ill patients [14].

Lactate is a physiological product of cell metabolism produced by various organs (muscles, brain, red blood cells, skin, intestine), and, under physiological conditions, its blood concentration is around 1 mEq/L. The liver and the kidneys are responsible of blood lactate metabolism, respectively, 60% and 30%, with the contribution of other organs too [14]. Even minor increases in lactate concentrations to >1.5 mEq/L are associated with higher mortality rates [15].

Hyperlactatemia is a consequence of impaired cellular metabolism, particularly cellular respiration. Lactate production occurs, in fact, when there is an increase in glycolysis and therefore in pyruvate. Lactate is produced according to the following cytoplasmic reaction:

$$Pyruvate + NADH + H^+ \leftrightarrow Lactate + NAD^+$$

Under aerobic conditions, pyruvate is primarily metabolized within mitochondria through Krebs cycle. The synthesis of lactate in the cell is dependent on the ATP/ADP and NADH/NAD ratios, which are both related to the oxygen use in mitochondria. In fact, under hypoxemic conditions, mitochondrial oxidative phosphorylation is inhibited, and this determines a decrease in the ATP/ADP ratio and an increase in the NADH/NAD ratio. This metabolic condition therefore inhibits both the pyruvate carboxylase (converting pyruvate into oxaloacetate) and the pyruvate dehydrogenase (converting pyruvate into acetyl-CoA) [16]. When the physiologic pathway of pyruvate use is affected by alterations in the redox potential of the cell, the excess of pyruvate concentration is shifted to lactate production and to the less efficient lactic fermentation.

Hyperlactatemia is a hallmark of shock states, and so the precise pathophysiologic mechanisms behind it have been widely discussed. In fact, increased blood lactate levels may have multiple sources that do not always reflect hypoperfusion but, in contrast, may be non-perfusion related especially in septic patients (e.g., hyperadrenergism, liver dysfunction, hyperinflammation, hypermetabolism). The interpretation of this parameter is particularly challenging in some cases, but the distinction between these two scenarios (hypoxic versus nonhypoxic hyperlactatemia) is essential because it may strongly impact the therapeutic management. In fact, treatment of a nonhypoxic-related hyperlactatemia with sustained efforts aimed at increasing oxygen delivery (DO_2) could lead to detrimental effects of excessive fluids or inotropes [12]. Nonetheless, high serum lactate levels (irrespective of the source) are associated with worse outcome, and so a lactate-guided resuscitation approach is still recommended by the Surviving Sepsis Campaign guidelines [17].

Recently published data showed that lactate >4 mmol/L associated with hypotension led to a mortality rate of 44.5% in ICU patients with severe sepsis or septic shock [17]. For instance, a large retrospective study showed that a subgroup of ICU patients with severe hyperlactatemia (lactate >10 mmol/L) had a 78.2% chance of mortality, which increased up to 95% if hyperlactatemia persisted for more than 24 h [18].

At the same time, normal lactate levels even under severe circulatory stress suggest an adequate physiologic reserve and are associated with a better prognosis [19]. A recent study by Hernandez et al. involving 302 septic shock patients supports this notion since patients with sepsis-related hypotension without hyperlactatemia exhibited a very low mortality of less than 8% [19]. In contrast, Puskarich et al. [20] in a large randomized control trial of early sepsis resuscitation found that the presence of hyperlactatemia even without hypotension (cryptic shock) is associated with a very high mortality risk. Differences between the trials may reflect differences in population. On the one hand, hyperlactatemia without hypotension likely characterizes less severe patients; however, in the absence of hypotension, shock may often be unrecognized, especially in areas where lactate sampling is not systematic, and physicians may also be less aggressive in resuscitating these patients. Finally, relevance to time at which lactate is sampled should be considered. Usually, lactate levels can be ascribed to hypoxia shortly after admission, while the nonhypoxic component becomes predominant already after 24 h in most cases [21]. Chasing lactate at later stages of sepsis may be useless. Indeed, a recent study showed that lactate remained elevated in 50% of a cohort of ultimately surviving septic shock patients, but flow-sensitive variables (such as peripheral perfusion, central venous O_2 saturation, and venous-arterial pCO_2 gradients) were normal in almost 80% of patients at 2 h [22].

Lactates remain an objective metabolic surrogate to guide fluid resuscitation with significantly reduced mortality as compared to resuscitation without lactate monitoring [23], but this means that pursuing lactate normalization with fluid resuscitation may thus increase the risk of fluid overload [24]. The foremost priority in overt or cryptic shock is to determine the cause of persistent hyperlactatemia. Therefore, lactate assessment should be the starting point for a multimodal perfusion monitoring approach [12].

However, because serum lactate is not a direct measure of tissue perfusion [25], it is important to consider the trend of lactate (sometimes misnomed lactate clearance) despite being a single value. Serum lactate normalization is indicative of shock reversal, whereas severe persistent hyperlactatemia despite resuscitation is associated with very poor outcomes. Importantly, lactate-guided resuscitation in the early, hypovolemic, phase of shock is effective and may be even superior to hemodynamic-guided resuscitation without measuring lactate. This is explained by the minimal coherence between lactate trends and static hemodynamic measures (such as blood pressure) because, as it happens for hyperlactatemia, impaired microcirculation is ubiquitous in shock and is evident even in the setting of hemodynamic compensation. Moreover, persistent microcirculatory derangement is associated with poor outcome and may reflect ongoing shock and/or long-lasting damage [26, 27].

9.3 Clinical Assessment of Peripheral Perfusion

The deterioration of peripheral circulation and the consequent alteration of peripheral tissue perfusion are frequently observed in critically ill patients, and, in some of them, severe and persistent peripheral hypoperfusion is associated with worse outcomes, independently of systemic hemodynamic parameters [26]. Interventions aimed at stabilizing systemic hemodynamics have an unpredictable effect on peripheral perfusion parameters, especially during hyperdynamic conditions. It is well known that hemodynamic instability, irrespectively of the cause, is associated with impaired peripheral tissue perfusion [28]. Moreover, in patients with severe sepsis, a combination of hypovolemia, massive vasodilation, and reduced ventricular function can lead to pronounced hypotension and inadequate peripheral perfusion that may persist despite adequate hemodynamic resuscitation. During circulatory shock, systemic hypotension stimulates a sympathetic neurohumoral response that leads to blood flow diversion from less noble tissues to vital organs [29]. The vasoconstriction induced by the enhanced sympathetic activity primarily involves skin and muscles that therefore are the first hypoperfused tissues during shock and the last reperfused during resuscitation [13]. This means that peripheral perfusion is more related to local vasomotor tone and less to systemic circulation and represents the rationale of peripheral circulation monitoring as an early marker of hemodynamic instability. Signs of impaired peripheral circulation can be easily and rapidly determined at bedside using simple clinical assessment without any other device [30]. Surely, in the next future, new reliable algorithms and grading scores will be developed further in order to offer a quick evaluation (even to minimally skilled operators), which requires only 2 min for calculation with good interrater consistency and agreement with traditional 45-min-long analysis [31].

9.3.1 Role of the Capillary Refill Time

Clinical examination of the peripheral circulation allows for rapid and repeated assessment of critically ill patients at the bedside because it only requires touching the skin or measuring capillary refill time (CRT). In particular, CRT has been advocated as a measure of abnormal skin perfusion that could be caused by either decreased skin blood flow or derangement of the cutaneous microcirculation.

CRT is defined as the time required for a distal piece of tissue (usually nail bed) to recolor after pressure is applied to cause blanching. It is not purely capillary, and it also encompasses arteriole and venule response.

CRT is a very attractive tool because it is costless, easy to learn, repeatable, and available in any circumstance (pre-ICU, ICU, resource-limited settings), but it depends on the extent and modality of the applied pressure and ambient and skin temperatures. To standardize the maneuver, Ait-Oufella et al. recommended to use just enough pressure to remove the blood at the tip of the physician's nail illustrated by the appearance of a thin white distal crescent under the nail, for 15 s [32].

Over the past 40 years, the definition of a delayed capillary refill time has been debated in the literature. The CRT concept was first introduced by Champion et al. in 1981 as a component of the international trauma severity score for the rapid and structured cardiopulmonary assessment of ICU patients [33]. In a healthy adult population, Schriger and Baraff defined the upper limit of an abnormal CRT as about 4 s [34]. This limit seems to be highly reproducible for critically ill patients admitted to the ICU despite high interobserver variability. CRT at 6 h after initial resuscitation was strongly predictive of 14-day mortality (area under the curve of 84% [IQR: 75–94]). Hernandez et al. reported that CRT <4 s, 6 h after resuscitation, was associated with resuscitation success, with normalization of lactate levels 24 h after the occurrence of severe sepsis/septic shock [35]. A prospective cohort study of 1320 adult patients with hypotension in the emergency room showed an association between CRT and in-hospital mortality [36]. More recently, the ANDROMEDA-SHOCK (a multicenter, randomized trial involving 28 intensive care units in 5 countries) assessed whether a normalized CRT could be superior to lactate as a target for early septic shock resuscitation. The normalized CRT was assessed by applying a fixed pressure to ventral surface of right index finger distal phalanx until skin was blanched and then maintained for 10 s, by using a glass microscope slide. The time for return for normal skin color was registered with a chronometer, assessed every 30 min, and considered abnormal if greater than 3 s. The resuscitation strategy targeting normalization of CRT, compared with a strategy targeting serum lactate levels, did not reduce all-cause 28-day mortality. However, peripheral perfusion-targeted resuscitation was associated with beneficial effects on the secondary outcome of SOFA score at 72 h and lower 28-day mortality in the predefined subgroup of patients with less severe organ dysfunction at baseline [37]. In addition, patients with a prolonged capillary refill time, even if hemodynamically stable, had significantly higher odds of developing worsening organ failure than patients with a normal capillary refill time [30]. Similar observations have been made during therapeutic hypothermia following cardiac arrest [38].

9.4 Peripheral Perfusion Assessed by Skin Functional and Clinical Assessment

9.4.1 Skin Temperature and Mottling

Skin is a non-vital organ involved in maintaining body's thermoregulation through its rich vascular bed. When hemodynamic instability occurs, the systemic response determines a redistribution of blood flow from skin and other non-vital organs to noble ones. This implies that when derangements of peripheral vasculature occur during shock, direct effects can be seen as cold, clammy, white, and mottled skin. However, clinical assessment of skin perfusion, despite being inexpensive, rapid, and easy to obtain, is not routinely used by the physicians as a trigger to guide fluid resuscitation, as confirmed by the results of the FENICE study [39]. For sure, peripheral perfusion can be influenced by ambient temperature, skin color, and inter-observer variability, but these limitations can be overcome, at least during the initial management, by the mentioned advantages.

Skin temperature is estimated using the dorsal surface of the hands or fingers of the medical examiner, as these areas are most sensitive to temperature perception. Patients are considered to have cool extremities if all examined extremities are perceived as cool by the examiner or if only the lower extremities are cool despite warm upper extremities in the absence of peripheral vascular occlusive disease [40]. It has been demonstrated that subjectively determined variations in skin temperature correspond to objective measures of peripheral skin perfusion. Similarly, fingertip temperature estimations correlated well with objective assessments of fingertip blood flow [41]. Accordingly, patients with a subjectively determined "abnormal" peripheral perfusion following initial hemodynamic resuscitation have been associated with higher lactate levels and more severe organ dysfunction.

Although the absolute cutaneous temperature itself represents a useful and easily accessible parameter for circulatory shock severity, it has been shown that body temperature gradient better reflects changes in peripheral blood flow [42]. Body temperature gradients are determined by the temperature difference between two measurement points, such as peripheral-to-ambient, central-to-toe, and forearm-to-fingertip (Tskin-diff). Increased vasoconstriction during circulatory shock leads to decreased skin temperature and a diminished ability of the core to regulate its temperature before hypothermia occurs. Consequently, core temperature is maintained at the cost of the periphery to maintain vital organ perfusion, resulting in an increased central-to-peripheral temperature difference, when vasoconstriction decreases fingertip blood flow. This concept permits the establishment of central-to-toe temperature difference as an indicator of peripheral perfusion in critically ill patients, and a normal temperature gradient of 3–7 °C occurs once the patient's hemodynamics have been optimized [43]. The use of Tskin-diff is based on the assumption that reference temperature is a skin site exposed to the same ambient temperature producing little change in the gradient. Experimental studies have suggested Tskin-diff thresholds of 0 °C for initiating vasoconstriction and 4 °C for severe vasoconstriction .[43, 44] In critically ill adult patients, the simultaneous clinical observation and Tskin-diff measurements have helped to address the reliability of subjective peripheral perfusion assessment and are able to indicate abnormal peripheral perfusion in the post-resuscitation period [38]. In fact, a recent prospective observational study showed that toe-to-room temperature gradient reflects tissue perfusion and correlates with prognosis in ICU patients with severe infections [45].

More than 50 years ago, the skin of a patient during a septic shock was described by Vic-Dupont et al. as "pale often covered with perspiration" [32]. Mottling of the skin is easily recognized and often encountered in critically ill patients, together with pallor and cyanosis. Mottling is the overt result of cutaneous capillary vaso-constriction, and it is defined as a bluish skin discoloration that typically manifests near the elbows or knees and has a distinct patchy pattern. The assessment of mottling skin as a semiquantitative approach based on mottling extension around the knee has been recently proposed by Ait-Oufella et al. [46]. This scoring system is very easy to learn, has good interobserver agreement, and can be used at the bedside. This score ranges from 0 (no mottling) to 5 (an extremely severe mottling area that goes beyond the fold of the groin): a score ≥4 and persistence of high values during the first 6 h from the ICU admission, independent of systemic hemodynamic variables, were both associated with worst outcomes and were strong predictors of 14-day mortality during septic shock. Moreover, the progression of skin mottling is associated with lactate levels and urinary output, but it does not correlate with CO values, confirming the functional decoupling between cardiac function and progression of shock [46, 47].

From these studies, it is evident that the clinical assessment of peripheral perfusion is a valuable adjunct for the hemodynamic monitoring of critically ill patients and should be considered in future multimodal monitoring strategies to adequately monitor optimal circulatory shock resuscitation.

9.5 Optical Monitoring

Optical monitoring techniques provide important information on peripheral circulation and are easy to obtain and interpret at the bedside and in acute settings. Optical methods directly apply light with different wavelengths to tissue components and use their scattering characteristics to assess different tissue states [26]. At physiologic concentrations, the molecules that absorb most of the light are hemoglobin, myoglobin, cytochrome, melanin, carotenes, and bilirubin. These substances can be quantified and measured in intact tissues, thanks to different available techniques that apply optical methods to visualize the microcirculation, assess oxygen availability, measure Pco_2, and assess microvascular function in different tissues. The assessment of tissue oxygenation is based on the specific absorption spectrum of oxygenated hemoglobin (Hb-O) and deoxygenated hemoglobin (Hb). Commonly used optical methods for peripheral circulation monitoring are pulse oximeter signaling (peripheral perfusion index), near-infrared spectroscopy (NIRS), and sidestream darkfield (SDF) imaging [48].

These techniques are particularly promising because numerical information can be obtained noninvasively within a couple of minutes, but the interpretation of these data should always be guided by the clinical examination and additional peripheral perfusion measurements [41, 49].

9.5.1 Peripheral Perfusion Index

The peripheral perfusion index (PPI) is a noninvasive, continuous, and easy-to-obtain parameter derived from the photoelectric plethysmographic signal of pulse oximetry used to measure peripheral circulation in critically ill, trauma, and surgical patients [48]. Pulse oximetry, a standard of care in the ICU, allows for the measurement of arterial hemoglobin oxygen saturation and pulse rate monitoring. The principle of this noninvasive tool is based on the emission of two wavelengths of light (red and infrared, 660 nm and 940 nm, respectively) that are transmitted through the cutaneous vascular bed of distal phalanx of the index finger or earlobe and adsorbed differently by blood and tissues; the result is the display of a pulsatile photoplethysmographic waveform from which several variables, such as the PPI, can be derived [48]. Pulse oximeter is able to distinguish between the pulsatile component of arterial blood and the non-pulsatile component of other tissues, and PPI is the ratio of the pulsatile part to the non-pulsatile part of the curve, expressed as a percentage, and it does not depend on the patient's oxygen saturation. Alterations in peripheral perfusion determine variations in the pulsatile component but do not affect the non-pulsatile one, and this causes changes in PPI. As a result, the value of PPI displayed on the monitor reflects changes in peripheral circulation, particularly in peripheral vasomotor tone. This was first demonstrated in patients undergoing hand surgery who received axillary-plexus block; the analgesic effect of this block could be predicted by an increase in PPI as a measure of concomitant vasodilatation [50]. Similarly, the PPI rapidly reduced following sympathetic response-induced vasoconstriction after the introduction of a nociceptive skin stimulus or an intravenous injection of epinephrine or norepinephrine [49, 51]. Furthermore, in a lower body negative pressure model, the PPI also rapidly decreased following sympathetic activation in healthy volunteers who underwent stepwise decreases in venous return [52]. In a large population of healthy volunteers, the median PPI value was 1.4%. In critically ill patients, the same value represents a very sensitive cutoff point for determining abnormal peripheral perfusion, as defined by a prolonged capillary refill time and an increased skin temperature difference [53].

9.5.2 Near-infrared Spectroscopy

Near-infrared spectroscopy (NIRS) is a noninvasive technique that enables the determination and continuous monitoring of tissue oxygenation based on the spectrophotometric quantitation of oxyhemoglobin (HB-O) and deoxyhemoglobin (HB-r) within a tissue. NIRS is based on the same principle as a pulse oximeter and utilizes NIR light (700–1000 nm) to monitor the different light absorption of oxyhemoglobin (HB-O) and deoxygenated hemoglobin (HB-r), and, unlike pulse oximeter, NIRS does not require a pulsatile blood flow [54]. The measurement obtained is reported as the tissue oxygen saturation (StO_2) and reflects oxygen uptake in the tissue bed. NIRS can continuously monitor oxygen consumption through cerebral and regional circulation such as splanchnic, renal, and muscle [55]. In fact, although this technique was historically used in neurocritical care to monitor cerebral perfusion, it is now primarily used to monitor peripheral oxygenation of muscle tissue in critically ill patients.

The use of NIRS in muscle poses an interesting problem because muscle has a considerable quantity of myoglobin in addition to hemoglobin. However, Boushel and Piantadosi [56] showed that NIRS primarily monitors the vascular hemoglobin oxygenation and deoxygenation and not the myoglobin. Muscle oxygenation is usually measured at thenar eminence, but lower extremities and brachioradialis muscle can be used for bedside NIRS monitoring. Although a universal agreement is lacking, thenar eminence seems to be the most reliable site if compared to others because differences in fat mass and muscle are minimized.

In the case of a hypoperfusion state, muscle perfusion decreases in order to favor the blood supply to vital organs. Decreased thenar oxygen saturation measured via NIRS suggests the presence of severe hypoperfusion, and it might be a useful tool to monitor tissue hypoxia and guide resuscitation in hemorrhagic shock [57]. Nowadays, there is a crescent interest to its application in septic shock states where oxygen utilization pathophysiology is distorted. Unfortunately, the significance of StO_2 in the setting of sepsis is not as straightforward as in hemorrhagic shock, and, despite efforts to establish a correlation between $ScvO_2$ and StO_2, there is still a lack of consensus in recommending its routinary use to guide resuscitation [54]. At the same time, Colin et al. [58] observed the dynamic response of StO_2 at different sites during the first 6 h of severe sepsis resuscitation and argued that StO_2 values measured at the masseter muscle may better relate to patient outcome and may be a more reliable indicator of resuscitation success, if compared with measurements taken at the thenar eminence.

Derived parameters obtained from NIRS using vascular occlusion test (VOT) can perhaps be more helpful. Shapiro et al. [59] demonstrated that the dynamic NIRS variables collected during a vascular occlusion test (VOT) were strongly associated with the severity of organ dysfunction and mortality in patients with septic shock. When measured at the thenar eminence, NIRS-derived measurements are influenced by the peripheral circulation condition [41]. It is important to understand what the VOT really investigates: VOT evaluates the maximal recruitability of microvascular perfusion and is also affected by other determinants of oxygen transport (in particular Hb levels) and local oxygen consumption. Accordingly, VOT is related to microvascular perfusion with endothelial function as a common denominator, but other factors may affect both VOT and microvascular perfusion so that these two measurements are not identical.

Nevertheless, when integrated with other indicators of peripheral perfusion, repeated StO_2 monitoring has the potential to assess the effect of therapeutic intervention on the peripheral microvascular circulation in various shock states [49].

Lima et al. [41] examined the relationship between NIRS and peripheral circulation derangements and demonstrated that changes in peripheral circulation in critically ill patients strongly influence StO_2 resting values and StO_2 reoxygenation rate. In addition, changes in NIRS-derived variables were not accompanied by any major changes in systemic hemodynamic variables, and this, again, confirms that macrocirculatory changes might not accurately reflect the tissue oxygenation status in the critical care setting.

To date, the utility of NIRS in the management of critically ill patients is still questionable. The fact that NIRS is a low-cost, noninvasive, monitoring modality improves the attractiveness of the technology. However, although NIRS can be a very powerful tool for tissue oxygenation and perfusion assessment, more studies that explore the relationship between $ScvO_2$ and StO_2 and the use of VOT-derived parameters may be warranted before recommending its routine use in the critical care setting [54].

9.5.3 Assessment of Microvascular Perfusion

Microcirculation is the ultimate portion of the vasculature, responsible for fine-tuning tissue perfusion in order to meet oxygen requirements. In experimental models of sepsis, multiple trials demonstrated that multiple capillaries present stopped flow or intermittent flow while others are adequately perfused.

In humans, the investigation of microcirculation has long been difficult due to the lack of adequate tools. With the development of small handheld microscopes, the investigation of microcirculation at bedside was made feasible. De Backer et al. [60] demonstrated that the microvascular perfusion was altered in septic patients, compared to ICU controls. These alterations consisted of a decrease in functional capillary density and increased heterogeneity between areas close by a few microns. These alterations were fully reversible by topical application of acetylcholine. Interestingly, the severity of these microvascular alterations was associated with organ dysfunction and mortality [61–63].

Quantifying the microcirculation remains challenging and is nicely described in consensus documents [64]. While semiquantitative assessment remains practical and may allow point-of-care evaluation of microcirculation, recent advances in technology have allowed advanced computer-assisted measurements which may provide some better classification of microcirculation [65].

The impact of various interventions has been reported, from fluids to various vasoactive agents. Basically, the response of microcirculation is variable and cannot be predicted from the analysis of systemic hemodynamics [66].

At this stage, it remains difficult to use microcirculatory assessment outside clinical research given the unpredictable effects of therapeutic interventions and the difficulties to assess microcirculation at the bedside 24/7. Nevertheless, understanding the specificities of microvascular derangements is crucial, as it may help to understand why interventions may fail to improve tissue perfusion and signs of dysoxia, despite improving systemic hemodynamics.

Summary

The resuscitation of patients with acute circulatory failure should be aimed at obtaining adequate tissue perfusion, not at strictly achieving predefined static hemodynamic parameters. The presence of impaired tissue perfusion despite adequate resuscitation in a shocked patient is usually associated with worse outcome. Thus, normalization of some perfusion indices has become one of the resuscitation targets in patients with septic shock. Although recent evidence has increasingly confirmed a clear relation between poor peripheral perfusion and mortality, the use of different perfusion indices as a resuscitation guide needs more research.

References

1. Reinhart K, et al. Recognizing sepsis as a global health priority—a WHO resolution. N Engl J Med. 2017;377(5):414–7.
2. Evans L, et al. Surviving sepsis campaign: international guidelines for management of sepsis and septic shock 2021. Intensive Care Med. 2021;47(11):1181–247.
3. Vincent JL, et al. Assessment of the worldwide burden of critical illness: the intensive care over nations (ICON) audit. Lancet Respir Med. 2014;2(5):380–6.
4. Kaukonen KM, et al. Mortality related to severe sepsis and septic shock among critically ill patients in Australia and New Zealand, 2000-2012. JAMA. 2014;311(13):1308–16.
5. De Backer D, et al. Comparison of dopamine and norepinephrine in the treatment of shock. N Engl J Med. 2010;362(9):779–89.
6. Venet F, Monneret G. Advances in the understanding and treatment of sepsis-induced immuno-suppression. Nat Rev Nephrol. 2018;14(2):121–37.
7. Nakamori Y, Park EJ, Shimaoka M. Immune deregulation in sepsis and septic shock: reversing immune paralysis by targeting PD-1/PD-L1 pathway. Front Immunol. 2020;11:624279.
8. Connett RJ, et al. Defining hypoxia: a systems view of VO2, glycolysis, energetics, and intracellular PO2. J Appl Physiol (1985). 1990;68(3):833–42.
9. Cecconi M, et al. Consensus on circulatory shock and hemodynamic monitoring. Task force of the European Society of Intensive Care Medicine. Intensive Care Med. 2014;40(12):1795–815.
10. Vincent JL, De Backer D. Circulatory shock. N Engl J Med. 2013;369(18):1726–34.
11. Hiemstra B, et al. Clinical examination for diagnosing circulatory shock. Curr Opin Crit Care. 2017;23(4):293–301.
12. Hernandez G, et al. The holistic view on perfusion monitoring in septic shock. Curr Opin Crit Care. 2012;18(3):280–6.
13. Poeze M, et al. Monitoring global volume-related hemodynamic or regional variables after initial resuscitation: what is a better predictor of outcome in critically ill septic patients? Crit Care Med. 2005;33(11):2494–500.
14. Vincent JL, et al. The value of blood lactate kinetics in critically ill patients: a systematic review. Crit Care. 2016;20(1):257.
15. Singer M, et al. The third international consensus definitions for sepsis and septic shock (Sepsis-3). JAMA. 2016;315(8):801–10.
16. Alberti KG. The biochemical consequences of hypoxia. J Clin Pathol Suppl (R Coll Pathol). 1977;11:14–20.
17. Casserly B, et al. Lactate measurements in sepsis-induced tissue hypoperfusion: results from the surviving sepsis campaign database. Crit Care Med. 2015;43(3):567–73.
18. Haas SA, et al. Severe hyperlactatemia, lactate clearance and mortality in unselected critically ill patients. Intensive Care Med. 2016;42(2):202–10.
19. Hernandez G, et al. Persistent sepsis-induced hypotension without hyperlactatemia: is it really septic shock? J Crit Care. 2011;26(4):435.e9–435.e14.
20. Puskarich MA, et al. Outcomes of patients undergoing early sepsis resuscitation for cryptic shock compared with overt shock. Resuscitation. 2011;82(10):1289–93.
21. Rimachi R, et al. Lactate/pyruvate ratio as a marker of tissue hypoxia in circulatory and septic shock. Anaesth Intensive Care. 2012;40(3):427–32.
22. Hernandez G, et al. When to stop septic shock resuscitation: clues from a dynamic perfusion monitoring. Ann Intensive Care. 2014;4:30.
23. Rhodes A, et al. Surviving sepsis campaign: international guidelines for management of sepsis and septic shock: 2016. Intensive Care Med. 2017;43(3):304–77.
24. Hernandez G, Bellomo R, Bakker J. The ten pitfalls of lactate clearance in sepsis. Intensive Care Med. 2019;45(1):82–5.
25. Levy B. Lactate and shock state: the metabolic view. Curr Opin Crit Care. 2006;12(4):315–21.
26. Kiyatkin ME, Bakker J. Lactate and microcirculation as suitable targets for hemodynamic optimization in resuscitation of circulatory shock. Curr Opin Crit Care. 2017;23(4):348–54.
27. Hernandez G, Teboul JL. Is the macrocirculation really dissociated from the microcirculation in septic shock? Intensive Care Med. 2016;42(10):1621–4.

28. Bonanno FG. Clinical pathology of the shock syndromes. J Emerg Trauma Shock. 2011;4(2):233–43.

29. Lima A, Bakker J. Noninvasive monitoring of peripheral perfusion. Intensive Care Med. 2005;31(10):1316–26.

30. Lima A, et al. The prognostic value of the subjective assessment of peripheral perfusion in critically ill patients. Crit Care Med. 2009;37(3):934–8.

31. Naumann DN, et al. Real-time point of care microcirculatory assessment of shock: design, rationale and application of the point of care microcirculation (POEM) tool. Crit Care. 2016;20(1):310.

32. Ait-Oufella H, et al. Capillary refill time exploration during septic shock. Intensive Care Med. 2014;40(7):958–64.

33. Champion HR, et al. Trauma score. Crit Care Med. 1981;9(9):672–6.

34. Schriger DL, Baraff L. Defining normal capillary refill: variation with age, sex, and temperature. Ann Emerg Med. 1988;17(9):932–5.

35. Hernandez G, et al. Evolution of peripheral vs metabolic perfusion parameters during septic shock resuscitation. A clinical-physiologic study. J Crit Care. 2012;27(3):283–8.

36. Londono J, et al. Association of clinical hypoperfusion variables with lactate clearance and hospital mortality. Shock. 2018;50(3):286–92.

37. Hernandez G, et al. Effect of a resuscitation strategy targeting peripheral perfusion status vs serum lactate levels on 28-day mortality among patients with septic shock: the ANDROMEDA-SHOCK randomized clinical trial. JAMA. 2019;321(7):654–64.

38. van Genderen ME, et al. Persistent peripheral and microcirculatory perfusion alterations after out-of-hospital cardiac arrest are associated with poor survival. Crit Care Med. 2012;40(8):2287–94.

39. Cecconi M, et al. Fluid challenges in intensive care: the FENICE study: a global inception cohort study. Intensive Care Med. 2015;41(9):1529–37.

40. De Backer D, Dubois MJ. Assessment of the microcirculatory flow in patients in the intensive care unit. Curr Opin Crit Care. 2001;7(3):200–3.

41. Lima A, et al. The relation of near-infrared spectroscopy with changes in peripheral circulation in critically ill patients. Crit Care Med. 2011;39(7):1649–54.

42. Rubinstein EH, Sessler DI. Skin-surface temperature gradients correlate with fingertip blood flow in humans. Anesthesiology. 1990;73(3):541–5.

43. Sessler DI. Skin-temperature gradients are a validated measure of fingertip perfusion. Eur J Appl Physiol. 2003;89(3–4):401–2; author reply 403–4.

44. House JR, Tipton MJ. Using skin temperature gradients or skin heat flux measurements to determine thresholds of vasoconstriction and vasodilatation. Eur J Appl Physiol. 2002;88(1–2):141–5.

45. Bourcier S, et al. Toe-to-room temperature gradient correlates with tissue perfusion and predicts outcome in selected critically ill patients with severe infections. Ann Intensive Care. 2016;6(1):63.

46. Ait-Oufella H, et al. Mottling score predicts survival in septic shock. Intensive Care Med. 2011;37(5):801–7.

47. Jouffroy R, et al. Skin mottling score and capillary refill time to assess mortality of septic shock since pre-hospital setting. Am J Emerg Med. 2019;37(4):664–71.

48. Vincent JL, SpringerLink. Annual update in intensive care and emergency medicine 2013. 1st ed. Annual update in intensive care and emergency medicine. Berlin: Springer: Imprint: Springer; 2013.

49. van Genderen ME, van Bommel J, Lima A. Monitoring peripheral perfusion in critically ill patients at the bedside. Curr Opin Crit Care. 2012;18(3):273–9.

50. Mowafi HA, et al. The efficacy of perfusion index as an indicator for intravascular injection of epinephrine-containing epidural test dose in propofol-anesthetized adults. Anesth Analg. 2009;108(2):549–53.

51. Biais M, et al. Impact of norepinephrine on the relationship between pleth variability index and pulse pressure variations in ICU adult patients. Crit Care. 2011;15(4):R168.

52. van Genderen ME, et al. Peripheral perfusion index as an early predictor for central hypovolemia in awake healthy volunteers. Anesth Analg. 2013;116(2):351–6.

53. Lima A, et al. Peripheral vasoconstriction influences thenar oxygen saturation as measured by near-infrared spectroscopy. Intensive Care Med. 2012;38(4):606–11.

54. Green MS, Sehgal S, Tariq R. Near-infrared spectroscopy: the new must have tool in the intensive care unit? Semin Cardiothorac Vasc Anesth. 2016;20(3):213–24.

9

55. Nioka S, et al. A novel method to measure regional muscle blood flow continuously using NIRS kinetics information. Dyn Med. 2006;5:5.

56. Boushel R, Piantadosi CA. Near-infrared spectroscopy for monitoring muscle oxygenation. Acta Physiol Scand. 2000;168(4):615–22.

57. Lima A, et al. Low tissue oxygen saturation at the end of early goal-directed therapy is associated with worse outcome in critically ill patients. Crit Care. 2009;13(Suppl 5):S13.

58. Colin G, et al. Masseter tissue oxygen saturation predicts normal central venous oxygen saturation during early goal-directed therapy and predicts mortality in patients with severe sepsis. Crit Care Med. 2012;40(2):435–40.

59. Shapiro NI, et al. The association of near-infrared spectroscopy-derived tissue oxygenation measurements with sepsis syndromes, organ dysfunction and mortality in emergency department patients with sepsis. Crit Care. 2011;15(5):R223.

60. De Backer D, et al. Microvascular blood flow is altered in patients with sepsis. Am J Respir Crit Care Med. 2002;166(1):98–104.

61. Sakr Y, et al. Persistent microcirculatory alterations are associated with organ failure and death in patients with septic shock. Crit Care Med. 2004;32(9):1825–31.

62. De Backer D, et al. Microcirculatory alterations in patients with severe sepsis: impact of time of assessment and relationship with outcome. Crit Care Med. 2013;41(3):791–9.

63. Edul VS, et al. Quantitative assessment of the microcirculation in healthy volunteers and in patients with septic shock. Crit Care Med. 2012;40(5):1443–8.

64. Ince C, et al. Second consensus on the assessment of sublingual microcirculation in critically ill patients: results from a task force of the European Society of Intensive Care Medicine. Intensive Care Med. 2018;44(3):281–99.

65. Hilty MP, et al. Automated algorithm analysis of sublingual microcirculation in an international multicentral database identifies alterations associated with disease and mechanism of resuscitation. Crit Care Med. 2020;48(10):e864–75.

66. De Backer D, et al. The effects of dobutamine on microcirculatory alterations in patients with septic shock are independent of its systemic effects. Crit Care Med. 2006;34(2):403–8.

Dysregulated Immune Response and Organ Dysfunction

Contents

Management of Dysregulated Immune Response in the Critically Ill: Heart and Circulation

Benjamin Deniau, Charles de Roquetaillade, Alexandre Mebazaa, and Benjamin Chousterman

Contents

© The Author(s), under exclusive license to Springer Nature Switzerland AG 2023
Z. Molnar et al. (eds.), *Management of Dysregulated Immune Response in the Critically Ill*, Lessons from the ICU, https://doi.org/10.1007/978-3-031-17572-5_10

Management of Dysregulated Immune Response in the Critically Ill: Heart...

173

10

⊜ Learning Objectives

In this chapter, we will elaborate the pathophysiology of inflammation in cardiovascular diseases, and notably the central role of cytokines in inflammation during cardiovascular diseases. Furthermore, we will discuss the pivotal and critical role of inflammasome in one of the most frequent cardiac diseases: acute myocardial infarction. Furthermore, inflammation in acute heart failure, cardiogenic shock, and vascular disease will be discussed. Main therapeutic approach of inflammation during cardiovascular diseases will be enumerated. After reading this chapter, you will understand the main pathophysiological basis of cardiovascular diseases and main therapeutic options currently being studied.

10.1 Inflammation in Cardiovascular Diseases

10.1.1 The Central Role of Cytokines in Inflammation During Cardiovascular Diseases

Inflammation is defined as the cellular and humoral response to infectious or noninfectious injury. Although inflammation is needed to fight against pathogens, dysregulated inflammation can trigger acute injury, maladaptive repair, and chronic disease [1]. The NLRP3 inflammasome is part of the innate immune response; it is a macromolecular protein complex that finely regulates the activation of caspase-1 and the subsequent production of proinflammatory cytokines such as IL-1β and IL-18. Cytokines, produced by monocytes and macrophages [2], are indicating proteins involved in the communication of immune cells regulating the inflammatory response.

Interleukin-1 (IL-1) is the leading and most studied proinflammatory cytokine. It is part of the complex IL-1–IL-1 receptor family whose production is finely regulated by the NLRP3 inflammasome.

The IL-1 family is composed of 11 cytokine members and 10 receptors [3]. IL-1 and IL-18 are synthesized as inactive precursors, and both require caspase-1 to become active molecules. IL-33 gets inactivated by caspase-1. Other members of the IL-1 family represented by IL-37 and IL-38 are involved in the limitation of inflammatory processes, by reducing the levels of IL-1, TNF-α, IL-6, and chemokines [1]. In addition, IL-37 inhibits the NLRP3 inflammasome.

IL-1 receptors are ubiquitous and present at the membrane of all nucleated cells. Two types of IL-1 receptors are described: ligand-binding chains (such as IL1-R1) and accessory chains (such as IL-1R3). The intracellular domain of receptors contains the Toll-IL-1-receptor (TIR) domain, nearly identical to the TIR domain of TLRs (Toll-like receptors) explaining the common mechanism inducing inflammation [1]. Both TLRs and IL-1R can trigger the activation of NF-κB leading to the transcription of the NLRP3 inflammasome component. To counteract the proinflammatory effect of IL-1 and limit systemic inflammation, other members act as anti-inflammatory actors. Binding the extracellular domain of IL-1R1, IL-1 receptor antagonist (RA) modifies the conformation of the receptor preventing the binding to IL1-R3 and the proinflammatory signal. In the same way, IL1-R2 binds to IL-1β preventing its binding to IL-1R1, inhibiting the proinflammatory signal.

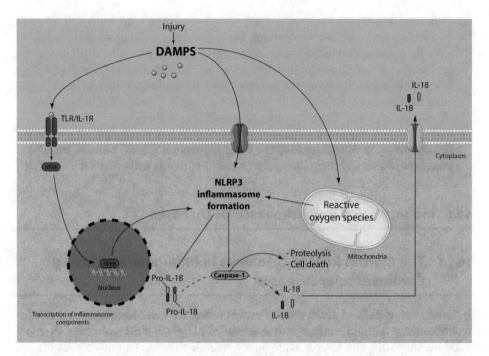

◘ Fig. 10.1 NLRP3 inflammasome formation following DAMP activation after injury. *DAMPs* damage-associated molecular patterns, *IL* interleukin, *NF-κB* nuclear factor-kappa B, *NLRP3* NACHT LRR and PYD domain-containing protein 3, *TLR* Toll-like receptor

Caspase-1 is a major enzyme involved in the inflammation process; its activation is regulated by an oligomeric macromolecular complex: the inflammasome [4]. NLRP3 (for NACHT, LRR, and PYD domain-containing protein 3) is the sensing component of the inflammasome and responds to various danger signals such as oxidative stress and lysosome destabilization (◘ Fig. 10.1) [1].

In response to stress, the extracellular release of DAMPs promotes the transcription of proinflammatory genes (such as pro-IL-1β and pro-IL-18) together with components of the inflammasome (NLRP3, ASC) (◘ Fig. 10.1) [1]. NLRP3, which may be activated by various intracellular signals (lysosomal destabilization, oxidative stress, failed mitophagy …), further oligomerizes and binds the protein adaptor ASC, which in turn activates pro-caspase-1 to active caspase-1. Caspase-1 cleaves pro-IL-1β and pro-IL-18 into active forms (◘ Fig. 10.1). Interleukin-18 is considered as a risk factor of cardiovascular events [1]. Interleukin-33 is another IL-1 cytokine member inactivated by caspase-1. Interleukin-33 reduces the T helper 1 response, favoring the resolution of inflammation [5, 6].

The fine interplay between the IL-1 family and NLRP3 inflammasome has been involved in the pathogenesis of multiple cardiovascular conditions [7, 8] and is now a target for various therapeutic interventions.

10.1.2 The Pivotal and Critical Role of NLRP3 Inflammasome in Acute Myocardial Infarction (AMI)

Acute myocardial infarction (AMI) corresponds to the myocardial ischemia induced by the reduction of coronary blood flow. The imbalance between the need and supply of oxygen leads to a critical energy failure, leading to inflammation and cell death [1]. The cornerstone of AMI management is based on the reperfusion strategy. However, AMI is followed by the release of cell content in the blood flow, e.g., DAMPs and cytokines, followed by local and systemic inflammation starting immediately after ischemia.

After a reduction of coronary blood flow, cell death quickly occurs. Cell content, e.g., DAMPs, is released in the systemic blood flow. DAMPs induce the expression of the inflammasome via TLR and IL-1R cell receptor activation, leading to the activation of NF-κB (◘ Fig. 10.1) [9]. Activation of the NLRP3 inflammasome amplifies the inflammatory response by activating the secretion of IL-1β and IL-18 (◘ Fig. 10.1) [10, 11]. These cytokines exit the cell via gasdermin D pores, a substrate of caspase-1, responsible for the extracellular release of IL-1β, IL-18, and active caspase-1 [10]. Preclinical studies had shown the detrimental effect of NLRP3 inflammasome on AMI by using *Nlrp3*-deficient mice. In a model of AMI induced by coronary ischemia-reperfusion, *Nlrp3*-deficient mice have a smaller infarct size and preserved cardiac function when compared to control mice [12, 13]. Similar results were observed in *Casp1*- or *ASC*-deficient mice, highlighting the pivotal and critical role of NLRP3 inflammasome in the development and maintenance of inflammation following AMI [4, 14]. For example, colchicine, a nonspecific inhibitor of the NLRP3 inflammasome, already evaluated in AMI mouse model, is associated with a significantly reduced infarct size, ventricular remodeling, and prolonged 7-day survival [15]. Moreover, in addition to cardiomyocytes, other types of cardiac cells are indirectly involved in cardiac dysfunction during AMI via the NLRP3 inflammasome.

10.2 Inflammation in Septic Cardiomyopathy

Sepsis is defined as a dysregulated host response to infection [16]. Its pathophysiology encompasses profound circulatory, metabolic, and cellular abnormalities. It is consistently associated with circulatory shock of peripheral origin, as well as hyperlactatemia, despite the absence of hypovolemia. The first identification of septic cardiomyopathy was made by Parker et al., who were the first to identify systolic dysfunction associated with sepsis using radionucleotides [17]. Pathophysiology of sepsis-induced cardiomyopathy is multifactorial involving humoral substances addressed as myocardial depressant factors, abnormalities in calcium handling, sarcomeric and mitochondrial dysfunction, as well as coronary microvascular changes [18] (◘ Fig. 10.2).

The existence of humoral factors driving myocardial depression in septic shock has been suggested since 1985 when Parillo et al. exposed mammalian myocardial cells in vitro to serum obtained from septic shock patients and observed a reversible reduction in shortening fraction [19]. Later observations highlighted the crucial role of IL-1β [18], TNF [20], and IL-8 [21] in myocardial depression syndrome. Cardiomyocytes activated by TNF or IL-1β secrete chemokines further responsible for the protraction

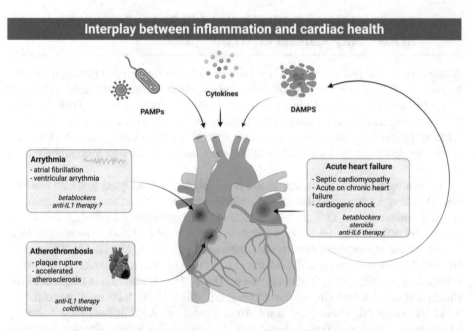

Fig. 10.2 Interplay between inflammation and cardiac health. *DAMPs* damage-associated molecular patterns, *IL* interleukin, *PAMPs* pathogen-associated molecular patterns

of neutrophils in the cardiac tissue, which could be detrimental in the acute phase [22]. In a mice model of sepsis, pharmacologic inhibition of the NLRP3 inflammasome by glyburide demonstrated attenuated myocardial dysfunction together with reduced mortality [23]. However, in the clinical setting, measurement of numerous circulating cytokines (IL-1β, IL-6, IL-8, IL-10, IL-18, TNF-α, and monocyte chemoattractant protein-1) together with repeated echocardiogram monitoring did not find any association between circulating cytokine levels and myocardial dysfunction [24].

From a therapeutic standpoint, studies evaluating the effect of recombinant human interleukin 1 receptor antagonist (rh-IL-1ra) on the outcome following septic shock found no effect on the resolution of shock nor on the reduction of mortality [25]. In their study, Fisher et al. [26] did not report the incidence of cardiac dysfunction syndrome; however, their results were in favor of a reduction in mortality among the most severe patients [26]. A recent reanalysis in patients harboring features of macrophage activation syndrome, a syndrome often qualified as a cytokine storm [27], confirmed the possible interest of rhIL-1ra in septic patients with high levels of circulating cytokines [28].

10.3 Inflammation and Cardiac Arrhythmias

Management of arrhythmia is a major problem in emergency and critical care medicine (○ Fig. 10.2). Depending on studies and definition criteria, 12–20% of patients may face sustained arrhythmia during their ICU stay [29, 30]. Atrial fibrillation (AF) is the most common rhythm disorder encountered in the ICU [31], which can be either prevalent (preexisting) or incident (new-onset). In the recent study of Moss et al. based on 8356 adult admissions, AF was observed in 1610 patients (16.6%), among whom 861 (53.4%) had a priori diagnosis and 749 (46.6%) had new-onset AF [32].

Inflammation undoubtedly plays a central role in the development of AF in the ICU (● Fig. 10.2) but also in chronic inflammation such as rheumatoid arthritis [33]. Incidence of AF has been shown to correlate with blood cell rise following surgery [34], and other inflammatory markers (C-reactive protein, tumor necrosis factor-α, IL-2, IL-6, and IL-8) have been linked with AF [35, 36]. Several studies reported an increase of macrophages in the atrium among patients suffering from AF [37, 38]. However, it is still unclear if leukocyte infiltration is responsible for the development of AF or part of the global inflammatory process responsible for remodeling and subsequent AF; however, emerging evidence from the preclinical field seems to confirm their causative role [39]. Although the relationship between systemic inflammation and AF among ICU patients is clear, no interventional study, to date, has proven its ability to reduce or prevent AF in this setting.

Conduction disorders may also occur in the atrioventricular node and ventricles giving rise to ventricular tachycardia and fibrillation, respectively. Those conditions are less frequent (2–3%) but life-threatening [29, 30]. Those arrhythmias often occur in patients with AMI, a situation that triggers emergency myelopoiesis and infiltration of myocardium by leukocytes [40]. Although excessive inflammation is associated with adverse remodeling after AMI [41], its role in the development of ventricular arrhythmia is more scarce. In a mice model of AMI, preexisting LPS injections lead to more arrhythmia including inducible non-sustained ventricular tachycardia suggesting inflammation as a key contributor of ventricular arrhythmia [42]. In another animal model of AMI, treatment with anti-IL1 (anakinra) could reduce inducible ventricular arrhythmia [42]. Further studies are warranted to confirm the possible benefit of anti-IL-1 therapy as antiarrhythmic therapy.

10.4 Inflammation in Acute Heart Failure and Cardiogenic Shock

Acute heart failure (AHF) is defined as a new or worsening symptom of heart failure (HF) [43]. The most severe form of AHF is cardiogenic shock (CS), a critical condition defined by the association of systolic blood pressure <90 mmHg for ≥30 min or the requirement for support to achieve adequate blood pressure and evidence of end-organ hypoperfusion defined by the presence of cool extremities, altered mental status, urine output <30 mL/h, or serum lactate >2.0 mmol/L [44, 45]. Etiologies of CS are numerous but are mainly represented by AMI (80% of cases) [45]. Despite recent advances in treatment and management, CS remains a high-mortality complication of AMI, with a mortality rate comprised between 38 and 65% [46–48].

Pathophysiology of CS is complex, but its understanding has substantially evolved over the past two decades [44]. The cornerstone of the pathophysiology of CS is a profound depression of myocardial contractility resulting in a downward circle of reduced cardiac output, low blood pressure, and coronary ischemia, leading to further reduction in myocardial contractility [44]. Simultaneously, several compensatory mechanisms are triggered to counteract the decrease in myocardial contractility. The main compensatory mechanism is systemic vasoconstriction followed by acute cardiac injury and ineffective stroke volume [49]. In addition, it is established that CS is followed by alteration of the entire circulatory system, including peripheral vasculature, and is not limited to the heart [44]. Even if the low stroke volume is the inciting event, inadequate circulatory compensation also contributes to shock [44]. The presence of inflammation during CS is undebatable. Among the numerous identified mediators, nitric oxide (NO), produced by the inducible NO synthase (iNOS) [50] and interleukins, can act as a myocardial depressant factor and plays an important role in CS. Inflammation seems to play a role in the development of multiple-organ failure (MOF) following CS. In their observational study among ICU patients with CS, Geppert et al. found that patients with CS exhibit very high levels of IL-6, similar as seen in septic shock [51]. Moreover, higher levels of IL-6 were associated with the development of subsequent MOF, suggesting a role of inflammation in the progression from CS to MOF. Several interventional studies aiming at mitigating immune response during AHF and CS are ongoing and should clarify the precise role of hyperinflammation in this setting.

10.5 Inflammation and Vascular System

For several decades, the endothelium has been recognized as an organ system involved in a multitude of physiological functions. Endothelial dysfunction following aggression is related to various causes, namely endothelial cell (EC) death, glycocalyx breakdown, and junction protein dysregulation [52].

10.5.1 Endothelial Dysfunction

Several types of aggression (release of DAMPs and PAMPs) can lead to the activation of inflammatory pathways especially NF-κB [53, 54] and activate endothelium, later altering its structure and function [55].

In response to inflammation, EC releases pro- and anti-inflammatory proteins, such as cytokines and chemokines. This response from EC aims at limiting a microbiological spread. Unfortunately, this phenotypical change can also lead to impaired microcirculation, tissue perfusion, and organ failure [52]. Activated myeloid cells also participate in systemic inflammation by the production of cytokines. Among them, IL-6, produced by both leukocytes and EC, can sustainably impair the endothelial barrier function [56].

Following aggression, impaired vascular tone can also be explained by the dysregulated production of nitric oxide (NO). It is demonstrated that sepsis downregulates endothelial NO synthase (eNOS) expression [57, 58]. Moreover, endotoxins lead to the overexpression of inducible NO synthase (iNOS), followed by amounts of vasodilating NO. In this perspective, several authors have proposed blocking iNOS activity during sepsis. However, to date, no intervention targeting at NO synthesis has yet proven its efficacy in terms of reduced mortality nor length of stay in the setting of critical care [59]. In addition, several authors have reported serious deleterious adverse effects such as altered macrohemodynamics [60, 61].

To counteract sepsis-induced endothelial dysfunction, therapeutics like vasodilating agents, namely Ilomedine, is under investigation [62, 63]. Statins present vascular anti-inflammatory properties and could be an interesting agent to use during sepsis. Ulinastatin was clinically tested in septic shock patients. Interestingly, main biomarkers of inflammation were decreased in treated patients, but no reduction of mortality was observed [64]. A recent meta-analysis concluded that statins had no benefit in septic shock [65, 66].

10.5.2 Glycocalyx Breakdown

The glycocalyx is a heparan layer of glycosaminoglycans and proteoglycans that covers vascular endothelium; it is involved in vascular integrity and cell trafficking [67, 68]. During sepsis, the thickness of glycocalyx is reduced by destruction [69], modifying the macromolecule permeability, leukocyte adhesion, blood flow, and organ perfusion [52]. Sepsis is not the only condition associated with glycocalyx destruction, and other conditions such as trauma and ischemia-reperfusion syndrome have demonstrated that they could reproduce glycocalyx damages [70]. In addition, the effects of sepsis on vascular tone are increased when the glycocalyx is damaged [71, 72]. To date, no intervention aiming at targeting specifically glycocalyx is under investigation, but adjunctive therapeutics, thought to have a beneficial effect on glycocalyx integrity, namely microparticles, carnitine, and vitamin C, are currently tested in clinical trials.

10.5.3 Junction Protein Dysregulation

Angiopoietin-1 and -2, two growth factors, and their tyrosine kinase receptors, Tie 1 and Tie 2, act as regulators of vascular homeostasis via signaling pathways, namely Akt and FOXO-1 [52]. Experimental studies observed a role in the prevention of vascular permeability of angiopoietin-1, whereas angiopoietin-2 could have a detrimental role in increasing vascular leakage and lung injury during sepsis [73, 74]. From these observations, therapies have been developed to target angiopoietin-1 and angiopoietin-2 activity. However, the promising perspectives demonstrated in animal models need to be confirmed in humans.

10.6 Long-Term Impact of Critical Care on Cardiovascular Health: Immune Scar

Along with the improvement in the management of critical care patients has emerged the concern of the quality of life and long-term outcomes associated with survival. Recent data suggest that critical care survivors (in particular sepsis survivors) have an increased risk of long-term mortality [75]. Cardiovascular health seems particularly vulnerable following critical care. Epidemiological studies have reported a higher long-term risk of heart failure, myocardial infarction, stroke, and atrial fibrillation up to several years after pneumonia and sepsis [76–78]. The interplay between systemic inflammation and cardiovascular diseases (CVD) is now well recognized [79] (◘ Fig. 10.2). Several studies have demonstrated that systemic inflammation could "inflame" the atherosclerotic plaque accelerating further atherosclerosis and making it more prone to rupture and subsequent vessel thrombosis [80]. However, to date, no intervention has demonstrated its benefit in the prevention of cardiovascular events among ICU survivors. The inflammatory hypothesis of atherothrombosis has remained unproved till the recent publication of the CANTOS trial in which patients with previous myocardial infarction and a high-sensitivity CRP (>2 mg per liter) were randomized to receive either canakinumab (an anti-inflammatory therapy targeting the interleukin-1β innate immunity pathway) or its placebo [81]. In this trial, targeting IL-1β led to a significantly lower rate of recurrent cardiovascular events than placebo, independent of lipid-level lowering. However, this reduction was associated with an increased rate of fatal infection, which led to a similar all-cause mortality rate between groups. The results of this encouraging trial have been challenged by the negative results of the CIRT trial in which anti-inflammatory therapy with low-dose methotrexate failed to show benefit in terms of cardiovascular events or mortality [82]. Several hypotheses may explain this discrepancy such as the absence of enrichment in recruiting patients with torpid inflammation in the CIRT trial, and the differences between targeted anti-cytokine therapies and broader spectrum anti-inflammatory therapies [83]. However, those trials paved the way to further RCT aiming at reducing inflammation among patients harboring marks of torpid inflammation for the prevention of CVD.

10.7   Therapeutic Approach of Inflammation During CVD

Inflammation is the cornerstone of the pathophysiology of CVD. From atherosclerosis to acute thrombotic complications leading to acute myocardial infarction (plaque rupture), inflammation is involved in each step of the process [84]. Therefore, a therapeutical approach focusing on inflammation in CVD, regardless of the etiology, needs to be global. In this part, we focus on the more encouraging therapeutical approaches focusing on inflammation control in CVD.

10.7.1   Anakinra

Anakinra inhibits the biological activity of IL-1α and IL-1β by blocking the link between IL-1 and its receptor IL-1R1 [1]. When administered in ischemic HF patients, anakinra reduces circulating levels of CRP and IL-6 [85]. Interestingly, when anakinra is initiated during the first 24 h after acute decompensated systolic HF, patients had reduced systemic inflammation and improved left ventricular ejection fraction 14 days after the beginning of the treatment. In 2017, Van Tassel et al. found in the REDHART trial that acutely decompensated HF patients treated with anakinra had decreased NT proBNP levels when compared to the control group [86]. Anakinra was tested in patients with HF with preserved ejection fraction (HFrEF) and was associated with an increased treadmill exercise, lower NT proBNP levels, and improved quality of life [86]. Recently, Abatte et al. performed a pooled analysis of three early-phase randomized clinical trials in which 14 days of anakinra's effect was evaluated on the incidence of HF in STEMI patients (VUCART, VCUART2, and VCUART3). Anakinra significantly reduced the incidence of all-cause death and HF hospitalization. Unfortunately, these studies include a low number of patients (including 129 patients) and must be confirmed by larger randomized clinical trials.

10.7.2   Colchicine

Anti-inflammatory Mechanisms

Colchicine, an alkaloid molecule extracted from Colchicum plants for the first time in 1820, has been one of the oldest drugs used for inflammatory systemic diseases for more than one century. Rheumatic diseases are its best-known use [87, 88]. By binding

Management of Dysregulated Immune Response in the Critically Ill: Heart...

181

10

tubulins and disturbing polymerization during cellular processes requiring dynamic tubulin heterodimer polymerization (cell division, migration, shape, intracellular protein trafficking, and ionic homeostasis), colchicine exerts various pleiotropic effects [87, 89–91], notably anti-inflammatory, antifibrotic, and immune system downregulation. Several mechanisms of action of colchicine at different steps of the pathophysiology of AMI make this molecule particularly interesting in the management of ischemic disease. Colchicine reduces the cleavage of pro-interleukin-1β to active interleukin 1β, an important proinflammatory cytokine implicated in the pathophysiology of AMI, and inhibits the NLRP-3 inflammasome [91, 92]. Interestingly, colchicine reduces the production of interleukin-1β by inhibiting the Ras homolog family member A (RhoA) signaling cascade [93, 94]. In addition, inhibition of proinflammatory cytokines, such as interleukin-1β, prevents local chemoattraction of inflammatory and systemic cells implicated in the inflammation process [89–92]. Colchicine reduces local production of monocyte chemoattractant protein-1 (MCP-1), an important cytokine implicated in the postischemic inflammatory response responsible for leukocyte recruitment, angiogenesis, inflammation activation, and resolution [84, 95]. Then, colchicine exerts interesting antifibrotic effects by transforming the growth factor β signaling pathway [93, 94]. Anti-atherosclerotic effects through inflammation and ischemic process of AMI of colchicine have been investigated since 1990. In laboratory studies, it is established that colchicine can decrease migratory and proliferative activities of smooth muscle cells in atherosclerotic plaques, underlining its potential anti-atherosclerotic effect [84]. Its effect could be mediated by a decrease of concentrations of plasma fibrinogen [96] and increased nitric oxide production [97]. In addition, colchicine exerts beneficial effects on the ischemic myocardium such as inhibition of apoptosis [98] and of ventricular hypertrophy [99], and fibrosis [100]. Recent animal studies described a reduction of the infarct size and better cardiac function thanks to colchicine [88]. Moreover, antiarrhythmic effects of colchicine are described at cellular levels by reducing fibrosis in a rabbit model of heart failure [101]. Due to its in vitro and in vivo pleiotropic effects, colchicine is an interesting candidate for the ischemic and inflammatory myocardium and an interesting potential candidate for the treatment of ischemic chronic heart failure.

Therapeutic Benefits

In practice, colchicine may have two main indications in CVD: prevention of plaque rupture in coronary artery disease (anti-inflammatory effects) and infarct size limitation in AMI and its consequences (anti-inflammatory and anti-fibrotic effects). Beneficial effects of colchicine on the prevention of cardiovascular events have been suggested since 1990 and were described for the first time in 2007 when Crittenden et al. [102] observed a reduction in the prevalence of myocardial infarction in patients with gout treated by colchicine. In 2013, the first randomized clinical trial comparing a low dose of colchicine versus a placebo in a stable coronary disease showed a reduction of cardiac events, namely coronary syndrome, cardiac arrest, and noncardioembolic ischemic stroke in the treated group by colchicine. For the ischemic myocardium, clinical data are relatively recent and heterogeneous. Based on anti-inflammatory effects and the potential reduction of infarct size of colchicine, the first randomized clinical trial evaluating the interest of the molecule in acute coronary syndrome or stroke was conducted in 2012 by Raju et al. [103]. Patients were treated by colchicine or placebo for 30 days since the cardiac event. Authors failed to demonstrate a reduction of systemic inflammation, assessed by CRP measurements at day 30. In 2015, Deftereos et al. evaluated in a randomized clinical trial the interest of early treatment by colchicine (since coronary reperfusion and continued just up to 5 days after) in patients admitted for AMI with ST-segment elevation [104]. The authors observed a reduced infarct size assessed by creatine kinase and cardiac magnetic resonance in the colchicine group. In the same way, in 2017, Akodad et al. conducted a clinical trial in which patients admitted for AMI with ST-segment elevation treated by percutaneous angioplasty were randomized to receive colchicine during 1 month in addition to optimal medical treatment or optimal medical treatment alone [105]. Unfortunately, the inflammation (assessed by the CRP peak) was not different between the two groups, probably explained by the delayed initiation of colchicine without loading dose [87]. The LoDoCo-MI study in 2019 included 237 patients with AMI and evaluated the effect of a low dose of colchicine during 1 month versus placebo [106]. Unfortunately, results were comparable to the study of Akodad et al., and inflammation was not reduced in the treatment group 1 month after AMI. At last, the COLCOT study, a randomized clinical trial including 4745 patients with AMI, evaluated a treatment by colchicine (0.5 mg per day) versus placebo after AMI on the occurrence of a composite criterion, including cardiovascular death, resuscitated cardiac arrest, acute myocardial infarction, stroke, or hospitalization for angina requiring coronary revascularization [107]. Interestingly, the risk of cardiovascular events was decreased 30 days after AMI in the colchicine group. To confirm these interesting results of colchicine on the occurrence of cardiovascular events after AMI, several studies are currently ongoing.

10.7.3 Steroids

Acute myocardial infarction is characterized by an initial phase of inflammation, rapidly following the ischemic phase. Based on this pathophysiology, some studies have focused on assessing the possible benefit of corticosteroids in AMI despite the potential risk of increased cardiac rupture and impaired wound healing. First signals of corticosteroid therapy were observed in animal AMI models treated [108–110]. After an ischemic injury, some authors observed a preserved systolic cardiac function after methylprednisolone injection in dogs [108] and a decreased myocyte necrosis [111], suggesting the potential positive effect of corticosteroid therapy. To date, only a few human studies are available. In 2003, a meta-analysis focused on corticosteroid treatment following AMI included 8 RCT ($n = 1535$ patients) and 5 prospective non-randomized unblinded ($n = 1199$ patients) studies [112]. Regarding mortality, the authors concluded with a benefit of corticosteroid therapy with an OR of 0.74 (IC 95% 0.59–0.34, $p = 0.015$). However, when restricting the analysis to RCT, the authors found no benefit (OR 0.95 (IC 95% 0.71–1.29, $p = 0.75$). In studies included in the meta-analysis, no difference in side effects of corticosteroid therapy was found (including cardiac rupture, aneurysms, and arrhythmias). These data need to be carefully handled regarding the design of studies included, but this intervention surely deserves further investigations in properly conducted trials.

Take-Home Message

- Inflammation is a cornerstone of initiation and maintenance of cardiovascular diseases, namely cytokines.
- No therapeutic approach targeting inflammation has shown superiority regarding mortality.
- The more encouraging therapeutical approaches focusing on inflammation in cardiovascular diseases are anakinra, colchicine, and steroids.
- Ongoing clinical trials will allow progress to be made and to continue to understand the pathophysiology of CVD of inflammatory origin.

Conclusion

Inflammation is a cornerstone in the initiation and maintenance of CVD (ischemic, septic, etc.). Cytokines play a pivotal role in the pathophysiology of the inflammation of cardiac and vascular diseases. However, no therapeutic approach has shown superiority in terms of survival in the management of patients with cardiovascular pathologies of inflammatory origin, notably in ICU. This is mainly due to the complexity of the pathophysiology (numerous pathways involved, different patient profiles, etc.), which also explains the lack of positive therapeutic trials, especially in patients in ICU. Much progress has been made in recent years in terms of understanding the pathophysiology, but many questions remain. Ongoing clinical trials will allow progress to be made and to continue to understand the pathophysiology of CVD of inflammatory origin.

References

1. Abbate A, Toldo S, Marchetti C, Kron J, Van Tassell BW, Dinarello CA. Interleukin-1 and the inflammasome as therapeutic targets in cardiovascular disease. Circ Res. 2020;126(9):1260–80.
2. Opal SM, DePalo VA. Anti-inflammatory cytokines. Chest. 2000;117(4):1162–72.
3. Boraschi D, Italiani P, Weil S, Martin MU. The family of the interleukin-1 receptors. Immunol Rev. 2018;281(1):197–232.
4. Toldo S, Abbate A. The NLRP3 inflammasome in acute myocardial infarction. Nat Rev Cardiol. 2018;15(4):203–14.
5. Dinarello CA. The IL-1 family of cytokines and receptors in rheumatic diseases. Nat Rev Rheumatol. 2019;15(10):612–32.
6. Ca D. Interleukin-1 in the pathogenesis and treatment of inflammatory diseases. Blood [Internet]. 2011 [cité 14 mars 2022];117(14):3720–32. https://pubmed.ncbi.nlm.nih.gov/21304099/.
7. Van Tassell BW, Toldo S, Mezzaroma E, Abbate A. Targeting interleukin-1 in heart disease. Circulation. 2013;128(17):1910–23.
8. Buckley LF, Abbate A. Interleukin-1 blockade in cardiovascular diseases: from bench to bedside. BioDrugs. 2018;32(2):111–8.
9. Toldo S, Mezzaroma E, McGeough MD, Peña CA, Marchetti C, Sonnino C, et al. Independent roles of the priming and the triggering of the NLRP3 inflammasome in the heart. Cardiovasc Res. 2015;105(2):203–12.
10. Mauro AG, Bonaventura A, Mezzaroma E, Quader M, Toldo S The NLRP3 inflammasome in acute myocardial infarction. Nat Rev Cardiol [Internet]. 2018 [cité 14 mars 2022];15(4). https://pubmed.ncbi.nlm.nih.gov/29143812/.

11. Mezzaroma E, Toldo S, Farkas D, Seropian IM, Van Tassell BW, Salloum FN, et al. The inflammasome promotes adverse cardiac remodeling following acute myocardial infarction in the mouse. Proc Natl Acad Sci U S A. 2011;108(49):19725–30.

12. Liu Y, Lian K, Zhang L, Wang R, Yi F, Gao C, et al. TXNIP mediates NLRP3 inflammasome activation in cardiac microvascular endothelial cells as a novel mechanism in myocardial ischemia/reperfusion injury. Basic Res Cardiol. 2014;109(5):415.

13. Sandanger Ø, Ranheim T, Vinge LE, Bliksøen M, Alfsnes K, Finsen AV, et al. The NLRP3 inflammasome is up-regulated in cardiac fibroblasts and mediates myocardial ischaemia-reperfusion injury. Cardiovasc Res. 2013;99(1):164–74.

14. Kawaguchi M, Takahashi M, Hata T, Kashima Y, Usui F, Morimoto H, et al. Inflammasome activation of cardiac fibroblasts is essential for myocardial ischemia/reperfusion injury. Circulation. 2011;123(6):594–604.

15. Fujisue K, Sugamura K, Kurokawa H, Matsubara J, Ishii M, Izumiya Y, et al. Colchicine improves survival, left ventricular remodeling, and chronic cardiac function after acute myocardial infarction. Circ J [Internet]. 2017 [cité 14 mars 2022];81(8):1174–1182. https://pubmed.ncbi.nlm.nih.gov/28420825/.

16. Singer M, Deutschman CS, Seymour CW, Shankar-Hari M, Annane D, Bauer M, et al. The third international consensus definitions for sepsis and septic shock (Sepsis-3). JAMA. 2016;315(8):801–10.

17. Parker MM, Shelhamer JH, Bacharach SL, Green MV, Natanson C, Frederick TM, et al. Profound but reversible myocardial depression in patients with septic shock. Ann Intern Med. 1984;100(4):483–90.

18. Hollenberg SM, Singer M. Pathophysiology of sepsis-induced cardiomyopathy. Nat Rev Cardiol. 2021;18(6):424–34.

19. Parrillo JE, Burch C, Shelhamer JH, Parker MM, Natanson C, Schuette W. A circulating myocardial depressant substance in humans with septic shock. Septic shock patients with a reduced ejection fraction have a circulating factor that depresses in vitro myocardial cell performance. J Clin Invest. 1985;76(4):1539–53.

20. Kumar A, Thota V, Dee L, Olson J, Uretz E, Parrillo JE. Tumor necrosis factor alpha and interleukin 1beta are responsible for in vitro myocardial cell depression induced by human septic shock serum. J Exp Med. 1996;183(3):949–58.

21. Hoffmann JN, Werdan K, Hartl WH, Jochum M, Faist E, Inthorn D. Hemofiltrate from patients with severe sepsis and depressed left ventricular contractility contains cardiotoxic compounds. Shock. 1999;12(3):174–80.

22. Madorin WS, Rui T, Sugimoto N, Handa O, Cepinskas G, Kvietys PR. Cardiac myocytes activated by septic plasma promote neutrophil transendothelial migration: role of platelet-activating factor and the chemokines LIX and KC. Circ Res. 2004;94(7):944–51.

23. Zhang W, Xu X, Kao R, Mele T, Kvietys P, Martin CM, et al. Cardiac fibroblasts contribute to myocardial dysfunction in mice with sepsis: the role of NLRP3 inflammasome activation. PLoS One. 2014;9(9):e107639.

24. Landesberg G, Levin PD, Gilon D, Goodman S, Georgieva M, Weissman C, et al. Myocardial dysfunction in severe sepsis and septic shock: no correlation with inflammatory cytokines in real-life clinical setting. Chest. 2015;148(1):93–102.

25. Opal SM, Fisher CJ, Dhainaut JF, Vincent JL, Brase R, Lowry SF, et al. Confirmatory interleukin-1 receptor antagonist trial in severe sepsis: a phase III, randomized, double-blind, placebo-controlled, multicenter trial. The Interleukin-1 Receptor Antagonist Sepsis Investigator Group. Crit Care Med. 1997;25(7):1115–24.

26. Fisher CJ, Dhainaut JF, Opal SM, Pribble JP, Balk RA, Slotman GJ, et al. Recombinant human interleukin 1 receptor antagonist in the treatment of patients with sepsis syndrome. Results from a randomized, double-blind, placebo-controlled trial. Phase III rhIL-1ra Sepsis Syndrome Study Group. JAMA. 1994;271(23):1836–43.

27. Raschke RA, Garcia-Orr R. Hemophagocytic lymphohistiocytosis: a potentially underrecognized association with systemic inflammatory response syndrome, severe sepsis, and septic shock in adults. Chest. 2011;140(4):933–8.

28. Shakoory B, Carcillo JA, Chatham WW, Amdur RL, Zhao H, Dinarello CA, et al. Interleukin-1 receptor blockade is associated with reduced mortality in sepsis patients with features of macro-

10

phage activation syndrome: reanalysis of a prior phase III trial. Crit Care Med. 2016;44(2):275–81.

29. Annane D, Sébille V, Duboc D, Le Heuzey J-Y, Sadoul N, Bouvier E, et al. Incidence and prognosis of sustained arrhythmias in critically ill patients. Am J Respir Crit Care Med. 2008;178(1):20–5.

30. Knotzer H, Mayr A, Ulmer H, Lederer W, Schobersberger W, Mutz N, et al. Tachyarrhythmias in a surgical intensive care unit: a case-controlled epidemiologic study. Intensive Care Med. 2000;26(7):908–14.

31. Bosch NA, Cimini J, Walkey AJ. Atrial fibrillation in the ICU. Chest. 2018;154(6):1424–34.

32. Moss TJ, Calland JF, Enfield KB, Gomez-Manjarres DC, Ruminski C, DiMarco JP, et al. New-onset atrial fibrillation in the critically ill. Crit Care Med. 2017;45(5):790–7.

33. Lazzerini PE, Capecchi PL, Laghi-Pasini F. Systemic inflammation and arrhythmic risk: lessons from rheumatoid arthritis. Eur Heart J. 2017;38(22):1717–27.

34. Abdelhadi RH, Gurm HS, Van Wagoner DR, Chung MK. Relation of an exaggerated rise in white blood cells after coronary bypass or cardiac valve surgery to development of atrial fibrillation postoperatively. Am J Cardiol. 2004;93(9):1176–8.

35. Marcus GM, Whooley MA, Glidden DV, Pawlikowska L, Zaroff JG, Olgin JE. Interleukin-6 and atrial fibrillation in patients with coronary artery disease: data from the Heart and Soul Study. Am Heart J. 2008;155(2):303–9.

36. Guo Y, Lip GYH, Apostolakis S. Inflammation in atrial fibrillation. J Am Coll Cardiol. 2012;60(22):2263–70.

37. Chen M-C, Chang J-P, Liu W-H, Yang C-H, Chen Y-L, Tsai T-H, et al. Increased inflammatory cell infiltration in the atrial myocardium of patients with atrial fibrillation. Am J Cardiol. 2008;102(7):861–5.

38. Smorodinova N, Bláha M, Melenovský V, Rozsívalová K, Přidal J, Ďurišová M, et al. Analysis of immune cell populations in atrial myocardium of patients with atrial fibrillation or sinus rhythm. PLoS One. 2017;12(2):e0172691.

39. Sun Z, Zhou D, Xie X, Wang S, Wang Z, Zhao W, et al. Cross-talk between macrophages and atrial myocytes in atrial fibrillation. Basic Res Cardiol. 2016;111(6):63.

40. Nahrendorf M, Swirski FK, Aikawa E, Stangenberg L, Wurdinger T, Figueiredo J-L, et al. The healing myocardium sequentially mobilizes two monocyte subsets with divergent and complementary functions. J Exp Med. 2007;204(12):3037–47.

41. Westman PC, Lipinski MJ, Luger D, Waksman R, Bonow RO, Wu E, et al. Inflammation as a driver of adverse left ventricular remodeling after acute myocardial infarction. J Am Coll Cardiol. 2016;67(17):2050–60.

42. De Jesus NM, Wang L, Lai J, Rigor RR, Francis Stuart SD, Bers DM, et al. Antiarrhythmic effects of interleukin 1 inhibition after myocardial infarction. Heart Rhythm. 2017;14(5):727–36.

43. Arrigo M, Jessup M, Mullens W, Reza N, Shah AM, Sliwa K, et al. Acute heart failure. Nat Rev Dis Primers. 2020;6(1):16.

44. van Diepen S, Katz JN, Albert NM, Henry TD, Jacobs AK, Kapur NK, et al. Contemporary management of cardiogenic shock: a scientific statement from the American Heart Association. Circulation. 2017;136(16):e232–68.

45. Brener MI, Rosenblum HR, Burkhoff D. Pathophysiology and advanced hemodynamic assessment of cardiogenic shock. Methodist Debakey Cardiovasc J. 2020;16(1):7–15.

46. Thiele H, Zeymer U, Neumann F-J, Ferenc M, Olbrich H-G, Hausleiter J, et al. Intraaortic balloon support for myocardial infarction with cardiogenic shock. N Engl J Med. 2012;367(14):1287–96.

47. Goldberg RJ, Spencer FA, Gore JM, Lessard D, Yarzebski J Thirty-year trends (1975 to 2005) in the magnitude of, management of, and hospital death rates associated with cardiogenic shock in patients with acute myocardial infarction: a population-based perspective. Circulation [Internet]. 2009 [cité 14 mars 2022];119(9):1211–9. https://pubmed.ncbi.nlm.nih.gov/19237658/.

48. De Luca G, Parodi G, Sciagrà R, Venditti F, Bellandi B, Vergara R, et al. Preprocedural TIMI flow and infarct size in STEMI undergoing primary angioplasty. J Thromb Thrombolysis. 2014;38(1):81–6.

49. Hollenberg SM, Kavinsky CJ, Parrillo JE. Cardiogenic shock. Ann Intern Med. 1999;131(1):47–59.

50. Hochman JS. Cardiogenic shock complicating acute myocardial infarction: expanding the paradigm. Circulation. 2003;107(24):2998–3002.

51. Geppert A, Steiner A, Zorn G, Delle-Karth G, Koreny M, Haumer M, et al. Multiple organ failure in patients with cardiogenic shock is associated with high plasma levels of interleukin-6. Crit Care Med. 2002;30(9):1987–94.

52. Joffre J, Hellman J, Ince C, Ait-Oufella H. Endothelial responses in sepsis. Am J Respir Crit Care Med. 2020;202(3):361–70.

53. Salvador B, Arranz A, Francisco S, Córdoba L, Punzón C, Llamas MÁ, et al. Modulation of endothelial function by Toll like receptors. Pharmacol Res [Internet]. 2016 [cité 14 mars 2022];108:46–56. https://pubmed.ncbi.nlm.nih.gov/27073018/.

54. Khakpour S, Wilhelmsen K, Hellman J Vascular endothelial cell Toll-like receptor pathways in sepsis. Innate Immun [Internet]. 2015 [cité 14 mars 2022];21(8):827–46. https://pubmed.ncbi.nlm.nih.gov/26403174/.

55. Ait-Oufella H, Maury E, Lehoux S, Guidet B, Offenstadt G. The endothelium: physiological functions and role in microcirculatory failure during severe sepsis. Intensive Care Med. 2010;36(8):1286–98.

56. Alsaffar H, Martino N, Garrett JP, Adam AP. Interleukin-6 promotes a sustained loss of endothelial barrier function via Janus kinase-mediated STAT3 phosphorylation and de novo protein synthesis. Am J Physiol Cell Physiol. 2018;314(5):C589–602.

57. Zhou M, Wang P, Chaudry IH. Endothelial nitric oxide synthase is downregulated during hyperdynamic sepsis. Biochim Biophys Acta. 1997;1335(1–2, 182):–90.

58. Wiel E, Pu Q, Corseaux D, Robin E, Bordet R, Lund N, et al. Effect of L-arginine on endothelial injury and hemostasis in rabbit endotoxin shock. J Appl Physiol (1985). 2000;89(5):1811–8.

59. Trzeciak S, Glaspey LJ, Dellinger RP, Durflinger P, Anderson K, Dezfulian C, et al. Randomized controlled trial of inhaled nitric oxide for the treatment of microcirculatory dysfunction in patients with sepsis*. Crit Care Med. 2014;42(12):2482–92.

60. López A, Lorente JA, Steingrub J, Bakker J, McLuckie A, Willatts S, et al. Multiple-center, randomized, placebo-controlled, double-blind study of the nitric oxide synthase inhibitor 546C88: effect on survival in patients with septic shock. Crit Care Med. 2004;32(1):21–30.

61. Sharma R, Joubert J, Malan SF. Recent developments in drug design of NO-donor hybrid compounds. Mini Rev Med Chem. 2018;18(14):1175–98.

62. Dépret F, Sitbon A, Soussi S, De Tymowski C, Blet A, Fratani A, et al. Intravenous iloprost to recruit the microcirculation in septic shock patients? Intensive Care Med. 2018;44(1):121–2.

63. Legrand M, Oufella HA, De Backer D, Duranteau J, Leone M, Levy B, et al. The I-MICRO trial, Ilomedin for treatment of septic shock with persistent microperfusion defects: a double-blind, randomized controlled trial-study protocol for a randomized controlled trial. Trials. 2020;21(1):601.

64. Singh RK, Agarwal V, Baronia AK, Kumar S, Poddar B, Azim A. The effects of atorvastatin on inflammatory responses and mortality in septic shock: a single-center, randomized controlled trial. Indian J Crit Care Med. 2017;21(10):646–54.

65. Wan Y-D, Sun T-W, Kan Q-C, Guan F-X, Zhang S-G. Effect of statin therapy on mortality from infection and sepsis: a meta-analysis of randomized and observational studies. Crit Care. 2014;18(2):R71.

66. Chen M, Ji M, Si X. The effects of statin therapy on mortality in patients with sepsis: a meta-analysis of randomized trials. Medicine. 2018;97(31):e11578.

67. Pillinger NL, Kam P. Endothelial glycocalyx: basic science and clinical implications. Anaesth Intensive Care. 2017;45(3):295–307.

68. Jacob M, Bruegger D, Rehm M, Stoeckelhuber M, Welsch U, Conzen P, et al. The endothelial glycocalyx affords compatibility of Starling's principle and high cardiac interstitial albumin levels. Cardiovasc Res. 2007;73(3):575–86.

69. Wiesinger A, Peters W, Chappell D, Kentrup D, Reuter S, Pavenstädt H, et al. Nanomechanics of the endothelial glycocalyx in experimental sepsis. PLoS One. 2013;8(11):e80905.

70. Grundmann S, Fink K, Rabadzhieva L, Bourgeois N, Schwab T, Moser M, et al. Perturbation of the endothelial glycocalyx in post cardiac arrest syndrome. Resuscitation. 2012;83(6):715–20.

71. Drake-Holland AJ, Noble MIM. Update on the important new drug target in cardiovascular medicine—the vascular glycocalyx. Cardiovasc Hematol Disord Drug Targets. 2012;12(1):76–81.

72. Broekhuizen LN, Mooij HL, Kastelein JJP, Stroes ESG, Vink H, Nieuwdorp M. Endothelial glycocalyx as potential diagnostic and therapeutic target in cardiovascular disease. Curr Opin Lipidol. 2009;20(1):57–62.
73. Ziegler T, Horstkotte J, Schwab C, Pfetsch V, Weinmann K, Dietzel S, et al. Angiopoietin 2 mediates microvascular and hemodynamic alterations in sepsis. J Clin Invest. 2013;123(8):3436–45.
74. David S, Park J-K, van Meurs M, Zijlstra JG, Koenecke C, Schrimpf C, et al. Acute administration of recombinant angiopoietin-1 ameliorates multiple-organ dysfunction syndrome and improves survival in murine sepsis. Cytokine. 2011;55(2):251–9.
75. Desai SV, Law TJ, Needham DM. Long-term complications of critical care. Crit Care Med. 2011;39(2):371–9.
76. Smeeth L, Thomas SL, Hall AJ, Hubbard R, Farrington P, Vallance P. Risk of myocardial infarction and stroke after acute infection or vaccination. N Engl J Med. 2004;351(25):2611–8.
77. Corrales-Medina VF, Alvarez KN, Weissfeld LA, Angus DC, Chirinos JA, Chang C-CH, et al. Association between hospitalization for pneumonia and subsequent risk of cardiovascular disease. JAMA. 2015;313(3):264–74.
78. Yende S, Iwashyna TJ, Angus DC. Interplay between sepsis and chronic health. Trends Mol Med. 2014;20(4):234–8.
79. Libby P, Nahrendorf M, Swirski FK. Leukocytes link local and systemic inflammation in ischemic cardiovascular disease: an expanded "cardiovascular continuum". J Am Coll Cardiol. 2016;67(9):1091–103.
80. Dutta P, Courties G, Wei Y, Leuschner F, Gorbatov R, Robbins CS, et al. Myocardial infarction accelerates atherosclerosis. Nature. 2012;487(7407):325–9.
81. Ridker PM, Everett BM, Thuren T, MacFadyen JG, Chang WH, Ballantyne C, et al. Antiinflammatory therapy with canakinumab for atherosclerotic disease. N Engl J Med. 2017;377(12):1119–31.
82. Ridker PM, Everett BM, Pradhan A, MacFadyen JG, Solomon DH, Zaharris E, et al. Low-dose methotrexate for the prevention of atherosclerotic events. N Engl J Med [Internet]. 2018 [cité 27 janv 2022]. https://www.nejm.org/doi/10.1056/NEJMoa1809798.
83. Ridker PM. Anti-inflammatory therapy for atherosclerosis: interpreting divergent results from the CANTOS and CIRT clinical trials. J Intern Med. 2019;285(5):503–9.
84. Akodad M, Sicard P, Fauconnier J, Roubille F. Colchicine and myocardial infarction: a review. Arch Cardiovasc Dis. 2020;113(10):652–9.
85. Van Tassell BW, Arena RA, Toldo S, Mezzaroma E, Azam T, Seropian IM, et al. Enhanced interleukin-1 activity contributes to exercise intolerance in patients with systolic heart failure. PLoS One. 2012;7(3):e33438.
86. Van Tassell BW, Canada J, Carbone S, Trankle C, Buckley L, Oddi Erdle C, et al. Interleukin-1 blockade in recently decompensated systolic heart failure: results from REDHART (Recently Decompensated Heart Failure Anakinra Response Trial). Circ Heart Fail. 2017;10(11):e004373.
87. Roubille F, Kritikou E, Busseuil D, Barrere-Lemaire S, Tardif J-C. Colchicine: an old wine in a new bottle? Antiinflamm Antiallergy Agents Med Chem. 2013;12(1):14–23.
88. Roubille F, Busseuil D, Merlet N, Kritikou EA, Rhéaume E, Tardif J-C. Investigational drugs targeting cardiac fibrosis. Expert Rev Cardiovasc Ther. 2014;12(1):111–25.
89. Bhattacharyya B, Panda D, Gupta S, Banerjee M. Anti-mitotic activity of colchicine and the structural basis for its interaction with tubulin. Med Res Rev. 2008;28(1):155–83.
90. Ravelli RBG, Gigant B, Curmi PA, Jourdain I, Lachkar S, Sobel A, et al. Insight into tubulin regulation from a complex with colchicine and a stathmin-like domain. Nature. 2004;428(6979):198–202.
91. Terkeltaub RA. Colchicine update: 2008. Semin Arthritis Rheum. 2009;38(6):411–9.
92. Pope RM, Tschopp J. The role of interleukin-1 and the inflammasome in gout: implications for therapy. Arthritis Rheum. 2007;56(10):3183–8.
93. Bozkurt D, Bicak S, Sipahi S, Taskin H, Hur E, Ertilav M, et al. The effects of colchicine on the progression and regression of encapsulating peritoneal sclerosis. Perit Dial Int. 2008;28 Suppl 5:S53–7.
94. Guan T, Gao B, Chen G, Chen X, Janssen M, Uttarwar L, et al. Colchicine attenuates renal injury in a model of hypertensive chronic kidney disease. Am J Physiol Renal Physiol. 2013;305(10):F1466–76.

95. Tucker B, Kurup R, Barraclough J, Henriquez R, Cartland S, Arnott C, et al. Colchicine as a novel therapy for suppressing chemokine production in patients with an acute coronary syndrome: a pilot study. Clin Ther. 2019;41(10):2172–81.

96. Wójcicki J, Hinek A, Jaworska M, Samochowiec L. The effect of colchicine on the development of experimental atherosclerosis in rabbits. Pol J Pharmacol Pharm. 1986;38(4):343–8.

97. Martínez GJ, Celermajer DS, Patel S. The NLRP3 inflammasome and the emerging role of colchicine to inhibit atherosclerosis-associated inflammation. Atherosclerosis. 2018;269:262–71.

98. Saji K, Fukumoto Y, Suzuki J, Fukui S, Nawata J, Shimokawa H. Colchicine, a microtubule depolymerizing agent, inhibits myocardial apoptosis in rats. Tohoku J Exp Med. 2007;213(2):139–48.

99. Prins KW, Tian L, Wu D, Thenappan T, Metzger JM, Archer SL. Colchicine depolymerizes microtubules, increases Junctophilin-2, and improves right ventricular function in experimental pulmonary arterial hypertension. J Am Heart Assoc. 2017;6(6):e006195.

100. Rennard SI, Bitterman PB, Ozaki T, Rom WN, Crystal RG. Colchicine suppresses the release of fibroblast growth factors from alveolar macrophages in vitro. The basis of a possible therapeutic approach ot the fibrotic disorders. Am Rev Respir Dis. 1988;137(1):181–5.

101. Lampidis TJ, Kolonias D, Savaraj N, Rubin RW. Cardiostimulatory and antiarrhythmic activity of tubulin-binding agents. Proc Natl Acad Sci U S A. 1992;89(4):1256–60.

102. Crittenden DB, Lehmann RA, Schneck L, Keenan RT, Shah B, Greenberg JD, et al. Colchicine use is associated with decreased prevalence of myocardial infarction in patients with gout. J Rheumatol. 2012;39(7):1458–64.

103. Raju NC, Yi Q, Nidorf M, Fagel ND, Hiralal R, Eikelboom JW. Effect of colchicine compared with placebo on high sensitivity C-reactive protein in patients with acute coronary syndrome or acute stroke: a pilot randomized controlled trial. J Thromb Thrombolysis. 2012;33(1):88–94.

104. Deftereos S, Giannopoulos G, Angelidis C, Alexopoulos N, Filippatos G, Papoutsidakis N, et al. Anti-inflammatory treatment with colchicine in acute myocardial infarction: a pilot study. Circulation. 2015;132(15):1395–403.

105. Akodad M, Fauconnier J, Sicard P, Huet F, Blandel F, Bourret A, et al. Interest of colchicine in the treatment of acute myocardial infarct responsible for heart failure in a mouse model. Int J Cardiol. 2017;240:347–53.

106. Hennessy T, Soh L, Bowman M, Kurup R, Schultz C, Patel S, et al. The Low Dose Colchicine after Myocardial Infarction (LoDoCo-MI) study: a pilot randomized placebo controlled trial of colchicine following acute myocardial infarction. Am Heart J. 2019;215:62–9.

107. Tardif J-C, Kouz S, Waters DD, Bertrand OF, Diaz R, Maggioni AP, et al. Efficacy and safety of low-dose colchicine after myocardial infarction. N Engl J Med. 2019;381(26):2497–505.

108. da Luz PL, Forrester JS, Wyatt HL, Diamond GA, Chag M, Swan HJ. Myocardial reperfusion in acute experimental ischemia. Beneficial effects of prior treatment with steroids. Circulation. 1976;53(5):847–52.

109. Mannisi JA, Weisman HF, Bush DE, Dudeck P, Healy B. Steroid administration after myocardial infarction promotes early infarct expansion. A study in the rat. J Clin Invest. 1987;79(5):1431–9.

110. Hammerman H, Kloner RA, Hale S, Schoen FJ, Braunwald E. Dose-dependent effects of short-term methylprednisolone on myocardial infarct extent, scar formation, and ventricular function. Circulation. 1983;68(2):446–52.

111. Libby P, Maroko PR, Bloor CM, Sobel BE, Braunwald E. Reduction of experimental myocardial infarct size by corticosteroid administration. J Clin Invest. 1973;52(3):599–607.

112. Giugliano GR, Giugliano RP, Gibson CM, Kuntz RE. Meta-analysis of corticosteroid treatment in acute myocardial infarction. Am J Cardiol. 2003;91(9):1055–9.

10

Brain

Annemieke M. Peters van Ton, Fabio Silvio Taccone, and Peter Pickkers

Contents

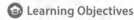 **Learning Objectives**

To learn about the pathophysiology and potential treatment options of cognitive decline and mental symptoms following critical illness

11.1 Introduction

Since its establishment during the polio epidemic in the 1950s, the relatively young specialty of intensive care medicine has been primarily focused on supporting vital functions of critically ill patients to improve short-term survival [1]. However, due to advancements in patient care and declining mortality rates over the last decennia [2], a shift in attention to long-term outcomes of critical illness and how to optimize them has also taken place [3, 4]. The expanding group of patients who survive critical illness demonstrates that surviving critical illness is associated with a range of long-lasting unfavorable health outcomes. Many intensive care unit (ICU) survivors are being hindered in their daily lives due to the physical, cognitive, or mental deficits that form the post-intensive care syndrome (PICS). This term describes the complex of "new or worsening impairments in physical, cognitive, or mental health status arising after critical illness and persisting beyond acute care hospitalization" [4]. It may occur after infections (including sepsis), surgery, or trauma, all conditions in which the brain initially may not appear to be involved. Still, these conditions may cause cerebral dysfunction, which includes acute problems such as delirium, or even persistent cognitive decline, dementia, or a deterioration in mental health status. Although the pathophysiology is likely multifactorial, the relevance of inflammation in the development of these cerebral complications is increasingly recognized. Of interest, also non-critically ill patients may be at risk of similar deficits related to cerebral dysfunction following states of (severe) systemic inflammation as has been shown by previous epidemiological studies [5–7]. Since these cerebral consequences may to a great extent influence the patients' quality of life and relate to an increased appeal on healthcare, increasing efforts are being made to advance the understanding of the pathophysiology of this association, in order to find modifiable factors for preventive or therapeutic interventions.

11.2 Epidemiology

During critical illness, acute encephalopathy occurs often [8], varying from sickness behavior, mild fluctuating cognitive dysfunction, and mental state changes (delirium) to coma. The delirium incidence in all ICU patients ranges from 11 to 89%, depending on ICU admission diagnoses and delirium subtype [9–13]. In patients with sepsis, in the absence of direct central nervous system (CNS) infection, structural brain abnormalities, or other types of encephalopathy, this is often called "sepsis-associated encephalopathy" (SAE) [14]. SAE is reported in up to 70% of patients suffering from sepsis [15]. Surgery is also associated with cerebral dysfunction in the acute postop-

11

erative phase, which may clinically appear as postoperative delirium. Although delirium was long regarded as a transient and reversible, and thus a benign, problem in the acute phase, it has now become evident that serious long-term sequelae may ensue.

Many patients who survive critical illness experience long-lasting negative effects on their health. The symptoms of PICS may vary in severity and persistence. A recent study demonstrated that overall, 50% of ICU survivors suffer from PICS based on questionnaires, with the highest incidence for physical and mental issues [16]. However, objective cognitive dysfunction has been established in over 50% of patients 3 months after ICU admission [17]. This incidence ranges from 10 to 78% at 12 months after ICU admission [17]. Overall, one out of four patients suffered from cognitive impairment 12 months after critical illness that was in severity similar to that of patients with mild Alzheimer's disease, and one out of three had an impairment severity which is typically associated with moderate traumatic brain injury [18]. Retrospectively, only 6% of patients had evidence of mild-to-moderate cognitive impairment before ICU admission, suggesting that the profound cognitive deficits were new in the majority of patients [18]. Interestingly, patients who survived severe sepsis were three times more likely to develop cognitive impairment than patients who were hospitalized for other reasons than sepsis [19]. Both mild and severe inflammatory events among over 10,000 patients admitted to the ICU could independently predict their risk of developing dementia within 3 years after ICU discharge [20]. However, longitudinal studies confirm that not only admission to the ICU but also every hospitalization may lead to a substantial cognitive decline in the elderly, also after controlling for disease severity and prehospital cognitive status [21, 22].

Long-term cognitive impairment may also occur in surgical patients and is described as postoperative cognitive dysfunction, or POCD. POCD is predominantly characterized by a deterioration in memory, attention, and speed of information processing. The incidence of such neurological complications increases with higher age and the extent and invasiveness of the surgical procedure. The prevalence of POCD after cardiac surgery ranges from 20 to 70% in the first week postoperatively. This decreases to 10–40% after 6 weeks and remains at this level thereafter [23]. In major noncardiac surgery, the prevalence is slightly lower [5, 6].

Not surprisingly, most studies in this field are limited by the lack of a baseline judgement of cognitive status or assessment of structural brain damage prior to ICU admission, which may predispose to the development of post-ICU cognitive deterioration. Comparison with a matched control group may not be sufficient if the cases who underwent the medical event already had more preexistent cognitive impairment, psychiatric symptoms, or brain damage. Attempts to estimate the baseline cognitive or psychiatric symptoms retrospectively by using subjective questionnaires are suboptimal since these often show discordance with objective measurements [24]. However, even a large population-based cohort including baseline and longitudinal follow-up assessments of both cognitive performance and cerebral MRI scans showed that each sepsis episode during follow-up was associated with an 82% increased risk to develop dementia within 10 years, irrespective of preexistent cognition or brain atrophy [25].

11.3 Pathophysiology

Presumed pathophysiological mechanisms related to cerebral dysfunction following (critical) illness or major surgery include inadequate oxygenation or ventilation, and hemodynamic alterations leading to hypoperfusion of the brain, watershed distribution infarcts, leukoencephalopathy, microembolization, and microbleeds. Moreover, cellular damage, mitochondrial and endothelial dysfunction, disturbances in neurotransmission and calcium homeostasis, and blood-brain barrier disruption have also been proposed as mechanisms involved in the pathophysiology. Often, sedatives and anesthetics are mentioned to play a role in the etiology of brain dysfunction; however, animal studies have shown that surgery itself, rather than anesthetics, triggers a neurocognitive decline [26, 27]. Since optimizing oxygenation, ventilation, hemodynamics, and pain management and targeting for the lightest possible level of sedation are already part of standard critical care [28, 29], there is probably not much more to gain on these issues to reduce the risk of developing cerebral dysfunction. Consequently, exploring other pathophysiological mechanisms, such as an immune-mediated pathway, could help to identify new therapeutic strategies against cerebral dysfunction after critical illness.

In practically all ICU patients, irrespective of their admission diagnosis, an exaggerated immune system activation may occur. Although the brain was long regarded as an immune-privileged organ, protected by the blood-brain barrier, there is increasing evidence that the peripheral immune system may interact with the immune cells of the brain. Microglia and astrocytes are the main resident innate immune cells in the CNS. Microglia share common features of peripheral myeloid lineage cells, such as the secretion of immunomodulatory molecules to signal neighboring and circulating cells. In the healthy brain, resting microglia monitor the brain environment. Upon CNS cell injury or systemic inflammatory stimuli, microglia and astrocytes are activated and undergo a transformation into an amoeboid morphology and present upregulation of surface molecules. Research in animals [30], molecular neuroimaging data from healthy humans [31–33], and postmortem brain tissue of patients suffering from severe systemic inflammation [34, 35] show that systemic inflammation is a potent trigger to activate the brain immune response. This activation and the subsequent inflammatory cascade in the brain parenchyma are called "neuroinflammation" [36] and presented in ◘ Fig. 11.1. Systemic inflammation affects the blood-brain barrier (BBB), enabling systemic inflammatory mediators to enter the brain tissue, which is also possible through several parts of the brain that lack a BBB [37]. Microglia and astrocytes are readily activated in response to these inflammatory cues. Depending on the integration of regulatory signals, microglia can acquire a more neurotoxic, pro-inflammatory phenotype (M1-like) upon activation, or a more neuroprotective, anti-inflammatory phenotype (M2-like) [38] (◘ Fig. 11.1). M1-like microglia produce pro-inflammatory cytokines and enzymes that promote sustained tissue inflammation, which may generate a detrimental microenvironment for neurons. In contrast, M2-like microglia secrete neurotrophic factors and anti-inflammatory mediators and are associated with the resolution of inflammation and tissue repair [39]. Clearly, this is an oversimplified representation of the in vivo situation, in which a continuous spectrum rather than a distinct phenotypical pattern is more likely [40].

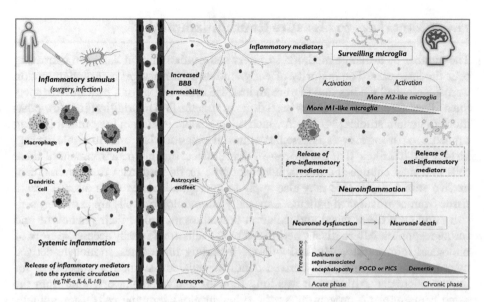

During aging, microglia can become sensitized by a primary inflammatory stimulus, which may induce overactivation of such primed microglia upon subsequent stimuli [41]. This may lead to an exaggerated neuroinflammatory cascade, which may disrupt homeostasis and cell function and could result in neuronal cell loss [42, 43]. This cascade is enhanced by the release of inflammatory mediators, which leads to changes in BBB permeability and infiltration of peripheral immune cells into the brain parenchyma [37]. Overactive microglia induce detrimental neurotoxic effects by the excessive secretion of many cytotoxic factors such as tumor necrosis factor-alpha (TNF-α), nitric oxide (NO), superoxide, and excesses of glutamate [42, 44]. Low-grade chronically activated microglia are present not only in normal aging [45], but also in neurodegenerative diseases [46]. The finding that overactivation of primed microglia can result in neurotoxicity corroborates with the fact that especially elderly and patients with preexisting cognitive failure, i.e., states associated with microglial priming, are most likely to suffer from long-term cognitive and functional decline following severe systemic inflammation [47].

While activation of microglia and astrocytes on the one hand may be crucial for host defense and neuronal survival, overactivation of these cells appears to account for detrimental and neurotoxic consequences on the other hand [41, 42, 44]. Therefore, further understanding of the pathophysiology of neuroinflammation in the development of cerebral dysfunction after critical illness has become an important focus of research in order to facilitate the discovery and development of novel therapeutic targets.

11.4   Biomarkers to Measure Neuroinflammation

The number of available methods to assess neuroinflammation has been increasing over the last years. The majority of early studies performed on neuroinflammation were histological studies that require an invasive brain biopsy or a postmortem specimen. Therefore, most work has been done in rodents [30] in addition to a few postmortem human studies [34, 35], in which microglial activation in the brain following exposure to pathogens was assessed. Postmortal isolation may result in viable microglia [48], but it is likely that the process of dying affects the microenvironment of these cells and may change the microglial phenotype or its responses upon subsequent ex vivo stimulations. This may also apply to microglia isolated from diseased brain tissue from neurosurgical patients. Especially immunological cells are extremely sensitive and even the surgical and isolation procedure may alter their phenotype and future responses. Alternatively, peripheral blood cells are an easily accessible store of biological information. Myeloid subsets, including monocytes, monocyte-derived macrophages, and monocyte-derived dendritic cells, are studied as substitutes for human microglia. Although it was long thought that microglia originate from the same hematopoietic progenitor as the other myeloid immune cells, they actually emerge from erythromyeloid progenitors from the embryonic yolk sac that populate the CNS during early development [49, 50]. Therefore, microglia and peripheral myeloid subsets are now regarded as distinct cell types, and a large phenotypic discrepancy between primary human microglia and currently used microglia-mimicking peripheral cell models has been demonstrated [51]. Additionally, this discrepancy with primary microglia was also found for commonly used cultured cell lines to study microglial biology (derived from microglia isolated from embryonic spinal cord and cortex, and human fetal microglia) [51]. Therefore, to acquire further understanding of mechanistic pathways, in vitro, animal, and autopsy studies alone are insufficient. Results should be translated to and verified in the human in vivo situation.

Due to the invasiveness to acquire brain tissue, in vivo human studies were, until recently, limited to the measurement of immune mediators in the cerebrospinal fluid (CSF). Although CSF sampling may be contraindicated in some patients, e.g., with coagulation disorders, CSF sampling is considered relatively noninvasive and well tolerated by adults [52]. Alternatively, instead of intermittent lumbar punctures, a lumbar drain can be used for continuous sampling, as is done in daily clinical practice in some neurosurgical or thoracic aortic aneurysm patients. Although CSF surrounds the brain and (waste) products of intracerebral biochemical pathways may end up in the CSF, it does not inform us about the origin of these products. Nevertheless, as brain tissue is almost inaccessible (apart from invasive biopsies), CSF is frequently used in neuroscience and in clinical practice of neurological diseases. Among other results, such studies have indicated that dysregulation of inflammatory processes, synapse pathology, and loss of homeostatic microglial control are involved in the pathophysiology of delirium [53, 54] and that these protein expression signatures in CSF of patients with delirium show similarities to those of patients with Alzheimer's disease [54]. Importantly, these findings could not be attributed to the presence of preclinical Alzheimer's disease pathology.

An alternative approach to investigate neuroinflammation is the use of positron-emission tomography (PET), which makes use of radioactively labelled molecules that can be specifically directed against a biological target. Clinical research applications of PET include the quantification of neuropathological markers or assessment of pharmacokinetic and pharmacodynamic properties of a therapeutic candidate in humans in vivo. One of such markers is the mitochondrial translocator protein (TSPO). TSPO is localized primarily in the outer mitochondrial membrane of steroid-synthesizing tissue, including the brain. One of its main functions is the transport of the substrate cholesterol into mitochondria, which is required for steroid synthesis [55]. TSPO expression is minimal in healthy brain, while activation of microglia and astrocytes is accompanied by markedly increased TSPO expression on these cells [55–59]. Therefore, TSPO is currently under investigation as a biomarker for neuroinflammation. Animal experiments have shown that different TSPO-binding tracers can sensitively image microglial and astrocytic activation [55]. In vitro and murine studies showed that TSPO expression is selectively increased in microglia and astrocytes with the pro-inflammatory M1-like phenotype, but not in the immune cells with the anti-inflammatory M2-like phenotype [60, 61]. In agreement, TSPO transcript levels were not induced in an anti-inflammatory brain environment [60]. It is therefore likely that nuclear imaging of neuroinflammation with a TSPO ligand measures the pro-inflammatory, deleterious activation of innate immune cells in the brain, although this needs confirmation in human in vivo studies.

The first in vivo study in humans using a TSPO tracer was published in 1995 [62]. Subsequently, several studies have been performed using TSPO tracers in humans. Increased microglial activation was found in numerous neurological diseases, such as mild cognitive impairment (MCI) [63], Alzheimer's [64–66] and Parkinson's disease [67, 68], stroke [69], traumatic brain injury [70], and amyotrophic lateral sclerosis (ALS) [71, 72], when compared to healthy controls. In addition, TSPO neuroimaging has shown associations between glial activity and psychiatric conditions such as major depression and psychotic disorders [73, 74]. This supports the role of neuroinflammation in the pathogenesis of these neurological and psychiatric conditions.

TSPO neuroimaging knows some practical challenges, and there is ongoing debate on which microglial phenotype and functional state the TSPO signal in the brain represents [60, 61, 75]. Given the challenges with TSPO neuroimaging, increasing effort is being put into the search for novel targets (receptors or enzymes) and tracers for PET imaging of microglial or astrocytic activation [76]. Such emerging biomarkers might allow more precise targeting of proteins involved in the cerebral immune response, which could help to delineate the mechanisms underlying systemic inflammation-induced cerebral dysfunction, as well as neurologic and psychiatric disorders.

11.5 Neuroinflammation in Systemic Inflammatory Conditions

Sepsis models in rodents demonstrate that peripheral inflammatory stimuli can induce microglial activation, concomitant with increases in inflammatory mediators in the brain. These peripheral stimuli result in deficits in cognitive performance of the animals on behavioral tests [77, 78]. Microglial activation is associated with an increase in mRNA expression or protein levels of Toll-like receptors (TLR-2 and TLR-4), TNF-α, and IL-1β [30]. Integrity of the BBB was assessed using different approaches in several animal studies, however with conflicting results [37]. Cecal ligation and puncture (CLP), a sepsis model in which animals develop an abdominal sepsis due to an induced fecal peritonitis, also results in a neuroinflammatory response accompanied by cognitive impairment in animals. Similar results are found in rodent studies exploring the effects of surgical procedures, which induce strong systemic inflammatory stimuli, on the brain and cognition. Postoperative microglial activation and increases in systemic and hippocampal pro-inflammatory cytokines are associated with postoperative impairment of spatial and contextual learning and memory [79]. Inhibition of central pro-inflammatory cytokine signaling attenuates postoperative memory impairment in these animals. Experiments in rats have shown that manipulation of the left coronary artery (mimicking cardiac surgery) or the mesenteric artery (mimicking abdominal surgery) affects different cognitive domains, suggesting that POCD after cardiac surgery may be more extended rather than more severe [79].

In humans, brain tissue of patients who deceased from sepsis shows a significant increase in activated microglia in grey matter compared to non-sepsis controls [34]. Hemorrhages, ischemia, micro-abscesses, hypercoagulability syndrome, and multifocal necrotizing leukoencephalopathy were discovered in postmortem brain tissue from patients who died from septic shock. Neuronal apoptosis is more pronounced in the autonomic nuclei of septic patients. Only occasional activated microglia and few reactive astrocytes are revealed by immunostaining in the small number of brain areas studied here [35].

In healthy volunteers participating in experimental human endotoxemia studies, an initial administration of endotoxin significantly increased tracer binding to TSPO with 30–70% compared to baseline [31, 33]. TSPO uptake is most pronounced in the cortical brain regions but presents diffuse throughout the brain. This demonstration of glial activation is accompanied by an increase in plasma levels of inflammatory cytokines, changes in vital signs, and sickness symptoms. Surprisingly, following a second challenge with endotoxin 7 days later, no increase but rather a decrease in cerebral TSPO binding was observed [33]. This may suggest reprogramming of the brain immune response following endotoxin-induced systemic inflammation in healthy young male volunteers, which could serve as a neuroprotective mechanism against excessive inflammation-induced neurotoxicity. Although immunotolerance is a familiar phenomenon in the peripheral immune system, research within the neuroinflammation field has thus far been mostly focused on trained immunity. In contrast, the concept of immunotolerance of the brain has been sparsely investigated. In vitro and animal experiments have shown that endotoxin-preconditioned microglia acquire an immune-suppressed phenotype [80]. Additionally, single peripheral administration of endotoxin in mice induced immune training, whereas repeated challenges induced immunotolerance [81]. Interestingly, immunotolerance alleviated cerebral β-amyloidosis load in a murine Alzheimer's disease model and resulted in less severe stroke pathology [81]. A study in patients undergoing prostatectomy was the first to explore the in vivo trajectory of microglial activation, and similar to the repeated experimental endotoxemia, results found a global downregulation of TSPO tracer binding at 3–4 days postoperatively, compared to baseline, which recovered again after 3 months [82]. This coincided with a transient reduction in immunoreactivity of peripheral blood cells, which is a well-known hallmark of an immunosuppressed state known as immunoparalysis. Immunoparalysis has been described in patients with sepsis and trauma and likely contributes to the high mortality in critically ill patients [83, 84]. These studies combined

discovered evidence for the existence of cerebral immunotolerance. One could argue that in those patients with brain dysfunction, e.g., delirium or long-term cognitive decline following a systemic inflammatory insult, the balance between pro- and anti-inflammatory responses is skewed to excessive pro-inflammation. A brain-specific intervention aimed at polarization towards a more immunosuppressive state could therefore have a therapeutic potential in certain patients. Future studies, including markers for cognitive and mental functioning, are warranted to validate these hypotheses.

11.6 Future Perspectives

Currently, the majority of the data related to neuroinflammation following systemic inflammation comes from animal studies. Important knowledge gaps within this area therefore remain. The trajectory of neuroinflammation after a systemic inflammatory stimulus in humans remains largely unclear, and its relation with clinical symptoms of cerebral dysfunction is far from elucidated. *In vivo* molecular imaging of microglial activity enables us to quantify the neuroinflammatory response noninvasively. However, the timing of PET data acquisition may be crucial especially when immunosuppression indeed plays a role in the cerebral compartment. In order to identify targets for novel interventions aimed at preventing or reducing cognitive decline post-critical illness, TSPO neuroimaging alone is insufficient as it only provides a global measurement of the state of activated cerebral immune cells and does not provide insights in important biochemical pathways. Although challenging in clinical in vivo studies, gaining further insights in the biochemical pathways involved in the cerebral immune response may direct future translational studies, to ultimately achieve precision medicine, which specifically targets the neuroinflammatory response appropriately in the right subset of patients.

The work performed in this field might also be a stepping stone for other systemic inflammatory conditions in which patients encounter unexplained cognitive or psychological deficits. Other inflammatory conditions in which neuroinflammation research could be meaningful include cancer, autoimmune disorders, COVID-19, chronic fatigue syndrome, Q-fever, and Lyme disease, and first investigations in some of these fields indeed have shown interesting and promising results [85, 86].

Although the step from bench to bedside still has to be made, there are already some things clinicians can do or consider in the follow-up of ICU survivors. Awareness and attention of physicians for the physical, cognitive, and mental impairments ICU survivors may face are of importance. Cognitive rehabilitation or treatment of psychiatric difficulties which could be driving the development of cognitive complaints could help to improve neuropsychological functioning [87]. Interestingly, preventing (chronic) sleep disturbance might be a feasible and attractive strategy, since sleep loss promotes astrocytic phagocytosis and microglial activation [88], which may result in synaptic loss and, through microglia priming, predispose the brain to further damage. Although appealing to consider, these approaches have not been properly studied in the context of cognitive impairment due to PICS. Clinically, physicians should be aware of the long-term impairments ICU survivors may face following their critical illness, and one may consider cognitive rehabilitation to improve neuropsychological functioning.

Summary

Over the last decades, there has been increasing clinical, scientific, but also societal awareness for the long-term consequences of (critical) illness. ICU survivors often experience symptoms related to the brain such as delirium during their admission, or longer lasting cognitive decline, mood disorders, or anxiety. Although the brain was long regarded as an immune-privileged organ, mounting evidence shows that peripheral inflammation interacts with the brain immune response and activates a cerebral inflammatory cascade. This so-called neuroinflammation is associated with neurotoxicity and development of neurodegenerative diseases and appears to be a potential modifiable mechanism to develop therapeutic interventions in order to reduce cerebral complaints following systemic inflammation.

Take-Home Messages

- Critical illness is associated with both acute and long-term cognitive and psychological sequelae.
- Systemic inflammation induces a neuroinflammatory response, which may play a role in the development of these long-term cerebral consequences.
- Nuclear neuroimaging can be used as a marker for microglial and astrocytic activity.

11

❓ Questions

1. What is PICS and how often does it occur?
2. What does delirium and Alzheimer's disease have in common?
3. How can you measure neuroinflammation in humans in vivo without damaging the brain parenchyma?
4. Could immunostimulatory therapy in an ICU patient with immunosuppression be harmful for the brain?

✔ Answers

1. PICS is the abbreviation for post-intensive care syndrome, which is the complex of new or worsening impairments in physical, cognitive, or mental health status arising after critical illness, persisting beyond acute care hospitalization. This occurs in 50% of patients one year after ICU discharge.
2. Delirium and Alzheimer's disease both occur predominantly in elderly patients. Delirium is an important risk factor to develop dementia (such as AD), and Alzheimer's patients are more at risk to develop delirium during illness. Finally, they share similar pathophysiological features in CSF proteins, which are involved in microglia-neuron communication and synapse functioning.
3. Studying proteins (and cells) in CSF or nuclear TSPO neuroimaging.
4. Theoretically yes, since stimulation of the immune system may result in excessive neuroinflammation with subsequent neurotoxicity and cerebral dysfunction. However, this has not been studied at all.

References

1. Kelly FE, Fong K, Hirsch N, Nolan JP. Intensive care medicine is 60 years old: the history and future of the intensive care unit. Clin Med. 2014;14(4):376.
2. Zimmerman JE, Kramer AA, Knaus WA. Changes in hospital mortality for United States intensive care unit admissions from 1988 to 2012. Crit Care. 2013;17(2):R81.
3. Desai SV, Law TJ, Needham DM. Long-term complications of critical care. Crit Care Med. 2011;39(2):371–9.
4. Needham DM, Davidson J, Cohen H, Hopkins RO, Weinert C, Wunsch H, et al. Improving long-term outcomes after discharge from intensive care unit: report from a stakeholders' conference. Crit Care Med. 2012;40(2):502–9.
5. Moller JT, Cluitmans P, Rasmussen LS, Houx P, Rasmussen H, Canet J, et al. Long-term postoperative cognitive dysfunction in the elderly ISPOCD1 study. ISPOCD investigators. International Study of Post-Operative Cognitive Dysfunction. Lancet. 1998;351(9106):857–61.
6. Monk TG, Weldon BC, Garvan CW, Dede DE, van der Aa MT, Heilman KM, et al. Predictors of cognitive dysfunction after major noncardiac surgery. Anesthesiology. 2008;108(1):18–30.
7. Shah FA, Pike F, Alvarez K, Angus D, Newman AB, Lopez O, et al. Bidirectional relationship between cognitive function and pneumonia. Am J Respir Crit Care Med. 2013;188(5):586–92.
8. Hughes CG, Patel MB, Pandharipande PP. Pathophysiology of acute brain dysfunction: what's the cause of all this confusion? Curr Opin Crit Care. 2012;18(5):518–26.
9. Aldemir M, Özen S, Kara IH, Sir A, Baç B. Predisposing factors for delirium in the surgical intensive care unit. Crit Care. 2001;5(5):265–70.
10. Dubois MJ, Bergeron N, Dumont M, Dial S, Skrobik Y. Delirium in an intensive care unit: a study of risk factors. Intensive Care Med. 2001;27(8):1297–304.
11. McNicoll L, Pisani MA, Zhang Y, Ely EW, Siegel MD, Inouye SK. Delirium in the intensive care unit: occurrence and clinical course in older patients. J Am Geriatr Soc. 2003;51(5):591–8.
12. Ouimet S, Kavanagh BP, Gottfried SB, Skrobik Y. Incidence, risk factors and consequences of ICU delirium. Intensive Care Med. 2007;33(1):66–73.
13. van den Boogaard M, Schoonhoven L, van der Hoeven JG, van Achterberg T, Pickkers P. Incidence and short-term consequences of delirium in critically ill patients: a prospective observational cohort study. Int J Nurs Stud. 2012;49(7):775–83.
14. Widmann CN, Heneka MT. Long-term cerebral consequences of sepsis. Lancet Neurol. 2014;13(6):630–6.
15. Gofton TE, Young GB. Sepsis-associated encephalopathy. Nat Rev Neurol. 2012;8(10):557–66.
16. Geense WW, Zegers M, Peters MAA, Ewalds E, Simons KS, Vermeulen H, et al. New physical, mental, and cognitive problems 1 year after ICU admission: a prospective multicenter study. Am J Respir Crit Care Med. 2021;203(12):1512–21.
17. Honarmand K, Lalli RS, Priestap F, Chen JL, McIntyre CW, Owen AM, et al. Natural history of cognitive impairment in critical illness survivors. A systematic review. Am J Respir Crit Care Med. 2020;202(2):193–201.
18. Pandharipande PP, Girard TD, Jackson JC, Morandi A, Thompson JL, Pun BT, et al. Long-term cognitive impairment after critical illness. N Engl J Med. 2013;369(14):1306–16.
19. Iwashyna TJ, Ely EW, Smith DM, Langa KM. Long-term cognitive impairment and functional disability among survivors of severe sepsis. JAMA. 2010;304(16):1787–94.
20. Guerra C, Hua M, Wunsch H. Risk of a diagnosis of dementia for elderly medicare beneficiaries after intensive care. Anesthesiology. 2015;123(5):1105–12.
21. Ehlenbach WJ, Hough CL, Crane PK, Haneuse SJ, Carson SS, Curtis JR, et al. Association between acute care and critical illness hospitalization and cognitive function in older adults. JAMA. 2010;303(8):763–70.
22. Wilson RS, Hebert LE, Scherr PA, Dong X, Leurgens SE, Evans DA. Cognitive decline after hospitalization in a community population of older persons. Neurology. 2012;78(13):950–6.
23. Bruce K, Smith JA, Yelland G, Robinson S. The impact of cardiac surgery on cognition. Stress Health. 2008;24(3):249–66.
24. Brück E, Larsson JW, Lasselin J, Bottai M, Hirvikoski T, Sundman E, et al. Lack of clinically relevant correlation between subjective and objective cognitive function in ICU survivors: a prospective 12-month follow-up study. Crit Care. 2019;23(1):253.

25. Peters van Ton AM, Meijer-van Leijsen EMC, Bergkamp MI, Bronkhorst EM, Pickkers P, de Leeuw FE, et al. Risk of dementia and structural brain changes following nonneurological infections during 9-year follow-up. Crit Care Med. 2022;50(4):554–64.

26. Cao XZ, Ma H, Wang JK, Liu F, Wu BY, Tian AY, et al. Postoperative cognitive deficits and neuroinflammation in the hippocampus triggered by surgical trauma are exacerbated in aged rats. Prog Neuro-Psychopharmacol Biol Psychiatry. 2010;34(8):1426–32.

27. Wan Y, Xu J, Ma D, Zeng Y, Cibelli M, Maze M. Postoperative impairment of cognitive function in rats: a possible role for cytokine-mediated inflammation in the hippocampus. Anesthesiology. 2007;106(3):436–43.

28. Devlin JW, Skrobik Y, Gélinas C, Needham DM, Slooter AJC, Pandharipande PP, et al. Clinical practice guidelines for the prevention and management of pain, agitation/sedation, delirium, immobility, and sleep disruption in adult patients in the ICU. Crit Care Med. 2018;46(9):e825–73.

29. Rhodes A, Evans LE, Alhazzani W, Levy MM, Antonelli M, Ferrer R, et al. Surviving sepsis campaign: international guidelines for management of sepsis and septic shock: 2016. Intensive Care Med. 2017;43(3):304–77.

30. Hoogland IC, Houbolt C, van Westerloo DJ, van Gool WA, van de Beek D. Systemic inflammation and microglial activation: systematic review of animal experiments. J Neuroinflammation. 2015;12:114.

31. Sandiego CM, Gallezot JD, Pittman B, Nabulsi N, Lim K, Lin SF, et al. Imaging robust microglial activation after lipopolysaccharide administration in humans with PET. Proc Natl Acad Sci U S A. 2015;112(40):12468–73.

32. Woodcock EA, Hillmer AT, Sandiego CM, Maruff P, Carson RE, Cosgrove KP, et al. Acute neuroimmune stimulation impairs verbal memory in adults: a PET brain imaging study. Brain Behav Immun. 2021;91:784–7.

33. Peters van Ton AM, Leijte GP, Franssen GM, Bruse N, Booij J, Doorduin J, et al. Human in vivo neuroimaging to detect reprogramming of the cerebral immune response following repeated systemic inflammation. Brain Behav Immun. 2021;95:321–9.

34. Lemstra AW, Groen in't Woud JC, Hoozemans JJ, van Haastert ES, Rozemuller AJ, Eikelenboom P, et al. Microglia activation in sepsis: a case-control study. J Neuroinflammation. 2007;4:4.

35. Sharshar T, Annane D, de la Grandmaison GL, Brouland JP, Hopkinson NS, Francoise G. The neuropathology of septic shock. Brain Pathol. 2004;14(1):21–33.

36. Rosenberg GA. Neuroinflammatory disease: IBC meeting on neuroinflammatory disease: research and treatment strategies London, UK, 17 and 18 September 1996. Mol Med Today. 1997;3(1):12–3.

37. Banks WA. Blood-brain barrier transport of cytokines: a mechanism for neuropathology. Curr Pharm Des. 2005;11(8):973–84.

38. Tang Y, Le W. Differential roles of M1 and M2 microglia in neurodegenerative diseases. Mol Neurobiol. 2016;53(2):1181–94.

39. Kettenmann H, Hanisch UK, Noda M, Verkhratsky A. Physiology of microglia. Physiol Rev. 2011;91(2):461–553.

40. Ransohoff RM. A polarizing question: do M1 and M2 microglia exist? Nat Neurosci. 2016;19(8):987–91.

41. Perry VH, Holmes C. Microglial priming in neurodegenerative disease. Nat Rev Neurol. 2014;10(4):217–24.

42. Block ML, Zecca L, Hong JS. Microglia-mediated neurotoxicity: uncovering the molecular mechanisms. Nat Rev Neurosci. 2007;8(1):57–69.

43. Godbout JP, Chen J, Abraham J, Richwine AF, Berg BM, Kelley KW, et al. Exaggerated neuroinflammation and sickness behavior in aged mice after activation of the peripheral innate immune system. FASEB J. 2005;19(10):1329–31.

44. Michels M, Steckert AV, Quevedo J, Barichello T, Dal-Pizzol F. Mechanisms of long-term cognitive dysfunction of sepsis: from blood-borne leukocytes to glial cells. Intensive Care Med Exp. 2015;3(1):30.

45. Matt SM, Johnson RW. Neuro-immune dysfunction during brain aging: new insights in microglial cell regulation. Curr Opin Pharmacol. 2016;26:96–101.

46. Heneka MT, Kummer MP, Latz E. Innate immune activation in neurodegenerative disease. Nat Rev Immunol. 2014;14(7):463–77.

11

47. Lee M, Kang J, Jeong YJ. Risk factors for post-intensive care syndrome: a systematic review and meta-analysis. Aust Crit Care. 2020;33(3):287–94.

48. Mizee MR, Miedema SS, van der Poel M, Adelia SKG, van Strien ME, et al. Isolation of primary microglia from the human post-mortem brain: effects of ante- and post-mortem variables. Acta Neuropathol Commun. 2017;5(1):16.

49. Ginhoux F, Greter M, Leboeuf M, Nandi S, See P, Gokhan S, et al. Fate mapping analysis reveals that adult microglia derive from primitive macrophages. Science. 2010;330(6005):841–5.

50. Gomez Perdiguero E, Klapproth K, Schulz C, Busch K, Azzoni E, Crozet L, et al. Tissue-resident macrophages originate from yolk-sac-derived erythro-myeloid progenitors. Nature. 2015;518(7540):547–51.

51. Melief J, Sneeboer MA, Litjens M, Ormel PR, Palmen SJ, Huitinga I, et al. Characterizing primary human microglia: a comparative study with myeloid subsets and culture models. Glia. 2016;64(11):1857–68.

52. Duits FH, Martinez-Lage P, Paquet C, Engelborghs S, Lleó A, Hausner L, et al. Performance and complications of lumbar puncture in memory clinics: results of the multicenter lumbar puncture feasibility study. Alzheimers Dement. 2016;12(2):154–63.

53. Poljak A, Hill M, Hall RJ, MacLullich AM, Raftery MJ, Tai J, et al. Quantitative proteomics of delirium cerebrospinal fluid. Transl Psychiatry. 2014;4:e477.

54. Peters van Ton AM, Verbeek MM, Alkema W, Pickkers P, Abdo WF. Downregulation of synapse-associated protein expression and loss of homeostatic microglial control in cerebrospinal fluid of infectious patients with delirium and patients with Alzheimer's disease. Brain Behav Immun. 2020;89:656–67.

55. Rupprecht R, Papadopoulos V, Rammes G, Baghai TC, Fan J, Akula N, et al. Translocator protein (18 kDa) (TSPO) as a therapeutic target for neurological and psychiatric disorders. Nat Rev Drug Discov. 2010;9(12):971–88.

56. Vowinckel E, Reutens D, Becher B, Verge G, Evans A, Owens T, et al. PK11195 binding to the peripheral benzodiazepine receptor as a marker of microglia activation in multiple sclerosis and experimental autoimmune encephalomyelitis. J Neurosci Res. 1997;50(2):345–53.

57. Kuhlmann AC, Guilarte TR. Cellular and subcellular localization of peripheral benzodiazepine receptors after trimethyltin neurotoxicity. J Neurochem. 2000;74(4):1694–704.

58. Wilms H, Claasen J, Röhl C, Sievers J, Deuschl G, Lucius R. Involvement of benzodiazepine receptors in neuroinflammatory and neurodegenerative diseases: evidence from activated microglial cells in vitro. Neurobiol Dis. 2003;14(3):417–24.

59. Lavisse S, Guillermier M, Hérard AS, Petit F, Delahaye M, Van Camp N, et al. Reactive astrocytes overexpress TSPO and are detected by TSPO positron emission tomography imaging. J Neurosci. 2012;32(32):10809–18.

60. Beckers L, Ory D, Geric I, Declercq L, Koole M, Kassiou M, et al. Increased expression of translocator protein (TSPO) Marks pro-inflammatory microglia but does not predict neurodegeneration. Mol Imaging Biol. 2018;20(1):94–102.

61. Pannell M, Economopoulos V, Wilson TC, Kersemans V, Isenegger PG, Larkin JR, et al. Imaging of translocator protein upregulation is selective for pro-inflammatory polarized astrocytes and microglia. Glia. 2020;68(2):280–97.

62. Groom GN, Junck L, Foster NL, Frey KA, Kuhl DE. PET of peripheral benzodiazepine binding sites in the microgliosis of Alzheimer's disease. J Nucl Med. 1995;36(12):2207–10.

63. Bradburn S, Murgatroyd C, Ray N. Neuroinflammation in mild cognitive impairment and Alzheimer's disease: a meta-analysis. Ageing Res Rev. 2019;50:1–8.

64. Hamelin L, Lagarde J, Dorothée G, Potier MC, Corlier F, Kuhnast B, et al. Distinct dynamic profiles of microglial activation are associated with progression of Alzheimer's disease. Brain. 2018;141(6):1855–70.

65. Kreisl WC, Lyoo CH, McGwier M, Snow J, Jenko KJ, Kimura N, et al. In vivo radioligand binding to translocator protein correlates with severity of Alzheimer's disease. Brain. 2013;136(Pt 7):2228–38.

66. Yasuno F, Ota M, Kosaka J, Ito H, Higuchi M, Doronbekov TK, et al. Increased binding of peripheral benzodiazepine receptor in Alzheimer's disease measured by positron emission tomography with [11C]DAA1106. Biol Psychiatry. 2008;64(10):835–41.

67. Terada T, Yokokura M, Yoshikawa E, Futatsubashi M, Kono S, Konishi T, et al. Extrastriatal spreading of microglial activation in Parkinson's disease: a positron emission tomography study. Ann Nucl Med. 2016;30(8):579–87.

68. Lavisse S, Goutal S, Wimberley C, Tonietto M, Bottlaender M, Gervais P, et al. Increased microglial activation in patients with Parkinson disease using [(18)F]-DPA714 TSPO PET imaging. Parkinsonism Relat Disord. 2020;82:29–36.

69. Ribeiro MJ, Vercouillie J, Debiais S, Cottier JP, Bonnaud I, Camus V, et al. Could (18) F-DPA-714 PET imaging be interesting to use in the early post-stroke period? EJNMMI Res. 2014;4:28.

70. Coughlin JM, Wang Y, Munro CA, Ma S, Yue C, Chen S, et al. Neuroinflammation and brain atrophy in former NFL players: an in vivo multimodal imaging pilot study. Neurobiol Dis. 2015;74:58–65.

71. Zurcher NR, Loggia ML, Lawson R, Chonde DB, Izquierdo-Garcia D, Yasek JE, et al. Increased in vivo glial activation in patients with amyotrophic lateral sclerosis: assessed with [(11)C]-PBR28. Neuroimage Clin. 2015;7:409–14.

72. Van Weehaeghe D, Van Schoor E, De Vocht J, Koole M, Attili B, Celen S, et al. TSPO versus P2X7 as a target for neuroinflammation: an in vitro and in vivo study. J Nucl Med. 2020;61(4):604–7.

73. Brites D, Fernandes A. Neuroinflammation and depression: microglia activation, extracellular microvesicles and microRNA dysregulation. Front Cell Neurosci. 2015;9:476.

74. Mondelli V, Vernon AC, Turkheimer F, Dazzan P, Pariante CM. Brain microglia in psychiatric disorders. Lancet Psychiatry. 2017;4(7):563–72.

75. Pozzo ED, Tremolanti C, Costa B, Giacomelli C, Milenkovic VM, Bader S, et al. Microglial pro-inflammatory and anti-inflammatory phenotypes are modulated by translocator protein activation. Int J Mol Sci. 2019;20(18):4467.

76. Jacobs AH, Tavitian B. Noninvasive molecular imaging of neuroinflammation. J Cereb Blood Flow Metab. 2012;32(7):1393–415.

77. Griffin ÉW, Skelly DT, Murray CL, Cunningham C. Cyclooxygenase-1-dependent prostaglandins mediate susceptibility to systemic inflammation-induced acute cognitive dysfunction. J Neurosci. 2013;33(38):15248–58.

78. Murray CL, Skelly DT, Cunningham C. Exacerbation of CNS inflammation and neurodegeneration by systemic LPS treatment is independent of circulating IL-1β and IL-6. J Neuroinflammation. 2011;8:50.

79. Hovens IB, van Leeuwen BL, Mariani MA, Kraneveld AD, Schoemaker RG. Postoperative cognitive dysfunction and neuroinflammation; cardiac surgery and abdominal surgery are not the same. Brain Behav Immun. 2016;54:178–93.

80. Schaafsma W, Zhang X, van Zomeren KC, Jacobs S, Georgieva PB, Wolf SA, et al. Long-lasting pro-inflammatory suppression of microglia by LPS-preconditioning is mediated by RelB-dependent epigenetic silencing. Brain Behav Immun. 2015;48:205–21.

81. Wendeln AC, Degenhardt K, Kaurani L, Gertig M, Ulas T, Jain G, et al. Innate immune memory in the brain shapes neurological disease hallmarks. Nature. 2018;556(7701):332–8.

82. Forsberg A, Cervenka S, Jonsson Fagerlund M, Rasmussen LS, Zetterberg H, Erlandsson Harris H, et al. The immune response of the human brain to abdominal surgery. Ann Neurol. 2017;81(4):572–82.

83. Hamers L, Kox M, Pickkers P. Sepsis-induced immunoparalysis: mechanisms, markers, and treatment options. Minerva Anestesiol. 2015;81(4):426–39.

84. Kox M, Pompe JC, Pickkers P, Hoedemaekers CW, van Vugt AB, van der Hoeven JG. Increased vagal tone accounts for the observed immune paralysis in patients with traumatic brain injury. Neurology. 2008;70(6):480–5.

85. Coughlin JM, Yang T, Rebman AW, Bechtold KT, Du Y, Mathews WB, et al. Imaging glial activation in patients with post-treatment Lyme disease symptoms: a pilot study using [(11)C]DPA-713 PET. J Neuroinflammation. 2018;15(1):346.

86. Nakatomi Y, Mizuno K, Ishii A, Wada Y, Tanaka M, Tazawa S, et al. Neuroinflammation in patients with chronic fatigue syndrome/myalgic encephalomyelitis: an [11]C-(R)-PK11195 PET study. J Nucl Med. 2014;55(6):945–50.

87. Jutte JE, Erb CT, Jackson JC. Physical, cognitive, and psychological disability following critical illness: what is the risk? Semin Respir Crit Care Med. 2015;36(6):943–58.

88. Bellesi M, de Vivo L, Chini M, Gilli F, Tononi G, Cirelli C. Sleep loss promotes astrocytic phagocytosis and microglial activation in mouse cerebral cortex. J Neurosci. 2017;37(21):5263.

11

Dysregulated Immune Response and Kidney Dysfunction

Nuttha Lumlertgul and Marlies Ostermann

Contents

© The Author(s), under exclusive license to Springer Nature Switzerland AG 2023
Z. Molnar et al. (eds.), *Management of Dysregulated Immune Response in the Critically Ill*,
Lessons from the ICU, https://doi.org/10.1007/978-3-031-17572-5_12

⊜ Learning Objectives
- To identify different pathophysiologic processes in acute kidney injury
- To recognise the roles of innate and adaptive immunity in the development, maintenance and recovery phase of acute kidney injury
- To appreciate different sub-types of acute kidney injury
- To recognise the consequence of acute kidney injury on remote organ dysfunction through dysregulated immunity

12.1 Introduction

Acute kidney injury (AKI) is a multifactorial syndrome characterised by a rapid (hours to days) deterioration of kidney function. Critically ill patients are particularly vulnerable. There is increasing evidence that AKI is associated with serious short- and long-term complications, including dysfunction of non-renal organs, development of chronic kidney disease (CKD) and an increased mortality risk. This chapter provides a review of the normal renal physiology and outlines the key pathophysiological processes that are involved in AKI and its sequelae.

12.2 Normal Physiology

The kidneys are vascular organs receiving ~20% of the cardiac output. Branches of the renal arteries terminate in glomerular afferent arterioles and form a capillary network responsible for glomerular filtration. Efferent arterioles emerging from the glomeruli either form a dense network of capillaries that run alongside the proximal and distal convoluted tubules or continue as vasa recta parallel to the loops of Henle. As a result, the oxygen tension between the renal cortex and the papillary tips gradually declines, resulting in a state of relative hypoxia within the renal medulla. Further, the counter-current arrangement of arteries and veins facilitates arterial-to-venous oxygen shunting in the renal cortex as well as between descending and ascending vasa recta in the renal medulla, both contributing to deoxygenation of the medulla.

In health, renal blood flow is maintained in a wide range of renal perfusion pressures (60–100 mmHg). Blood flow to the outer cortex is approximately 5–6 mL/g tissue/min, whereas the outer and inner medullas only receive approximately 1 and 0.5 mL/g/min, respectively. In the outer cortex, much of the blood flow is directed toward glomerular filtration. In contrast, the main roles of the peritubular microcirculation are to offload oxygen, deliver nutrients, return reabsorbed solutes and water to the systemic circulation and participate in the counter-current mechanisms that permit the reabsorption of water.

Tubuloglomerular feedback (TGF) is responsible for altering the pre-glomerular vascular tone of the afferent arterioles in response to changes in NaCl concentration in the tubular fluid. This directly impacts glomerular filtration rate (GFR) and renal blood flow. Various neurohormonal factors contribute, in particular, the sympathetic nervous system, vasodilators such as nitric oxide (NO) and prostaglandin E2, and vasoconstrictors like endothelin, angiotensin II and adenosine.

The proximal tubule Na/K ATPase is responsible for active reabsorption of solutes and is a major determinant of the oxygen requirement of the kidney (~80%). This renders tubular epithelial cells particularly vulnerable to changes in microcirculation. Further, tubular cells are continuously at the frontline of exposure to waste products, toxic metabolites and inflammatory mediators like cytokines, damage-associated molecular patterns (DAMPs) and pathogen-associated molecular patterns (PAMPs).

12.3 Acute Kidney Injury

Acute kidney injury (AKI) is a frequent complication during critical illness. It is often multifactorial with sepsis, inflammation and nephrotoxicity being the most common contributors. Following an injurious trigger, various pathophysiologic processes occur simultaneously and in sequence, including endothelial dysfunction, activation of inflammatory pathways, alteration of the microcirculation, tubular injury and potentially arterial occlusion and venous congestion [1].

12.3.1 Endothelial Dysfunction

Endothelial dysfunction is a characteristic feature in sepsis and inflammation leading to altered microcirculation in most organs. Following exposure to inflammatory mediators, the endothelium undergoes structural changes with loss of cell-to-cell contact and disruption of the glycocalyx, resulting in increased vascular permeability. Adhesion molecules may also be up-regulated leading to enhanced leukocyte-endothelium interactions and leukocyte transmigration. Within the kidney, these changes contribute to microcirculatory dysfunction, tubular injury and leukocyte migration toward the renal interstitium [2].

12.3.2 Microcirculatory Dysfunction

Sepsis typically results in systemic vasodilation impacting organ-specific microcirculation. Within the kidneys, this can lead to heterogenous blood flow distribution with areas of hyperperfusion next to areas of hypoperfusion [3]. Interactions between focal zones of micro-ischaemia and regions with preserved tissue oxygenation are thought to be associated with the generation of reactive oxygen species (ROS). Altered vascular tone, endothelial dysfunction and increased capillary permeability can lead to interstitial oedema, which may compromise microcapillary flow further. In addition, intra-renal shunting contributes to microcirculatory dysfunction by redistributing flow from the renal medulla to the renal cortex [3–5].

The formation of intravascular microthrombi is a feature of systemic inflammation and sepsis. Under physiological conditions, endothelial cells inhibit blood coagulation through their interaction with protein C and thrombomodulin. However, during inflammation, many of the natural anticoagulants, including protein C, are degraded or not generated at the usual rate leading to a procoagulant state. This disturbance of the procoagulant–anticoagulant balance triggers the formation of intravascular microthrombi, which is often associated with further influx of inflammatory cells [1, 6].

12.3.3 Tubular Cell Injury

Tubular epithelial cells are vulnerable to microcirculatory dysfunction and hypoperfusion. Further, they are continuously at the frontline of filtered exogenous and endogenous substances such as metabolic waste products, drug metabolites, cytokines, DAMPs and PAMPs [7]. During cardiac surgery with cardiopulmonary bypass, free haemoglobin may also be released and contribute to tubular damage through direct toxicity as well as intratubular crystal formation [8]. Further, leukocytes that have transmigrated into the interstitial space can directly induce tubular cell injury. Independent of the exact trigger, injured tubular and endothelial cells respond by releasing pro-inflammatory cytokines such as interleukin (IL)-1, IL-2, IL-6, IL-8 IL-12, IL-18, transforming growth factor-β (TGF-β), tumour necrosis factor (TNF), interferon (IFN) γ, C-C chemokine ligand 2 (CCL2) and CCL5 [9, 10]. This may trigger the recruitment of peritubular inflammatory cells (neutrophils, monocytes, macrophages and lymphocytes) and aggravate the inflammatory process. The responses of the tubular cells to this inflammatory milieu involve autophagy, mitochondrial dysfunction, necroptosis and apoptosis, all of which can lead to sustained AKI.

Histologically, tubular cell injury often manifests itself in structural changes including apical membrane blebbing, opening of tight junctions, loss of polarity, cell detachment from the basement membrane and cell swelling. Mitochondrial damage may also occur [11]. Increased mitochondrial fragmentation promotes the excess production of ROS, release of cytokines and cellular death, all of which contribute to the progression of AKI. At its extreme, tubular cell injury will result in cell death.

As a form of protection, injured tubular epithelial cells can trigger an oxidative outburst that is protective against further oxidative damage. Paracrine signals may also be triggered, including the release of cell cycle arrest markers aimed at protecting neighbouring tubular cells [12]. Therefore, tubular cells can be the victims as well as promoters of inflammatory processes and protectors.

12.3.4 Intrarenal Inflammation

AKI is considered as a pro-inflammatory condition with activated leukocytes acting as key mediators of all phases of endothelial and tubular cell injury in the initiation and maintenance phase of AKI. The kidneys also host a wide variety of resident immune cells, natural killer cells, macrophage/monocytes, neutrophils and small quantities of classical dendritic cells and B cells [13]. Immediately after endothelial or tubular epithelial cell injury, these resident inflammatory cells are activated, triggering further recruitment and invasion of leukocytes. Virtually all immune cells have been implicated in these pathophysiological processes. Most invading cells are thought to be deleterious (i.e., neutrophils, monocytes, dendritic cells), but some are likely protective (i.e., T regulatory cells). There are also circulating cells whose role varies depending on the phase of the disease process. For instance, resident M1 macrophages are involved in the initial response to injury and are targeted to the sites of injury through the release of DAMPs and hypoxia inducible factors (HIFs) from injured renal tubular epithelial cells. Subsequently, these recruited macrophages perpetuate the inflammatory response by recruiting other leukocytes including bone marrow-derived macrophages, neutrophils and lymphocytes through the secretion of pro-inflammatory mediators, such as TNF-α. Following this process, a shift in macrophage subtype from M1 macrophages to the M2 sub-type occurs which promotes tissue repair [14].

12.4 Additional Factors Contributing to Inflammation in AKI

12.4.1 Haemodynamic Instability

Systemic hypotension is associated with risk and progression of AKI [15]. However, the optimal blood pressure target to prevent AKI in individual patients with sepsis is unknown. Further, certain types of surgery are associated with a higher risk of renal hypoperfusion, in particular, surgical procedures that involve cross-clamping of the aorta above the renal arteries, or cardiac surgery using non-pulsatile flow during cardiopulmonary bypass. Finally, both degree and duration of hypotension impact the risk of AKI [15, 16].

12.4.2 Renal Venous Congestion

The kidney is an encapsulated organ. Elevated central venous pressure (CVP) and resultant increased backward pressure negatively impact renal function, mainly due to increased intra-renal pressure leading to compression of tubules and decrease of GFR.

12.4.3 Tubular Obstruction

Obstruction at any level from the tubules to urethra can cause AKI. Renal stones, crystal-forming drugs, myoglobinuria and also haemoglobinuria can cause intratubular obstruction, which is typically followed by activation of inflammatory processes.

12.4.4 Hypersensitivity Immune Reactions

The high blood flow to the kidneys exposes the tubular cells to large volumes of endogenous and exogenous substances that may induce hypersensitivity reactions and cause acute tubulo-interstitial inflammation. In the first phase, either the resident peritubular interstitial cells or the injured tubular epithelial cells can function as antigen presenters. When exposed to antigens or damage signals, the normally quiescent resident dendritic cells are activated and endocytose, process and express the incriminated antigenic components as peptides located on their surface. Once activated, dendritic cells migrate through the renal lymphatic vessels to regional lymph nodes where they present the antigen to the residual naïve T cells, which are then activated and migrate to the antigenic source or injury emitting the danger signal. Dendritic cells have also been shown to take up small potentially antigenic molecules directly from the tubular lumen. Acute tubulo-interstitial nephritis (AIN) is typically caused by a reaction to drugs but can also occur in the context of inflammatory diseases like sarcoidosis, Sjögren's syndrome or neoplastic diseases.

12.5 AKI Sub-types

Whilst AKI is considered a pro-inflammatory condition, there is increasing recognition that different triggers induce different responses, including activation of distinct inflammatory pathways and different molecular, cellular and functional changes [17, 18]. For instance, using ribonucleic acid (RNA) sequencing in two mouse models of AKI, one caused by arterial ischaemia and the other by severe hypovolaemia, it was demonstrated that the two types of AKI shared less than 10% of genetic pathways despite similar serum creatinine values. Volume depletion activated metabolic pathways related to starvation (i.e. lipid metabolism and gluconeogenesis) and anti-inflammatory responses, whereas ischaemic injury activated genes related to inflammation, coagulation and epithelial repair. Furthermore, the responses to volume loss occurred mainly in the inner medulla, whilst ischaemia-related changes were predominantly seen in the outer medulla.

Complement factors are over-activated in thrombotic microangiopathy (TMA), causing endothelial injury and microvascular thrombosis (immunothrombosis). In sepsis, bacterial endotoxins trigger endothelial dysfunction and vascular leakage, subsequently inducing the release of pro-inflammatory cytokines, leukocyte recruitment and tubular injury. Released histones from neutrophil extracellular traps (NETs) in the bloodstream or injured tubular cells also have pro-inflammatory effects.

Infection-induced AIN is triggered through the activation of resident dendritic cells, which then stimulate secondary immune response. In contrast, AIN in the context of exposure to immune checkpoint inhibitors is caused by the loss of self-tolerance and an autoimmune response against the kidney. AKI in glomerular diseases involves immune complex- or autoantibody-associated vascular injury driven by neutrophil necrosis, release of NETs and histones, complement activation and recruitment of professional phagocytic cells and T cells. Finally, persistent obstructive nephropathy is associated with mild activation of innate immunity and recruitment of anti-inflammatory and pro-fibrotic immune cells [19].

Using new technologies to identify specific sub-types of AKI will improve our understanding of the pathophysiology and also provide potential opportunities for targeted therapies and individualised management [20].

12.6 Organ Crosstalk

Injury to the kidneys can have distant effects on other organs through both cellular and circulating biochemical mediators [21, 22]. Clinical and translational studies have demonstrated interactions and complex mechanisms of crosstalk between injured kidneys and remote organs such as the lungs, liver, heart, gut, brain and hematologic system. These processes involve cells of the innate and adaptive immune system, activated leukocytes and lymphocytes, circulating biochemical mediators, pro-inflammatory cytokines/chemokines, ROS and altered transcriptional events in remote organs.

AKI itself has an immunosuppressive effect. Cytokine haemostasis is profoundly altered due to a reduction in cytokine clearance and ensuing increase in plasma cytokine concentrations, e.g. IL-6, IL-8 and TNF-α. Neutrophil dysfunction, including impaired rolling, impaired migration, impaired killing function and reduced recruitment into remote organs, also plays a key role in the link between AKI and subsequent infection. Plasma resistin, a 12-kDa uraemic toxin, correlates directly with the degree of neutrophil dysfunction in patients with septic shock and AKI. Consequently, AKI is associated with an increased risk of short-term and long-term infections [23]. However, renal replacement therapy has not been shown to improve neutrophil dysfunction nor resistin clearance [24].

12.7 Renal Repair/Progression

After the initial injury, surviving tubular cells undergo a process of de-differentiation and proliferation to replace damaged cells and restore integrity [25]. A time-dependent release of pro-inflammatory mediators in the early injury stage is accompanied by anti-inflammatory factors secreted by recruited and resident cells, resulting in injury resolution and healing [26]. Pro-inflammatory macrophages (M1 sub-type) inhibit repair and promote further injury, whilst anti-inflammatory macrophages (M2 subtype) and T regulatory cells support healing process. It is still unclear what causes functional shift between each phenotype of macrophage. In addition, tubular epithelial cells induce IL-22 secretion from interstitial myeloid cells to endorse tubular integrity, along with clonal expansion of renal progenitor cells (RPC) to regenerate some of the de-differentiated tubular epithelial cells [19]. However, abnormal and persistent inflammation coupled with protracted release of factors, such as TGF-β, can cause maladaptive tubular repair processes [25]. Damaged tubules, as well as immune cell-derived myofibroblasts, are a source of pro-fibrotic factors and contribute to progressive renal disease.

12.8 Management

To date, there is no specific therapy to reverse AKI or prevent progression to CKD. Management is supportive consisting of timely optimisation of fluid and haemodynamic status and avoidance of further nephrotoxic harm. Various anti-inflammatory drugs have been investigated and not been shown to be effective. The results of studies exploring new anti-inflammatory strategies in specific AKI types are awaited.

Summary

AKI is a pro-inflammatory syndrome with a multifactorial aetiology. Various pathophysiologic processes contribute, including tubular injury, endothelial dysfunction, inflammation, alteration of the microcirculatory, focal ischaemia and potentially arterial occlusion and venous congestion. Virtually, all immune cells have been implicated in the pathophysiology of AKI. Activated leukocytes are key mediators in the initiation and maintenance phase of AKI, together with resident immune cells, natural killer cells, macrophage/monocytes, neutrophils, dendritic cells and B cells. Following the initial injury, anti-inflammatory processes contribute to injury resolution and healing. Dysfunction of remote non-renal organs is common as a result of activated immune cells, complex cell interactions and release of inflammatory mediators. Management of AKI is supportive (◙ Fig. 12.1).

Take-Home Message

- AKI is a pro-inflammatory syndrome caused by different immunopathologic processes.
- Innate and adaptive immune responses play important roles in the mediation and repair phase of AKI.
- Different sub-types of AKI with unique pathophysiological characteristics have been identified offering opportunities for targeted interventions.
- AKI is associated with remote organ injuries as well as increased risk of infection due to reduced cytokine clearance and immune cell dysfunction, especially neutrophils.

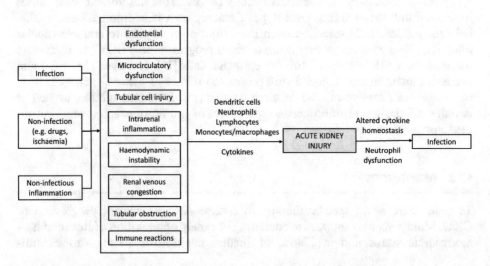

◙ **Fig. 12.1** Immune dysregulation as part of pathogenesis and consequence of acute kidney injury

References

1. Ostermann M, Liu K. Pathophysiology of AKI. Best Pract Res Clin Anaesthesiol. 2017;31(3):305–14.
2. Verma SK, Molitoris BA. Renal endothelial injury and microvascular dysfunction in acute kidney injury. Semin Nephrol. 2015;35(1):96–107.
3. Zafrani L, Payen D, Azoulay E, Ince C. The microcirculation of the septic kidney. Semin Nephrol. 2015;35(1):75–84.
4. Bellomo R, Kellum JA, Ronco C, Wald R, Martensson J, Maiden M, et al. Acute kidney injury in sepsis. Intensive Care Med. 2017;43(6):816–28.
5. Calzavacca P, Evans RG, Bailey M, Bellomo R, May CN. Cortical and medullary tissue perfusion and oxygenation in experimental septic acute kidney injury. Crit Care Med. 2015;43(10):e431–9.
6. Molitoris BA, Sandoval RM. Kidney endothelial dysfunction: ischemia, localized infections and sepsis. Contrib Nephrol. 2011;174:108–18.
7. Gomez H, Ince C, De Backer D, Pickkers P, Payen D, Hotchkiss J, et al. A unified theory of sepsis-induced acute kidney injury: inflammation, microcirculatory dysfunction, bioenergetics, and the tubular cell adaptation to injury. Shock. 2014;41(1):3–11.
8. Nadim MK, Forni LG, Bihorac A, Hobson C, Koyner JL, Shaw A, et al. Cardiac and vascular surgery-associated acute kidney injury: the 20th international consensus conference of the ADQI (Acute Disease Quality Initiative) Group. J Am Heart Assoc. 2018;7(11):e008834.
9. Zuk A, Bonventre JV. Recent advances in acute kidney injury and its consequences and impact on chronic kidney disease. Curr Opin Nephrol Hypertens. 2019;28(4):397–405.
10. McWilliam SJ, Wright RD, Welsh GI, Tuffin J, Budge KL, Swan L, et al. The complex interplay between kidney injury and inflammation. Clin Kidney J. 2021;14(3):780–8.
11. Ishimoto Y, Inagi R. Mitochondria: a therapeutic target in acute kidney injury. Nephrol Dial Transplant. 2016;31(7):1062–9.
12. Cantaluppi V, Quercia AD, Dellepiane S, Ferrario S, Camussi G, Biancone L. Interaction between systemic inflammation and renal tubular epithelial cells. Nephrol Dial Transplant. 2014;29(11):2004–11.
13. Turner JE, Becker M, Mittrücker HW, Panzer U. Tissue-resident lymphocytes in the kidney. J Am Soc Nephrol. 2018;29(2):389–99.
14. Jang HR, Rabb H. Immune cells in experimental acute kidney injury. Nat Rev Nephrol. 2015;11(2):88–101.
15. Gregory A, Stapelfeldt WH, Khanna AK, Smischney NJ, Boero IJ, Chen Q, et al. Intraoperative hypotension is associated with adverse clinical outcomes after noncardiac surgery. Anesth Analg. 2021;132(6):1654–65.
16. Poukkanen M, Wilkman E, Vaara ST, Pettilä V, Kaukonen KM, Korhonen AM, et al. Hemodynamic variables and progression of acute kidney injury in critically ill patients with severe sepsis: data from the prospective observational FINNAKI study. Crit Care. 2013;17(6):R295.
17. De Oliveira BD, Xu K, Shen TH, Callahan M, Kiryluk K, D'Agati VD, et al. Molecular nephrology: types of acute tubular injury. Nat Rev Nephrol. 2019;15(10):599–612.
18. Scholz H, Boivin FJ, Schmidt-Ott KM, Bachmann S, Eckardt KU, Scholl UI, et al. Kidney physiology and susceptibility to acute kidney injury: implications for renoprotection. Nat Rev Nephrol. 2021;17(5):335–49.
19. Anders HJ, Wilkens L, Schraml B, Marschner J. One concept does not fit all: the immune system in different forms of acute kidney injury. Nephrol Dial Transplant. 2021;36(1):29–38.
20. Ostermann M, Wu V, Sokolov D, Lumlertgul N. Definitions of acute renal dysfunction: an evolving clinical and biomarker paradigm. Curr Opin Crit Care. 2021;27(6):553–9.
21. Pickkers P, Darmon M, Hoste E, Joannidis M, Legrand M, Ostermann M, et al. Acute kidney injury in the critically ill: an updated review on pathophysiology and management. Intensive Care Med. 2021;47(8):835–50.
22. Doi K, Rabb H. Impact of acute kidney injury on distant organ function: recent findings and potential therapeutic targets. Kidney Int. 2016;89(3):555–64.
23. Mehta RL, Bouchard J, Soroko SB, Ikizler TA, Paganini EP, Chertow GM, et al. Sepsis as a cause and consequence of acute kidney injury: program to improve care in acute renal disease. Intensive Care Med. 2011;37(2):241–8.

24. Singbartl K, Miller L, Ruiz-Velasco V, Kellum JA. Reversal of acute kidney injury-induced neutrophil dysfunction: a critical role for resistin. Crit Care Med. 2016;44(7):e492–501.
25. Forni LG, Darmon M, Ostermann M, Oudemans-van Straaten HM, Pettilä V, Prowle JR, et al. Renal recovery after acute kidney injury. Intensive Care Med. 2017;43(6):855–66.
26. Andrade-Oliveira V, Foresto-Neto O, Watanabe IKM, Zatz R, Câmara NOS. Inflammation in renal diseases: new and old players. Front Pharmacol. 2019;10:1192.

Dysregulated Immune Response and Organ Dysfunction: Liver

Adrian T. Press and Michael Bauer

Contents

Illustrations are supported by Margit Leitner.

© The Author(s), under exclusive license to Springer Nature Switzerland AG 2023
Z. Molnar et al. (eds.), *Management of Dysregulated Immune Response in the Critically Ill*,
Lessons from the ICU, https://doi.org/10.1007/978-3-031-17572-5_13

> **Learning Objectives**
> - Role of different immunocompetent cells in the liver
> - The liver is critically ill (sepsis)
> - Importance of liver failure for the prognosis in critical ill
> - Current management and limitation of liver failure

13.1 Introduction

As an immunologically complex organ, the liver contains multiple tissue-resident immune cells, including lymphocytes, macrophages, and specialized endothelial cells. Lastly, the ability of parenchymal hepatocytes to control inflammation and infection through modulation of nutrition and hormone milieu and the availability of acute-phase proteins contribute significantly to the body's immune function. In health, the immune and parenchymal cells create a complex surveillance system programmed to tolerate microbes and microbial products typically originating from the intestines. This tolerogenic liver environment is vital for the immune homeostasis of the body. However, the thresholds are lowered in critical illness, mainly if liver comorbidities are in place. Consequently, slight dysregulations and even otherwise expected amounts of microbial material may trigger the liver to signal a systemic immune reaction, interfering and impairing its physiologic function such as detoxification or protein synthesis. Targeting the hepatic immune response is thus a promising avenue for novel therapeutics with the possibility to improve the body's control over the immune function, thus reducing tissue damage, lowering the risk for organ failure, and mobilizing the body's own immunological and regulatory capacities to fight illness.

13.2 Immune Competent Cells of the Liver and Their Function

The liver is supplied with blood from two significant vascular beds: The hepatic artery contributing to approximately 30% of the liver's blood inflow supplies the liver with up to 80–90% of the required oxygen. The portal vein provides a more significant part of its blood inflow, which carries low-oxygen but nutrient-rich blood from the intestines. The blood flows through sinusoids, the liver's capillaries lined by endothelial cells (liver-specific endothelial cells, LSECs) and hepatocytes into the central vein, draining the blood from the liver into the vena cava inferior (◘ Fig. 13.1). Hepatocytes take up nutrients and xenobiotics to metabolize, biotransform, and eliminate harmful molecules into the bile. While the bile was first discovered as amphiphilic fluid supporting the digestion of fatty acids, other regulatory, defense, and organ cross talk (enterohepatic cycle) are also described. The liver fulfills critical metabolic functions at the interface of the host and microbiome during health and disease. Together with different resident immune cell populations, the liver surveils all molecules absorbed in the intestine and creates a robust line of defense against any material that may be potentially harmful to the body. Under normal circumstances, the liver cells promote a tolerogenic environment that enables its cells to deal with

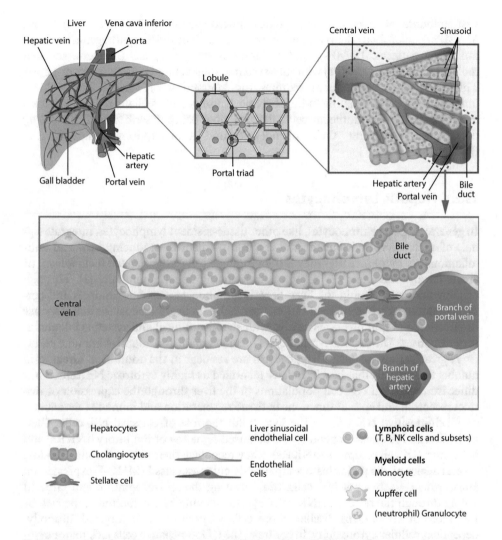

◘ Fig. 13.1 Liver functional anatomy and distribution of its cells. The hepatic artery and portal vein, supplying the liver with oxygen and nutrients. The sinusoids drain into the hepatic veins, ending in the inferior vena cava. Further, hepatocytes eliminate molecules that they synthesize or metabolize after absorption from the sinusoids into the canaliculi that drain into smaller bile ducts and the gallbladder towards their gastrointestinal recycling or elimination. The liver shows a "lobular" organization, which can be conceptualized as a hexagonal structure around each central vein. In this organization, referred to as lobule, blood flows from the portal triad (branch of the hepatic artery, portal vein, and bile duct) towards the central vein, while bile flows through canaliculi, formed by hepatocytes, from the central vein towards the corners of the lobule into the bile duct. Functional units with highly differentiated cells are established between the afferent and the efferent blood vessels of the liver. The hepatocytes, LSECs, endothelial cells, contractile hepatic stellate cells, and cholangiocytes build the framework in which tissue-resident Kupffer cells (liver macrophages) are localized. In addition, various other myeloid and lymphoid cells are localized in the tissue and constantly patrol the sinusoids, which are crucial for the liver's tolerogenic signaling and immune function

vast amounts of microbial metabolites (microbe-associated molecular patterns, MAMPs), microbial debris and immunogenic molecules (pathogen-associated molecular patterns, PAMPs), and endogenous danger signals (danger-associated molecular patterns, DAMPs) without a systemic spillover and inflammatory response. This tolerogenic environment requires the interaction of various liver-resident immune-competent cells, including hepatic lymphocytes, stellate cells, specialized macrophages, and endothelial cells, that are now being described with increasing detailedness regarding their phenotypic and transcriptional characteristics (◘ Fig. 13.1).

13.2.1 Hepatic Lymphocytes

In general, hepatic lymphocytes, like other tissue-resident lymphocytes, integrate signals of their microenvironment and respond to them in producing pro- and anti-inflammatory cytokines that may attract immune cells, alter hepatic metabolism, or create an anti-inflammatory response, modulating hepatic immunity [1]. Through residing and patrolling in the liver, hepatic lymphocytes serve as sentinels and perform immunosurveillance. In addition, they maintain liver homeostasis and response to infection and noninfectious insults, with significant local and systemic inflammatory responses. The hepatic lymphocytes include innate and adaptive immune cells.

A great variety of **innate lymphocytes** are resident in the adult liver. Greatest in number are pit cells that had been later identified as highly cytotoxic **NK cells.** They differ from classical NK cell populations in the liver through the expression of distinct receptors and special functions in tissue regeneration and immune tolerance.

CD56-positive NK cells in the liver fulfill the role of classical NK cells. Their activation and response depend on the balanced signaling of inhibitory (iNKRs) and activating NK cell receptors (aNKRs). They recognize their targets through binding several alleles of the major histocompatibility complex class I (MHC-I) expressed on autologous cells, but not NK cells, thus ensuring the self-recognition and targeted killing through the release of NK cells' cytotoxic granules. Furthermore, the lack of Fcγ receptor III (CD16) disables those cells to perform their targeted antibody-dependent cellular cytotoxicity. In contrast, the CD56-negative cells lack major cyto-toxic NK cell elements, i.e., perforin and granzyme A-B-positive cytotoxic granules required for targeted killing.

The CD56-negative population fulfills critical immune-regulatory functions in the liver and is present in equal concentrations as the CD56-positive NK population. Notably, the characteristics and markers of NK cells widely differ between species and are, for instance, more diverse in humans than mice. Despite an agreement on the importance of cholangiocyte, LSEC, KC, and even hepatocyte chemokines for their homing, little is known about their biology and function.

The predominant **adaptive lymphocytes** in the liver are **conventional T cells** (MHC-restricted), **CD4⁺** and **CD8⁺ T cells, and B cells.**

Unconventional T cells are differentiated through the tissue environment. This class comprises mainly three types of T cells, **NKT cells, MAIT cells,** and **γδ T cells,** all present with distinctive functions in the liver [2].

CD4⁺ and **CD8⁺ T cells** are considered the conventional T cell populations in the liver [3].

In the liver, conventional CD8$^+$ T cells dominate the T cell population relatively to CD4$^+$ T cells and CD3$^+$ T cells that co-express CD56, otherwise found on NK cells. As a result, T cells invade and proliferate in the liver, where a large amount undergoes apoptosis. This observation had led to the *graveyard model*. This model describes the liver as the "final destination" of T cells, cleared in the hepatic tolerogenic environment at the end of their life. However, recent evidence depicts that liver T cells are also retained and involved in clearing liver infections, which can be reprogrammed in the liver to support the tolerogenic environment.

Cytotoxic CD8$^+$ T cells are considered the primary effector cells in the liver. Upon antigen presentation on MHC I by any liver cell, they release cell-directed cytokines, perforins, and granzymes, eliminating, e.g., infected or malignant cells. Conversely, blocking CD8$^+$ T cells through neutralizing antibodies decreases liver inflammation, associated steatosis, and tissue damage, thus indicating their essential but not exclusive function in liver inflammation and injury. Another class of hepatic CD8$^+$ T cells necessary for the hepatic immune response is the CD8$^+$ memory T cells (TRM). TRM residing in the liver tissue and patrolling the sinusoids are potent effectors to known antigens reaching the liver, initiating a quick response to prevent reinfection with a previously encountered pathogen.

B cells are another significant population of lymphocytes in the liver. Blood-borne, they immigrate in the liver, and if not encountering their cognate antigen, they move back to the periphery, where they die after a few days. However, if they recognize their antibody, they either differentiate to short-lived IgM-producing plasma cells or migrate to lymphoid tissues where they interact with T cells. B cells co-stimulated by T cells undergo a transformation, and class-switch recombination of epitopes, producing neutralizing antibodies before they may reside as terminally differentiated memory B cells or as precursors to long-lived plasma cells in the body.

B cells in the liver exhibit pro-fibrotic features in experimental liver fibrosis through IL-6 signaling. Studies suggest a similar mechanism in humans. Epstein-Barr virus (EBV) infections constitute up to 70% of the B cell posttransplant lymphoproliferative disorders. Such patients receive immunosuppressive agents. Consequently, EBV remains uncontrolled and transforms many B cells, resulting in fibrosis and other complications.

NKT cells are enriched in the liver microvascular where they scout and react to self- and microbial lipid antigens through Toll-like receptors and MHC-like molecule (CD1d). In response to receptor activation, they secrete pro- or anti-inflammatory cytokines and critically determine the immune pro- or anti-inflammatory milieu for the different immune responses in the liver. Importantly, two NKT cell populations (type I and type II) with widely opposing functions had been characterized in hepatocytes. Type I NKT cells contribute to the control over the induction or prevention of immunological responses and critically determine the progression of liver diseases. Counteracting the type I inflammatory response signaling the tolerogenic liver environment, type II NKT cells are the larger population of NKT cells in humans. Their anti-inflammatory phenotype may further provide them with an essential function in the resolution of liver inflammation that studies could confirm for different liver pathologies.

MAIT cells are considered "innate-like" T cells that recognize conserved antigens from microbial riboflavin synthesis. Constituting circa 50% of the livers' T cells, they may be the most significant local T cell population present. MAIT cells provide the fundamental of the liver immune surveillance system responding to both inflammatory cytokines and MAMPs but are also present throughout the whole gastrointestinal tract. They are pro-fibrinogenic and accumulate in the liver during liver cirrhosis but are found to counteract different bacterial infections. MAIT cells' versatility and ability to promote inflammation and even dysbiosis resulting in obesity make them an exciting target for lipid metabolism-associated therapies.

γδ T cells significantly accumulate in the liver upon inflammation. They had been recently characterized in mice as antagonists to metabolic-driven inflammatory processes and keepers of glucose homeostasis. Research indicates a diverse position in regulating hepatic inflammation beyond its function at the interphase of metabolism and inflammation. They can modulate inflammation and active CD4$^+$ and NKT but also possess the function to downregulate similar cells mediating anti-inflammatory effects. Which pathway might be taken depends highly on the immunopathology and the differentiation of an acute or chronic status, but the underlying mechanism to date is ongoing research.

Understanding the complex interactions between different liver-resident cell types and the microenvironment with lymphocytes in the future will be vital to research and utilize therapeutic strategies directed to hepatic lymphocyte signaling.

13.2.2 Myeloid Cells in the Liver

The hepatic macrophages, termed **Kupffer cells**, reside within the sinusoids of the liver, serving as gatekeepers responding to foreign molecules entering the liver. They are the largest population of the liver's myeloid cell population and have the power to stimulate pro- and anti-inflammatory reactions. KCs account for as much as 90% of all resident macrophage populations in the body. Pattern recognition receptors (PRRs), e.g., Toll-like receptors, complement receptors, and Fc receptors, are ubiquitously expressed on the surface of myeloid liver cells. Kupffer cells respond to their activation with increased phagocytosis rates and cytokine synthesis. This immune mechanism in Kupffer cells had increasingly become the focus for liver regeneration [4]. However, their regeneration might be impaired through metabolic dysregulation, particularly a lipid overload, resulting in a disease-accelerating phenotype.

Myeloid and plasmacytoid dendritic cell (DC) populations are phenotypically immature despite the vigorous immune-modulatory activity essential in the liver's T cell response facilitating tolerance [5]. Thus, the hepatic DCs may be an inducible phenotype, and specific subpopulation changes quickly during infection or liver injury.

Myeloid-derived suppressor cells (MDSCs) regulate the immune system and present heterogeneous myeloid immune cells that expand during various pathological conditions [6]. MDSCs suppress T cell activation in response to pro-inflammatory cytokines secreting immunosuppressors such as IL-10, TGF-β, and arginase. Their exhaustion in liver injury may cause the dysregulated immune response during acute and chronic liver injury enhancing severity. However, a comprehensive characterization, differentiation, and road map of myeloid cell interaction are not conceptualized to date.

13.2.3 Liver Sinusoidal Endothelial Cells

The **liver sinusoidal endothelial cells** (LSECs) form a unique population lining the low-shear-stress liver capillaries (sinusoids) lacking a basement membrane. LSECs include an irregular open fenestration, i.e., transcellular pores, termed sieve plates, due to their appearance in small, clustered groups of fenestration with circa 110 nm in diameter. They form a unique filtration layer with vital physiologic and immunological functions. As a filter, they are characterized as excellent scavengers and first-line defense against multiple viral and bacterial infections with a remarkable capacity for endocytosis, antigen presentation, and leukocyte recruitment. Their ability to clear antigens modulates the systemic inflammatory signaling and modulation of the tolerogenic state within the liver [7]. They further act as antigen-presenting cells in the liver, thereby being another class of immune-competent cells regulating inflammation by releasing cytokines and activating immune cell signaling pathways. LSEC additionally engages in the active clearance and lysosomal degradation of pathogens, particularly viruses, also indicating the active immunological function of the livers' endothelial cells. In response to nosocomial bacteria, LSECs can lose their porosity. In turn, this tightening of the barrier is an important pathophysiological event resulting in impaired lipoprotein and chylomicron uptake by hepatocytes. In favor, the increased serum concentration of both becomes apparent in clinical hyperlipidemia, a strong confounder found in sepsis describing tissue lipoprotein lipase inhibition and increased hepatic triglyceride delivery. Ultimately, they take part in the immune cell homing, e.g., through the expression of CXCL6 supporting the recruitment of $CXCR6^+$ T cells.

13.2.4 Hepatic Stellate Cells

The hepatic stellate cells (HSCs) are a contractile cellular population that physiologically regulates microcirculation, i.e., blood flow in the liver. They deposit collagen, the most prominent extracellular matrix protein in the liver, giving the lobular structure. Further, they inherit a unique metabolic function by regulating the circulating vitamin A concentration and delivery through their ability of need-independent, receptor-mediated vitamin A uptake and storage. HLCs themselves are reactive cells and subject to many hepatic cytokines and metabolites. Upon activation through cytokines and metabolites, HSC transdifferentiates to myofibroblasts. As a result, the contract loses its ability to store vitamin A, proliferate, and inherit an increased collagen synthesis rate during this process. Altogether, they change the extracellular matrix and may even cause microischemic events, resulting in cell death and release of pro-inflammatory molecules. Thus, while in the healthy liver induction of regulatory T cells (Treg), T cell apoptosis (via B7-H1, PDL-1), or inhibition of cytotoxic $CD8^+$ T cells contributes to an HSC-anti-inflammatory phenotype during inflammation, the indirect pathophysiological mechanism may contribute significantly to the amplification of a pro-immune response in the liver.

13.2.5 **Hepatocytes**

Hepatocytes are the metabolic cells of the liver. They are involved in the small-molecule and protein synthesis of the organism, storage, and biotransformation. Hepatocytes are differentiated among oxygen, nutrition, and hormonal gradients within the liver lobule between the portal and central veins, sharing metabolic functions in an assembly-line fashion exchanging small molecules through gap junctions. Despite being no classical immune cells, hepatocytes significantly control systemic inflammatory processes through their ability to take up and eliminate MAMPs, DAMPs, and PAMPS, reducing their systemic activity on other cells. Further, hepatocytes adapt their protein synthesis, secreting various acute-phase proteins that control inflammation, restrain bacterial growth, and alter. Another critical feature of hepatocytes is their metabolic adaptation and distinct metabolic response to injury and infection, which may directly or indirectly affect inflammatory reactions and might even be directly antimicrobial. Those features are tightly controlled during inflammation by the presence of inflammatory mediators and hormones released, e.g., by liver immune cells and LSECs that hepatocytes recognize through different immune receptors.

13.3   **Liver Impairment in Patients with Critical Illness**

The liver, with its various immune-competent cells, not only regulates the body's nutritional and hormonal supply but is also powerful yet at the same time a vulnerable modulator of inflammation and infection.

The healthy liver environment is tolerogenic, regulated through myeloid suppressor cells harboring immune-suppressive capacities and activated through macrophage infiltration to the liver. Once activated, they exert tolerogenic regulatory action through, e.g., secretion of IL-10 and TGF-β or production of arginase and myeloid suppressor and immune checkpoint indoleamine-pyrrole 2,3-dioxygenase [8, 9].

Typically, the liver would synthesize most plasma proteins, including fibrinogen, transport proteins such as albumin, retinol-binding protein, lipoproteins, and immune factors, i.e., complement factor protease inhibitors. When the tolerogenic threshold passes, the liver rapidly responds to circulating cytokines from extrahepatic sources, with an acute-phase response (APR) dictating the innate immune response. Consequently, the synthesis of acute-phase proteins massively increases. Firstly, pro-inflammatory IL-6, phospholipase A2, and C-reactive proteins are among the most noted acute-phase proteins and, when secreted, can maintain and amplify the acute-phase response. Additionally, complement proteins (e.g., C3, C4, C9), enhancing phagocytosis, acting as a chemoattractant, anaphylactic, and enhancers of vascular permeability, are secreted. Furthermore, the increased release of iron-binding proteins (haptoglobin, hemopexin, ferritin, hepcidin) reduces the concentration of free iron, otherwise a readily available and utilized source of vital nutrition for pathogens. Finally, the synthesis of clotting factors (e.g., fibrinogen, factor VIII, IX, von Willebrand factor, prothrombin) enhances the coagulation to an extent that spontaneous life-threatening clotting events may occur.

13

However, all those mechanisms act directly on the immune cells and follow one central goal: their activation, migration to the site of infection, and promotion of pathogen clearance. Secondary and less immediate effects of the APR are the induction of bone marrow leukocytosis to refuel the immune cell populations and neuronal changes resulting in pyrexia. In contrast, acute-phase proteins also exhibit anti-inflammatory properties to limit excessive inflammation. CRP, for instance, triggers the TNF-α production in KCs; however, at the same time, released protease inhibitors may cleave CRP, rendering it inactive and carrying out even anti-inflammatory effects recruiting and activating MDSC.

The significance of the vast immunological and immune-metabolic functions carried out in the liver for the outcome of critical illness is demonstrated in clinical trials for various diseases [10, 11]. The role of preexisting liver injury or dysfunction, most notably liver cirrhosis, is associated with a poor outcome in patients admitted to intensive care units. Thus, mechanical ventilation in patients with liver cirrhosis is associated with a 1-year mortality rate of 89%. Furthermore, ICU patients frequently have a chronic liver injury that decompensates, resulting in "acute-on-chronic liver failure" (ACLF) [12, 13]. In addition, critically ill ACLF patients often develop progressive multiple-organ dysfunction syndromes (MODS) due to the incapability of liver cells to control inflammation and related metabolism. Thus, even after the development of MODS, preexisting impaired liver function worsens the prognosis further [14].

While liver failure and severe liver injury are considered independent risk factors for the prognosis in critical illness, the knowledge about the effects of a mild-to-moderate liver dysfunction on the outcome is not yet understood well.

The sequential organ failure assessment (SOFA) score is routinely applied to assess organ dysfunction in the intensive care unit. Liver function is exclusively evaluated here through the accumulation of bilirubin in plasma. Bilirubin, a hemoglobin degradation product, is metabolized and eliminated in the liver. Therefore, the livers' inability to clear bilirubin and a bilirubin overload, e.g., due to hemolytic bacteria or extracorporeal circuits, such as dialysis, increases "indirect (unconjugated) bilirubin." After hepatocellular metabolization (e.g., glucuronidation), the water solubility increases, historically rendering the molecule easier accessible to biochemical measurement, leading to the term of "direct" bilirubin. In the SOFA liver subscore, a (total) bilirubin concentration of up to 1.9 mg/dL (32 µmol/L) is considered moderate organ dysfunction, with further cutoffs for increased severity for bilirubin concentrations between 2.0–5.9 mg/dL (33–101 µmol/L; SOFA 2) and 6.0–11.9 mg/dL (102–204 µmol/L; SOFA 3). Plasma bilirubin above 12.0 mg/dL (204 µmol/L) reflects overt liver failure at a SOFA of 4 points [15].

Two different pathologies can be distinguished from their clinical appearance and laboratory markers. The first prominent phenotype, termed ischemic hepatitis [16], results from shock/hypoxemia frequently triggered by a reduced arterial blood supply in circa 5–10% of critically ill patients increasing mortality [17, 18]. The resulting pericentral or diffuse necrosis causes an elevation of various hepatic enzymes, particularly transaminases, and in late stages metabolic markers, e.g., bilirubin. More common (circa 20% of all critical ill [18]) is cholestatic liver dysfunction, defined by a metabolic phenotype with impaired bile formation or elimination. The origin of this injury may be further differentiated into an extrahepatic injury characterized by a posthepatic obstruction (a rare event during ICU stay) or an "intrahepatic type" where complex molecular rearrangements in hepatocytes result in the loss of function of the metabolic or excretory machinery [19–22]. Regardless of the kind of injury, cholestatic dysfunction is variably defined, e.g., by a rise in bilirubin (>2 mg dL^{-1} bilirubin [23]) that is frequently accompanied by an increase of alkaline phosphatase (ALP) plasma levels [24].

Despite the frequent occurrence of hepatic dysfunction in 11–31% of critically ill patients [23, 25], it still did not receive as much attention as, e.g., respiratory or cardiac failure. One reason might be that liver failure does not result in an immediate life-threatening complication as other organ failures; however, looking at the long-term mortality of patients with a liver complication in the ICU, this assumption seems treacherous.

Kramer and coworkers were among the first to address the role of hepatic impairment utilizing bilirubin to analyze the liver impairment in 4146 patients in the ICU with early hepatic dysfunction [23], highlighting the correlation between liver dysfunction, detected by increased bilirubin levels and hospital mortality [26]. Further, Kramer and colleges identified a significantly increased incidence of sepsis among patients with liver dysfunction. However, the cause-effect relationship between infection and liver dysfunction has yet to be elucidated; that is, it is still a matter of research to decipher whether liver dysfunction increases susceptibility for infection or the other way around. Experimental studies from the last decades suggest, in contrast to clinical data restricted to hyperbilirubinemia, early and frequent impairment of the liver excretory machinery in sepsis, highlighting the importance of liver for metabolism and inflammation control [27].

13.4　The Liver in Systemic Inflammation and Sepsis

After the gut mucosa with its immune system and microbiome, the liver is the second line of defense against potentially harmful molecules or pathogens deriving from the gut microbiome. Thus, maintaining liver function is essential for the immune homeostasis of the body. The immunological functions of the liver depend on various highly specialized immune cells and liver parenchyma that forms a complex cellular network modulating a systemic immune response towards pathogens, leading to tolerance and the "net" anti- or pro-inflammatory host response.

The organization of the fenestrated liver sinusoidal endothelial cells lining as a single layer of the space of Disse surrounding hepatocytes results in a vast interaction surface of gut-derived blood-borne molecules, called microbe-associated molecular patterns (MAMPs) with the parenchyma. These molecules interact with pattern recognition receptors (PRRs) ubiquitously expressed on hepatocytes and Kupffer cells and are subsequently engulfed through endocytosis (hepatocytes) or phagocytosis (Kupffer cells) and degraded. In synergy with PRR signaling, the breakdown of MAMPs does not result in the systemic release of inflammatory mediators and thus efficient detoxification, hindering a detrimental systemic immune reaction.

The liver responds to pathogens and infectious stimuli that reach via the bloodstream not as a trigger for the systemic host response to blood-borne pathogens but as a filter capable of eliminating pathogens, pathogen-associated molecular patterns, and debris as well as cytokines and other pro-inflammatory factors.

The liver responds to blood-borne pathogens within its vast sinusoidal network lined by LSECs that house the Kupffer cells (liver-resident macrophages), hepatic stellate cells, and lymphocytes. LSECs act as sentinel and antigen-presenting cells after endocytosis, PAMPs, and other debris to stimulate and recruit particularly lymphocytes of the adaptive immune system. Various immune receptors and co-stimulatory, PRR, and adhesion molecules on a large surface accomplish a great capacity to filter PAMPs and pathogens. These factors shield Kupffer cells and hepatocytes from significant exposure to those xenobiotics that otherwise would excessively recruit neutrophils. Neutrophils in the liver had been depicted to undergo NETosis, a cell death mechanism during which the nuclear DNA is released to form neutrophil extracellular traps (NETs). These NETs hold histones and proteases that, like a spider web, can capture, damage, or even kill bacteria. Through phago-cytosis, protease-containing granules, and NETs, the hepatic microcirculation might be constrained, resulting in localized ischemic events potentiating injury and recruit-ment of neutrophils to cope with the increased amount of cellular debris. A vicious circle might occur if the system fails to compensate for the increasing amount of infiltrating immune cells and subsequent tissue damage, which can attract more neutrophils again. Ultimately, these processes are discussed as significant factors leading to fibrotic sequelae in chronic liver disease but also after recovering from critical illness [28].

Kupffer cells and monocyte-derived macrophages directly kill circulating bacteria after engulfing them through phagocytosis. For the recognition and phagocytosis of pathogens, Kupffer cells express high concentrations of scavenger receptors, Toll-like receptors, complement, and antibody Fcγ receptors. In addition, the activation of Kupffer cells results in the expression and secretion of various pro-inflammatory and chemoattractant cytokines, including TNF-α, IL-6, and IL-1β. However, the secre-tion of Kupffer cell-derived cytokines also modifies hepatic metabolic function. Hepatocytes respond to the inflammatory stimulation through Kupffer cell-derived cytokines, particularly IL-6, by synthesizing factors that decrease iron mobilization into the blood to reduce bacterial nutritional sources and secretion of acute-phase proteins (APPs) such as C-reactive protein, which rises from nearly not detectable plasma levels to 80–400 mg/dL within a few hours upon stimulation [29]. CRP and other acute-phase proteins are central regulators of the antimicrobial response by opsonizing pathogens for macrophages and potentiating immune signals. The mas-sive synthesis of APPs, however, requires a vast amount of metabolic resources; thus, as a consequence, housekeeping proteins from hepatocytes, such as serum albumin synthesis and bile formation, are significantly reduced [30].

The complexity of the interactions between parenchymal and non-parenchymal cells and other immune cells, cytokines, APPs, and other humoral factors determine the inflammatory processes in the liver and distant organs. However, the complexity of this intercellular network reaches a complexity that till today has not yet been wholly conceptualized.

The importance of hepatocytes, the liver parenchyma, as a nonspecialized immune cell with no phagocytic activity for immune control is astonishing. Hepatocytes in the liver serve as a bacterial scavenger, detoxifying cells for all xeno-biotics, the primary source for APPs, and producing inflammatory cytokines. However, all those effects modulate the systemic immune response at the expense of liver damage due to the overwhelming inflammation, immune cell recruitment, and cell death. Liver damage is often aggravated by hypoxic events resulting from cardiac, circulatory, or respiratory failure, and NETs primarily meant to capture and defeat pathogens can result in microthrombus formation resulting in reduced sinusoidal perfusion. The inflammatory signaling in LSECs includes the induction of iNOS and simultaneously increased secretion of endothelin (ET)-1 acting on stellate cells, which are situated around the sinusoids, contracting and torching the capillaries restricting blood flow additionally.

On the level of hepatocytes, the internalization and downregulation of biliary transporters that are eliminating bile acids, bilirubin, drugs, and other xenobiotics through the hepatobiliary route reflect a hallmark of sepsis, resulting in cholestasis [31, 32]. Furthermore, even cholangiocytes themselves release in such a situation pro-inflammatory cytokines, predominantly TNF-α and IFN-γ. This expansion of the periductal inflammation further impedes chloride and bicarbonate secretion by cholangiocytes and, due to the resulting loss of otherwise passively excreted water, restricts bile flow.

In summary, a complex immune response and local and often diffuse hypoxic events together with metabolic reprogramming of hepatocytes and ductal inflammation and cholestasis may lead to liver dysfunction, an underestimated and early poor prognostic event in sepsis.

13.5 Management of Liver Failure in Critical Illness

The management of liver failure in critical illness is restricted mainly to source control and supportive care. However, particularly in the light of the vast immunological function of liver cells, exerted directly by local immune cells through, e.g., cytokine secretion or indirectly by hepatocytes that control the elimination of immunogenic debris and the energy delivery to the periphery, a targeted therapy of the liver would be desirable.

The guidelines recommend hemodynamic stabilization, optimizing perfusion, and adequate treatment for infection. In case infections are suspected, a targeted initiation as early as possible and a subsequent culture-dependent adaptation of the antimicrobial therapy are indicated [33]. Early enteral nutrition is a recommended standard in managing critical illness when feasible [34]. Reasons for a delayed beginning of enteral nutrition may be an uncontrolled shock, hyperlactatemia, hypoxemia, acidosis, increased gastric residual volume, abdominal obstruction, or abdominal compartment syndrome [35]. Further, managing metabolic function through glucose control by insulin therapy reduces the events of cholestatic dysfunction in critical illness [36]. Specific interventions into remote or systemic inflammatory response are not supported by current evidence [37].

Hemofiltration by resins or oral sequestrants lowers serum bile acid concentration and the associated cholestasis-induced immune dysregulation that may be pro-inflammatory or anti-inflammatory depending on the cell type and bile acid composition. Farnesoid-X-receptor ligands are already available, interfering with bile acid homeostasis in hepatocytes and promoting gut integrity. However, their usefulness in sepsis and critical illness is not yet determined. The use of ursodeoxycholic acid (UDCA) has cytoprotective effects on cholangiocytes. It may act by causing a switch in the bile acid pool, reducing concentrations of cytotoxic, hydrophobic bile acids, and therefore is commonly used in the treatment of cholestatic liver diseases. However, none of these interventions is currently supported by high-quality evidence and will be considered in the post-acute phase if signs of cholestatic injury persist.

Advanced extracorporeal systems, i.e., albumin dialysis, have the power to remove albumin-bound molecules such as bile acids and other water-soluble molecules. However, in randomized controlled studies, the albumin dialysis reduced serum bile acids and significantly improved hepatic encephalopathy and systemic hemodynamics, while an overall survival benefit could not be observed.

The human body harbors a vast microbiome, and for understanding infectious disease and the impact of antibiotics, the host should be viewed as "holobiont," particularly in the gut, where the gut-liver axis reflects a most powerful interface that determines prognosis in the critically ill, which should prompt research into manipulating this interface for therapeutic interventions. Beyond any doubt, cross talk between gut and liver is essential for metabolism and immune response in health and disease. Hepatocytes, for example, remove bacterial products in bloodstream infection. Preexisting liver conditions and presumably evolving impairment of liver function in the critically ill are often associated with dysbiosis, a term summarizing a disruption of microbiota homeostasis due to altered functional composition and metabolic activities. Interaction of the gut microbiome with the function of parenchymal and non-parenchymal liver cells has also been demonstrated in various liver diseases in general and for septic complications in chronic liver disease in particular [38]. Therapeutic manipulation of the gut microbiome, such as selective digestive decontamination or fecal transplantation and administration of probiotics, has shown promising results for modulation of the gut microbiome in preventing and treating bacterial infections and organ dysfunctions and reducing the length of ICU stays. Interestingly, the best-defined intervention affecting the gut microbiome, i.e., selective decontamination of the digestive tract (SDD), has clinically been almost exclusively studied regarding the prevention of nosocomial lung infection and antibiotic resistance patterns. In contrast, albeit plausible, its impact on liver function has not been evaluated.

13.6 Targeting Immune Dysregulation in Liver Disease

The dysregulated host response in the critically ill might be significant in the liver. The various interactions and regulatory functions of the innate and adaptive immune system and other immune-competent cells in the liver on the hepatocellular function may be essential for targeted drugs. The body's incapability to resolve liver inflammation causes chronic liver injury and fibrosis, leading to liver failure and affecting metabolism, fostering oncogenesis and dysregulation of other organ systems.

Since inflammatory processes depend on multiple immune cell types in the liver and their specific involvement depends on the inflammatory insult, targeting interventions to key mediators in a personalized manner may be indicated. One approach to attenuate liver inflammation's consequences and driving forces is to target the HSC population. HSCs respond to various cytokines with activation and transdifferentiation to myofibroblasts. The accompanying chronic inflammation further reduces the NK cell-dependent induction of myofibroblast apoptosis. Myofibroblasts synthesize and secrete vast amounts of collagen and cytokines that provide the basis of liver fibrosis. Nanotherapies against collagen production, activation [39], and differentiation of HSCs are explored preclinically with promising results. Additionally to HSC-directed therapeutics, antagonizing pathophysiological attraction of inflammatory monocyte-derived macrophages into the liver may further present a druggable target since those macrophages directly promote fibrosis and hinder KC to stimulate anti-fibrotic regulatory T cell differentiation.

Another approach to increase the tolerogenic capacity of the liver is the modulation of biotransformation and support of hepatocytes during critical illness. Hepatocytes sequester cytokines, MAMPs, DAMPs, and PAMPs, and metabolize and eliminate them. The failure of hepatocytes to biotransform and excrete small molecules is often the cause for pro-inflammatory cholestatic phenotype, cytokine secretion, and cell death and impairs the liver homeostasis significantly. Key enzymes such as PI3K-γ and protein kinases are involved in many intracellular pathways responsible for trafficking molecules keeping up the biotransformation and elimination. The disturbances of kinase signaling in the liver had been associated with cholestasis in various experimental conditions such as sepsis or ischemia-reperfusion injury. However, the bottleneck of these targets is their different off-target effects on the immune system. It can compromise their success in sepsis by inhibiting the immune system and thus bacterial defense. Therefore, tissue-specific drug application is a promising avenue, and various nanocarriers allow a liver-directed application of small molecules, oligonucleotides, or genes developed to overcome side effects from the uptake of a drug in unwanted tissues. The restoration of liver function in the critically ill utilizing such targeted kinase inhibitors has been promising in experimental settings and provides an indirect but sufficient way to modulate the liver's immune response.

Interventions targeting cell interaction or metabolism in the liver may resolve pathophysiological changes that reduce the tolerogenic capacity and make the liver more vulnerable to decompensation due to infection and other inflammatory stimuli.

In such a vulnerable setting, the threshold to be overcome, resulting in a liver-driven cytokine storm, is significantly lowered, increasing the risk of decompensation and multiple-organ failure [40].

In liver transplants and autoimmune disorders, immunosuppressive drugs are applied to suppress inflammation and thus increase tolerogenic signaling pathways that support the resolution of inflammation, reduce subsequent fibrosis, and foster liver regeneration. However, the risk of infections increases under such circumstances due to the systemic side effects on the immune system. To harbor the tissue-specific immune modulation, targeted immune-modulatory medicines such as a combination of TGF-β and erythropoietin to increase liver regeneration had been applied successfully. In addition, in case of underlying genetic variations that result in a vulnerable tolerogenic liver phenotype, personalized medicines, as developed for type I interferonopathies, may be applied [41].

In sepsis, corticosteroids such as methylprednisolone, dexamethasone, or hydrocortisone were employed to suppress inflammation, albeit their positive effect on outcome remains controversial. However, recent clinical trials, supported by experimental data, would support a role for IFN-γ-to-IL-10 ratio, a measure for the body's control over the immune response, including the liver's innate immune response [42], and may be applied as a theranostic biomarker for a personalized, successful use of corticosteroids in critical illness [43].

A more pronounced cytokine storm, as it occurs in critical courses of SARS-CoV-2 infections, may be controlled through targeted neutralizing anti-cytokine antibodies, additionally to the use of corticosteroids as general immune regulators [44]. Compounds such as the IFN-γ inhibitor emapalumab and the TNF-α inhibitor adalimumab attenuate neutrophil-triggered inflammation but may attenuate pathogen clearance. In addition, positive regulatory cytokines of inflammation or their receptors are neutralized to counteract high levels of IL-6 (e.g., tocilizumab) or IL-1 (e.g., anakinra). JAK inhibitors were also further approved in such scenarios as immunosuppressive agents (e.g., ruxolitinib). More invasive approach might be utilizing blood purification therapy, but such interventions' clinical benefit is controversial. Also, the use of mesenchymal stem cells, which can modulate immune cells and may act as a source to enhance regeneration, seems promising [45].

The long hyperinflammatory phase causes immune suppression in the liver, and immune-stimulating cytokines and antibodies were developed to reverse those effects [46]. Another example highlighting the value of immune-modulatory therapies is the use of tremelimumab, a cytotoxic T-lymphocyte-associated protein (CTLA) 4 (CD152) inhibitor in patients with HCV infection and hepatocellular carcinoma [47]. CD152 is an immune checkpoint, and its expression efficiently blocks its ability to kill cancer cells. The blockage of CD152 in phase II clinical trial resulted in a favorable antitumor and antiviral response [48]. However, different immune checkpoint inhibitors might result in other clinical observations. For example, atezolizumab infiltrated conventional T cells to the liver parenchyma and was associated with liver fibrosis [49, 50]. The complexity of the immune-modulatory mechanism makes therapies and generalization of such results challenging.

Summary

The liver is the largest immunological organ in the body. It comprises specialized immune cells and a vast population of metabolic active cells, namely hepatocytes. Together with endothelial cells and contractile stellate cells, this network controls the body's metabolism, protein and molecule synthesis, storage, and immune reactions in health and disease. In health, the liver maintains a tolerogenic environment and operates in an anti-inflammatory mode that allows the organ to inactivate microbial compounds and potential harmful pathogens entering the body on a daily basis mostly through the gut. However, inflammatory stimuli and circulation failure in patients on intensive care units often trigger a complex immune response and local and often diffuse hypoxic events. Together with metabolic reprogramming of hepatocytes, ductal inflammation, and cholestasis, those changes may lead to liver dysfunction, an underestimated and early poor prognostic event in sepsis. Various studies depicted that the disturbance of this delicate balance between pro- and anti-inflammatory reactions makes the body vulnerable translating into an increased short- and long-term mortality in intensive care units in patients who have experienced a liver failure throughout the course of disease.

> **Take-Home Messages**
>
> ▬ The liver encounters foreign material from the gut and signals in a tolerogenic environment an anti-inflammatory reaction.
> ▬ All liver cells create an immunological network that serves as a surveillance system and first line of defense against danger signals and pathogens.
> ▬ The liver is an immunological organ that controls the host's response to inflammatory stimuli and infection.
> ▬ The immune response is modulated through resident immune cells, such as specialized T cells, natural killer cells, and Kupffer cells, plus the endothelial and metabolic active hepatocytes through the removal of endo- and xenobiotics and secretion of inflammatory molecules such as acute-phase proteins.
> ▬ Comorbidities of the liver reduce the tolerogenic capacity, thus reducing the body's ability to counteract inflammatory stimuli and worsen the course of disease in the critically ill.
> ▬ Liver failure occurs early in critically ill and is an independent risk factor for mortality in critically ill.
> ▬ The human body is a holobiont, and the interaction between microbiome and host is critically controlled in the gut-liver axis, reflecting a most powerful interface that determines prognosis in the critically ill.
> ▬ The immune signaling in the liver depends on the genetic pre-deposition, comorbidities, and type of injury, and therapy requires a personalized approach for an efficient treatment.
> ▬ Nanomedicine and other targeted approaches are promising avenues to selectively interfere with the liver's immunology and restore the tolerogenic environment that supports the host to control the systemic host response and fight a disease efficiently.

13

References

1. Wang Y, Zhang C. The roles of liver-resident lymphocytes in liver diseases. Front Immunol. 2019;10:1582.
2. Scoville SD, Freud AG, Caligiuri MA. Modeling human natural killer cell development in the era of innate lymphoid cells. Front Immunol [Internet]. 2017 [cited 2021 Dec 28];8:360. https://pubmed.ncbi.nlm.nih.gov/28396671/.
3. Mikulak J, Bruni E, Oriolo F, Di Vito C, Mavilio D. Hepatic natural killer cells: organ-specific sentinels of liver immune homeostasis and physiopathology. Front Immunol. 2019;10:946.
4. Mellergård J, Edström M, Jenmalm MC, Dahle C, Vrethem M, Ernerudh J. Increased B cell and cytotoxic NK cell proportions and increased T cell responsiveness in blood of natalizumab-treated multiple sclerosis patients. PLoS One [Internet]. 2013 [cited 2021 Dec 28];8(12):e81685. https://pubmed.ncbi.nlm.nih.gov/24312575/.
5. Pellicci DG, Koay HF, Berzins SP. Thymic development of unconventional T cells: how NKT cells, MAIT cells and γδ T cells emerge. Nat Rev Immunol [Internet]. 2020 [cited 2021 Dec 28];20(12):756–70. https://www.nature.com/articles/s41577-020-0345-y.
6. Ficht X, Iannacone M. Immune surveillance of the liver by T cells. Sci Immunol [Internet]. 2020 [cited 2021 Dec 28];5(51):eaba2351. https://www.science.org/doi/abs/10.1126/sciimmunol.aba2351.
7. Wen Y, Lambrecht J, Ju C, Tacke F. Hepatic macrophages in liver homeostasis and diseases-diversity, plasticity and therapeutic opportunities. Cell Mol Immunol [Internet]. 2020 [cited 2021 Dec 28];18(1):45–56. https://www.nature.com/articles/s41423-020-00558-8.

8. Thomson AW, Knolle PA. Antigen-presenting cell function in the tolerogenic liver environment. Nat Rev Immunol [Internet]. 2010 [cited 2021 Dec 28];10(11):753–66. https://www.nature.com/articles/nri2858.

9. Gabrilovich DI, Nagaraj S. Myeloid-derived suppressor cells as regulators of the immune system. Nat Rev Immunol [Internet]. 2009 [cited 2021 Dec 28];9(3):162–74. https://www.nature.com/articles/nri2506.

10. Crispe IN. Liver antigen-presenting cells. J Hepatol [Internet]. 2011 [cited 2021 Dec 29];54(2):357–65. https://pubmed.ncbi.nlm.nih.gov/21084131/.

11. Dou L, Ono Y, Chen YF, Thomson AW, Chen XP. Hepatic dendritic cells, the tolerogenic liver environment, and liver disease. Semin Liver Dis [Internet]. 2018 [cited 2021 Dec 29];38(2):170–80. https://pubmed.ncbi.nlm.nih.gov/29871022/.

12. Zheng M, Tian Z. Liver-mediated adaptive immune tolerance. Front Immunol. 2019;5(10):2525.

13. Bacher A, Zimpfer M. Hot topics in liver intensive care. Transplant Proc [Internet]. 2008 [cited 2021 Dec 29];40(4):1179–82. https://pubmed.ncbi.nlm.nih.gov/18555143/.

14. Olson JC, Wendon JA, Kramer DJ, Arroyo V, Jalan R, Garcia-Tsao G, et al. Intensive care of the patient with cirrhosis. Hepatology [Internet]. 2011 [cited 2021 Dec 29];54(5):1864–72. https://pubmed.ncbi.nlm.nih.gov/21898477/.

15. Levesque E, Saliba F, Ichaï P, Samuel D. Outcome of patients with cirrhosis requiring mechanical ventilation in ICU. J Hepatol [Internet]. 2014 [cited 2021 Dec 29];60(3):570–8. https://pubmed.ncbi.nlm.nih.gov/24280294/.

16. Weil D, Levesque E, McPhail M, Cavallazzi R, Theocharidou E, Cholongitas E, et al. Prognosis of cirrhotic patients admitted to intensive care unit: a meta-analysis. Ann Intensive Care [Internet]. 2017 [cited 2021 Dec 29];7(1):33. /pmc/articles/PMC5359266/.

17. Meersseman P, Langouche L, du Plessis J, Korf H, Mekeirele M, Laleman W, et al. The intensive care unit course and outcome in acute-on-chronic liver failure are comparable to other populations. J Hepatol [Internet]. 2018 [cited 2021 Dec 29];69(4):803–9. https://pubmed.ncbi.nlm.nih.gov/29730473/.

18. Koch C, Edinger F, Fischer T, Brenck F, Hecker A, Katzer C, et al. Comparison of qSOFA score, SOFA score, and SIRS criteria for the prediction of infection and mortality among surgical intermediate and intensive care patients. World J Emerg Surg [Internet]. 2020 [cited 2021 Dec 29];15(1):63. /pmc/articles/PMC7687806/.

19. Lightsey JM, Rockey DC. Current concepts in ischemic hepatitis. Curr Opin Gastroenterol [Internet]. 2017 [cited 2021 Dec 29];33(3):158–63. https://pubmed.ncbi.nlm.nih.gov/28346236/.

20. Fuhrmann V, Kneidinger N, Herkner H, Heinz G, Nikfardjam M, Bojic A, et al. Hypoxic hepatitis: underlying conditions and risk factors for mortality in critically ill patients. Intensive Care Med [Internet]. 2009 [cited 2021 Dec 29];35(8):1397–405. https://pubmed.ncbi.nlm.nih.gov/19506833/.

21. Jenniskens M, Langouche L, Vanwijngaerden YM, Mesotten D, Van den Berghe G. Cholestatic liver (dys)function during sepsis and other critical illnesses. Intensive Care Med [Internet]. 2016 [cited 2021 Dec 29];42(1):16–27. https://pubmed.ncbi.nlm.nih.gov/26392257/.

22. Horvatits T, Drolz A, Trauner M, Fuhrmann V. Liver injury and failure in critical illness. Hepatology [Internet]. 2019 [cited 2021 Dec 29];70(6):2204–15. https://onlinelibrary.wiley.com/doi/full/10.1002/hep.30824.

23. Shah R, John S. Cholestatic jaundice. StatPearls [Internet]. 2018 [cited 2021 Dec 29]. http://europepmc.org/books/NBK482279.

24. Wijarnpreecha K, Thongprayoon C, Sanguankeo A, Upala S, Ungprasert P, Cheungpasitporn W. Hepatitis C infection and intrahepatic cholestasis of pregnancy: a systematic review and meta-analysis. Clin Res Hepatol Gastroenterol. 2017;41(1):39–45.

25. Delemos AS, Friedman LS. Systemic causes of cholestasis. Clin Liver Dis [Internet]. 2013 [cited 2021 Dec 29];17(2):301. /pmc/articles/PMC4378837/.

26. Kramer L, Jordan B, Druml W, Bauer P, Metnitz PGH. Incidence and prognosis of early hepatic dysfunction in critically ill patients—a prospective multicenter study. Crit Care Med [Internet]. 2007 [cited 2021 Dec 29];35(4):1099–104. https://pubmed.ncbi.nlm.nih.gov/17334250/.

27. Mesotten D, Wauters J, Van Den Berghe G, Wouters PJ, Milants I, Wilmer A. The effect of strict blood glucose control on biliary sludge and cholestasis in critically ill patients. J Clin Endocrinol Metab [Internet]. 2009 [cited 2021 Dec 29];94(7):2345–52. https://pubmed.ncbi.nlm.nih.gov/19366849/.

28. Brienza N, Dalfino L, Cinnella G, Diele C, Bruno F, Fiore T. Jaundice in critical illness: promoting factors of a concealed reality. Intensive Care Med [Internet]. 2006 [cited 2021 Dec 29];32(2):267–74. https://pubmed.ncbi.nlm.nih.gov/16450099/.

29. Zhang J, Xu M, Chen T, Zhou Y. Correlation between liver stiffness and diastolic function, left ventricular hypertrophy, and right cardiac function in patients with ejection fraction preserved heart failure. Front Cardiovasc Med. 2021;8:748173.

30. Marshall JC. New translational research provides insights into liver dysfunction in sepsis. PLoS Med [Internet]. 2012 [cited 2021 Dec 29];9(11):e1001341. https://journals.plos.org/plosmedicine/article?id=10.1371/journal.pmed.1001341.

31. Liu K, Wang FS, Xu R. Neutrophils in liver diseases: pathogenesis and therapeutic targets. Cell Mol Immunol [Internet]. 2020 [cited 2021 Dec 29];18(1):38–44. https://www.nature.com/articles/s41423-020-00560-0.

32. Schmidt-Arras D, Rose-John S. IL-6 pathway in the liver: from physiopathology to therapy. J Hepatol. 2016;64(6):1403–15.

33. Gulhar R, Ashraf MA, Jialal I. Physiology, acute phase reactants. StatPearls [Internet]. 2021 [cited 2021 Dec 29]. https://www.ncbi.nlm.nih.gov/books/NBK519570/.

34. Schaarschmidt B, Vlaic S, Medyukhina A, Neugebauer S, Nietzsche S, Gonnert FA, et al. Molecular signatures of liver dysfunction are distinct in fungal and bacterial infections in mice. Theranostics. 2018;8(14):3766–80.

35. Yan J, Li S, Li S. The role of the liver in sepsis [Internet]. vol. 33. International Reviews of Immunology. Informa Healthcare; 2014 [cited 2020 Dec 29]. p. 498–510. /pmc/articles/PMC4160418/?report=abstract.

36. Vincent JL, Lefrant JY, Kotfis K, Nanchal R, Martin-Loeches I, Wittebole X, et al. Comparison of European ICU patients in 2012 (ICON) versus 2002 (SOAP). Intensive Care Med [Internet]. 2018 [cited 2021 Dec 29];44(3):337–44. https://pubmed.ncbi.nlm.nih.gov/29450593/.

37. Peter JV, Woran JL, Phillips-Hughes J. A metaanalysis of treatment outcomes of early enteral versus early parenteral nutrition in hospitalized patients. Crit Care Med [Internet]. 2005 [cited 2021 Dec 29];33(1):213–20. https://pubmed.ncbi.nlm.nih.gov/15644672/.

38. Reintam Blaser A, Starkopf J, Alhazzani W, Berger MM, Casaer MP, Deane AM, et al. Early enteral nutrition in critically ill patients: ESICM clinical practice guidelines. Intensive Care Med [Internet]. 2017 [cited 2021 Dec 29];43(3):380–98. https://pubmed.ncbi.nlm.nih.gov/28168570/.

39. Van den Berghe G, Wilmer A, Hermans G, Meersseman W, Wouters PJ, Milants I, et al. Intensive insulin therapy in the medical ICU. N Engl J Med [Internet]. 2006 [cited 2021 Dec 29];354(5):449–61. https://www.nejm.org/doi/full/10.1056/nejmoa052521.

40. Fuhrmann V, Bauer M, Wilmer A. The persistent potential of extracorporeal therapies in liver failure. Intensive Care Med [Internet]. 2020 [cited 2021 Dec 29];46(3):528–30. https://pubmed.ncbi.nlm.nih.gov/31822935/.

41. Leonhardt J, Haider RS, Sponholz C, Leonhardt S, Drube J, Spengler K, et al. Circulating bile acids in liver failure activate TGR5 and induce monocyte dysfunction. Cell Mol Gastroenterol Hepatol. 2021;12(1):25–40.

42. Hassan R, Tammam SN, El Safy S, Abdel-Halim M, Asimakopoulou A, Weiskirchen R, et al. Prevention of hepatic stellate cell activation using JQ1- and atorvastatin-loaded chitosan nanoparticles as a promising approach in therapy of liver fibrosis. Eur J Pharm Biopharm. 2019;(134):96–106.

43. Van Der Poll T, Van De Veerdonk FL, Scicluna BP, Netea MG. The immunopathology of sepsis and potential therapeutic targets. Nat Rev Immunol [Internet]. 2017 [cited 2021 Dec 29];17(7):407–20. https://pubmed.ncbi.nlm.nih.gov/28436424/.

44. Bernardi M, Moreau R, Angeli P, Schnabl B, Arroyo V. Mechanisms of decompensation and organ failure in cirrhosis: from peripheral arterial vasodilation to systemic inflammation hypothesis. J Hepatol. 2015;63(5):1272–84.

45. Melki I, Frémond ML. Type I interferonopathies: from a novel concept to targeted therapeutics. Curr Rheumatol Rep [Internet]. 2020 [cited 2021 Dec 29];22(7):1–14. https://link.springer.com/article/10.1007/s11926-020-00909-4.

46. Sommerfeld O, Medyukhina A, Neugebauer S, Ghait M, Ulferts S, Lupp A, et al. Targeting complement C5a receptor 1 for the treatment of immunosuppression in sepsis. Mol Ther [Internet]. 2020 [cited 2020 Dec 29]. https://pubmed.ncbi.nlm.nih.gov/32966769/.

13

47. Sangro B, Gomez-Martin C, De La Mata M, Iñarrairaegui M, Garralda E, Barrera P, et al. A clinical trial of CTLA-4 blockade with tremelimumab in patients with hepatocellular carcinoma and chronic hepatitis C. J Hepatol [Internet]. 2013 [cited 2021 Dec 29];59(1):81–8. https://pubmed.ncbi.nlm.nih.gov/23466307/.

48. Tang L, Yin Z, Hu Y, Mei H. Controlling cytokine storm is vital in COVID-19. Front Immunol. 2020;11:3158.

49. Gazdic M, Arsenijevic A, Markovic BS, Volarevic A, Dimova I, Djonov V, et al. Mesenchymal stem cell-dependent modulation of liver diseases. Int J Biol Sci. 2017;13(9):1109–17.

50. Cohen J V., Dougan M, Zubiri L, Reynolds KL, Sullivan RJ, Misdraji J. Liver biopsy findings in patients on immune checkpoint inhibitors. Mod Pathol [Internet]. 2020 [cited 2021 Dec 29];34(2):426–37. https://www.nature.com/articles/s41379-020-00653-1.

Hemostasis

Romein W. G. Dujardin, Derek J. B. Kleinveld, and Nicole P. Juffermans

Contents

Hemostasis

Learning Objectives
- Describe the pathophysiology of inflammation-induced coagulopathy
- Identify patients at risk for inflammation-induced coagulopathy
- Know the different scoring systems used to diagnose DIC/SIC
- Understand the clinical consequences of inflammation-induced coagulopathy and DIC, including both bleeding and thrombosis
- Be familiar with the methods to prevent bleeding in patients with inflammation-induced coagulopathy
- Know anticoagulant strategies in patients with inflammation-induced coagulopathy and DIC

14.1 Introduction

An inflammatory host response is invariably accompanied by disturbances in the coagulation system. A procoagulant response exists in which coagulation factors and platelets are consumed in the formation of (micro)thrombi. Coagulation disorders range from mildly decreased platelet count to disseminated intravascular coagulation (DIC). Whereas DIC is a recognized entity with a strong association with adverse outcome, less attention has been given to the broader concept of inflammatory-driven consumption coagulopathy. However, DIC most likely is not an "on or off phenomenon," but rather reflects a continuum. In line with this, a linear relationship exists between platelet count and mortality in patients on the intensive care unit (ICU), suggesting that even modestly decreased platelet counts are associated with harm [1].

In this chapter, we refer to this condition as inflammation-induced coagulopathy. The associated mortality of coagulation alterations in the ICU is probably mediated via increased risk of both bleeding and macro- and micro-thromboembolic events, which contribute to organ failure. Thereby, the management of inflammation-induced coagulopathy is a challenge. Interventions to diminish the risk of bleeding may aggravate thrombosis and vice versa, anticoagulant strategies increase the risk of bleeding. Of importance, there does not seem to be a safe platelet threshold, because also patients with a mildly disturbed platelet count have an increased risk of bleeding [1].

Here, we describe the pathophysiology underlying the coagulation derangements that occur during a dysregulated immune response in ICU patients, as well as incidence, risk factors, and outcome of inflammation-induced coagulopathy. In addition, we discuss management strategies of patients who are (at risk for) bleeding and developing thrombosis.

14.2 The Pathophysiology of Inflammation-Induced Coagulopathy

14.2.1 Normal Hemostasis

In normal hemostasis, damage to the endothelium exposes the subendothelial collagen layer [2]. Circulating platelets become activated and adhere to the site of injury [3]. This adhesion is strengthened by von Willebrand Factor (vWF) and its interconnection with platelet glycoprotein domains (i.e., GPIb) [4]. The localization of plate-lets promotes interaction with collagen. These activated platelets in response to injury and adhesion release contents of stored granules (i.e., ADP, platelet-activating factor, thromboxane) into the circulation, thereby activating additional platelets [5]. The contents of these granules also increase calcium levels within platelets increasing the affinity of glycoprotein IIb/IIIa to bind fibrinogen [6, 7]. Together with shape changes in platelets, the aggregation of platelets completes the primary hemostasis.

Secondary hemostasis includes the formation of a cross-linked fibrin network [8]. Regardless of this name, the processes of primary and secondary hemostasis occur simultaneously. Secondary hemostasis starts by exposure of tissue factor (TF) from damaged endothelium, leading to the activation of coagulation factors. TF first acti-vates factor VII, serving as an activator of the common pathways Xa, Va, and throm-bin (IIa) [3]. Thrombin orchestrates many processes, including activation of factor XII and VIII, which are part of the contact activation pathway. Thrombin most impor-tantly results in conversion of fibrinogen to fibrin [9]. Fibrin cross-linking occurs due to factor XIII activation, resulting in an increase in stability of the clot [10]. Together with the primary platelet plug, this process finalizes the secondary hemostasis.

A procoagulant response will always generate an anticoagulant response, to counterbalance vessel obstruction due to excessive coagulation. Anticoagulant pro-teases come into play, such as antithrombin, protein C, and tissue factor pathway inhibitor (TFPI) [11]. Antithrombin inhibits thrombin and inactivates factor X (FXa), reducing the capacity to form fibrin [8, 12]. Protein C is a vitamin K-dependent protease and is converted to activated protein C by thrombin, a process that is accel-erated during complex formation of thrombin with thrombomodulin [13, 14]. Furthermore, protein S functions as a cofactor of activated protein C, leading to inactivation of factor Va and factor VIIIa [15]. TFPI is produced from endothelial cells and can be found on the surface of endothelial cells as well as circulating in the plasma [16]. TFPI inhibits the tissue factor pathway. First, TFPI binds to factor Xa and then subsequently adheres to the TF-FVIIa complex, forming a new complex in which factor VIIa and factor Xa are inhibited. Protein S enhances the interaction of TFPI with factor Xa [16].

Next to the anticoagulant pathways, the fibrinolytic system actively degrades (excessive) fibrin formation, keeping the procoagulant system in check [17, 18]. Plasmin is the main enzyme of the fibrinolytic system. It is synthesized by the liver in the form of its proenzyme plasminogen. Plasminogen does not cleave fibrin but binds to fibrin and is therefore incorporated into the clot. Both tissue plasminogen activa-tor (tPA) and urokinase-type plasminogen activator (uPa) can activate plasmin. tPA is released into the blood by damaged endothelial cells [19]. tPA has the capacity to bind to fibrin where it converts clot-bound plasminogen into plasmin. Plasmin then cleaves fibrin into fibrin degradation products (FDP, D-dimers). These end products of lysis can be measured in clinical practice.

Fibrinolysis is also counterbalanced, by several inhibitors, acting on different proteins. Plasminogen activator inhibitors (PAIs) inhibit tPA. Plasmin is inhibited by inhibitors such as a2-antiplasmin and a2-macroglobulin. Finally, thrombin activat-able fibrinolysis inhibitor (TAFI) removes the C-terminal of fibrin, making it a less potent cofactor for tPA-mediated plasminogen activation [20, 21].

In summary, the normal hemostatic response is promoted by endothelial cells, platelets, and coagulation factors with the end product being a stable fibrin clot. A coagulation response is kept in balance by anticoagulant proteins and the fibrinolytic system, with the aim to maintain vascular patency.

14.2.2 Inflammation-Induced Alterations in the Coagulation System

Inflammation and coagulation are closely related systems, and both play pivotal roles in the pathogenesis of critical illness [22, 23]. The development of coagulopathy is associated with the need of transfusion and mortality [24]. The phenotypes of the coagulopathy are wide, ranging from isolated thrombocytopenia to more complex coagulation defects [25, 26].

The similarity in many underlying pathologies in critically ill patients is a highly activated host-immune response to either pathogens (i.e., sepsis) or tissue damage (i.e., trauma, surgery, and ischemia). The difficulty lies within the balance of the immune and coagulation response in response to these pathologies. For example, immunothrombosis may be beneficial in case of a local barrier loss. However, in systemic inflammatory illness, immunothrombotic dysregulation results in a systemic coagulopathy with microvascular obstructions, which hamper oxygen and nutrient supply to organs.

The main drivers of immunothrombosis are platelets and innate immune cells (i.e., neutrophils, monocytes, and macrophages) [27]. The activation and interconnected processes between platelets and immune cells are mediated by the coagulation and complement systems [28]. Pathogen- and/or damage-associated molecular patterns (PAMPs and/or DAMPs) trigger both platelets and neutrophils, via toll-like receptors, NOD-like receptors, and c-type lectin receptors [29]. Platelets can present the PAMPs and DAMPs to neutrophils, thereby promoting the activation of neutrophils resulting in neutrophil extracellular trap (NET) formation [30]. NETs are composed of DNA, histones, and contents from neutrophil granules (i.e., myeloperoxidase, neutrophil elastase) [31]. These NETs have high platelet binding potential, thereby forming microthrombosis.

The complement system contributes to a bidirectional interplay between inflammation and a procoagulant response with thrombosis during critical illness [32]. Several complement factors (i.e., C1q, C3a, C5a, and MAC) can activate platelets. Vice versa, platelets provide a surface for complement activation. Pro-inflammatory mediators can also activate platelets. Histamine and interleukins lead to a release of ultralarge von Willebrand factor multimers from the endothelium [33]. These vWF multimers promote platelet thrombi. Normally, these vWF multimers are cleaved by ADAMTS13 activity into smaller fragments with less affinity to bind to platelets; however, as ADAMTS13 levels decrease during inflammatory conditions, its capacity to cleave vWF fails to meet the excessive release of vWF. Causes for this imbalance probably are multifactorial, including interleukins, coagulation factors, and plasmin activity, as all of these can inhibit ADAMTS13 activity or potentially degrade parts of ADAMTS13.

The anticoagulant system also fails in acute critical illness in which antithrombin and protein C pathways are downregulated, thereby increasing thrombin generation, promoting microthrombosis. Thereby, the fibrinolytic pathway becomes less active, probably due to an upregulation of plasminogen activator inhibitor.

Taken together, during acute critical illness, a shift in balance towards a more procoagulant response is observed, while anticoagulant responses are downregulated.

14.3 Specific Forms of Inflammation-Induced Coagulopathy

The first and most frequent alteration that is apparent in laboratory testing of coagulation disorders in ICU patients is a decrease in platelet count. There is a wide variance in estimates of the incidence of thrombocytopenia, ranging from 10 to 65% of ICU patients [34]. This is mainly due to varying definitions of thrombocytopenia. Thrombocytopenia also complicates critical illness in younger age groups: 20–50% of critically ill neonates develop thrombocytopenia, including 5–10% with platelet counts less than 50×10^9/L [35].

A prolonged PT is supposedly somewhat less common, although still a frequent finding, occurring in 10–30% of ICU patients [36]. Of note, only a proportion of patients with these abnormalities go on to develop end-stage coagulation abnormalities, which is overt disseminated intravascular coagulation (DIC).

14.3.1 Disseminated Intravascular Coagulation

DIC is defined as a systemic intravascular activation of coagulation with a loss of localization, leading to access generation of thrombin and deposition of fibrin, with formation of widespread microvascular thrombosis. These microthrombi are thought to impair organ perfusion and to contribute to organ failure. During the coagulation process, consumption of coagulation factors and aggregation of platelets occur, as reviewed earlier in this chapter.

DIC never occurs by itself as a specific illness. It is always secondary to an underlying disorder. DIC is associated with several clinical conditions that generally involve activation of systemic inflammation. These are listed in ◘ Table 14.1.

14

◘ **Table 14.1** Clinical conditions associated with DIC

Severe infection and sepsis
Solid tumors
Hematologic malignancies
Obstetrical complications (HELLP, fluid embolism, eclampsia)
Acute pancreatitis
Trauma
Severe transfusion reactions
Snake venom or other severe toxic reactions
Heat stroke and hyperthermia

Epidemiology of DIC has recently been summarized [37], but studies are >20 years old, and they differ in diagnostic criteria and study population. What is apparent though is that DIC is a frequent complication of sepsis, occurring in 30–60% of cases, whereas only 5–10% of patients with solid cancer develop DIC [37]. These epidemiologic figures corroborate with inflammatory pathways driving DIC pathogenesis.

It has been suggested that these different causes of DIC trigger the coagulation response differently, potentially yielding different phenotypes with differential risks of bleeding and thrombosis.

14.3.2 Sepsis-Induced Coagulopathy (SIC)

The most common cause of DIC is sepsis, accounting for 80% of all critically ill adult and pediatric patients with DIC [37, 38]. The concept of immunothrombosis has been put forward, reflecting tight interactions between the innate immune system and the coagulation response. A hallmark of sepsis-associated coagulation alterations is overproduction of PAI-1, leading to suppression of fibrinolysis. Thereby, this phenotype may present with a high risk of thromboembolic events. The ensuing widespread deposition of fibrin is thought to contribute to microthrombi, which obstruct the microcirculation and contribute to organ failure. The implication of this may be that antifibrinolytic therapy should be avoided while patients may benefit from procoagulant interventions.

14.3.3 Malignancy-Associated DIC

Some hematological diseases are characterized by a DIC form with a hyper-fibrinolytic phenotype [39]. Acute promyelocytic cells can express a co-receptor for plasminogen and tPA, which leads to plasmin activation and fibrinolysis. Thereby, bleeding is a much more frequent problem, necessitating antifibrinolytic therapy, while thrombosis and organ failure are less frequently observed.

14.3.4 Obstetric Associated DIC

Obstetric complications associated with DIC occur in 1 per 20,000 patients undergoing delivery and consist of abruptio placentae, amniotic fluid embolism, and preeclampsia [40]. In patients with abruptio placentae, the cause of the activation of the coagulation system most likely lies in the leakage of tissue factor from the placental system into the maternal circulation. In case of amniotic fluid embolism, the release of procoagulant phosphatidylserine and tissue factor exposing extracellular vesicles may be of importance in developing DIC.

14.3.5 COVID-Associated Coagulopathy: An Exception to this Chapter

Of note, COVID is an inflammatory driven procoagulant phenotype, but it is entirely different from SIC and does not fall under the term inflammation-induced coagulopathy as used in this chapter. In COVID, the procoagulant response is driven by endothelial activation, exemplified by high activity of vWF and of sTM derived from the endothelium. Platelet counts, however, largely remain normal and only become decreased when patients are about to die [41].

14.3.6 Trauma-Induced Coagulopathy (TIC)

TIC occurs in 25% of trauma patients and contributes to mortality [42]. Following tissue injury, coagulation factors are activated, resulting in a thrombin burst, which depletes fibrinogen. Injured cells release tPA, resulting in a fibrinolytic response. In addition to a loss of coagulation factors, shock results in increased soluble thrombomodulin, which complexes with thrombin and leads to activation of protein C, leading to further inhibition of coagulation factors and increased lysis. All of this contributes to an increased bleeding risk. TIC differs from septic DIC, as fibrinogen levels are low and aPC levels are high. However, the time course in TIC is of importance. After the bleeding has stopped, an endogenous ongoing procoagulant response remains, which may induce microthrombi and mediate organ failure [43]. This late response may in some ways resemble DIC, but for the sake of clarity should not be termed as such.

14.4 Diagnosis of Inflammation-Induced Coagulopathy

A mildly decreased platelet count or a mildly prolonged PT that does not fulfill a diagnosis of DIC is currently not regarded as relevant, because these laboratory tests do not trigger an intervention. However, given the association between even mildly reduced platelet counts and mortality in the ICU, we propose to refer to these phenomena as inflammation-induced coagulopathy [1]. Even though specific therapy is currently lacking, the use of a proper term can be useful for defining patient groups for future research aiming at improved monitoring of the risks of bleeding and thrombosis or aimed to study specific pro- or anticoagulant interventions.

14.4.1 Disseminated Intravascular Coagulation

None of the laboratory values (platelet count, PT, APTT, fibrinogen, and fibrinogen degradation products) alone is specific enough to determine whether DIC is present or not. Therefore, scoring systems have been developed to assess the diagnosis. The International Society on Thrombosis and Haemostasis (ISTH) DIC score is widely used to diagnose patients with *overt* DIC (◻ Table 14.2). For the ISTH DIC score, four laboratory values (platelet count, PT, D-dimer or another fibrin degradation marker, and fibrinogen) are required in order to score between 0 and 8 points. An ISTH DIC score ≥5 confirms the diagnosis of DIC.

While this scoring remains the main method of establishing a diagnosis of DIC, it is often not sensitive enough to detect its presence; 50% of cases of DIC have a normal PT for example. Low or rapidly decreasing platelet levels are the most common abnormal hematological feature, though these too may be normal in some cases [44].

As anticoagulant therapy may potentially improve outcomes in patients with coagulation alterations, it is important to identify sepsis patients with DIC at an earlier stage in order to include them into trials investigating anticoagulant interventions. This necessitates a simple stratification tool. The Japanese Association for Acute Medicine (JAAM) definition is specifically designed for inflammation-induced coagulopathy as it consists of a systemic inflammatory response syndrome criteria score (SIRS criteria) and three laboratory values (platelet count, PT, and fibrin degradation marker). A JAAM DIC score of ≥4 confirms the diagnosis of DIC and may also be useful to identify *non-overt* DIC (ISTH score 1–4). However, a potential limitation of the JAAM score is that SIRS has become obsolete in the most recent sepsis definition. In line with this, the term sepsis-induced coagulopathy (SIC) was proposed, which (consistent with the sepsis definition) includes SOFA score next to both international normalized ratio (INR) and platelet count. See ◻ Table 14.2.

◻ **Table 14.2** Inflammation-induced coagulopathy scoring systems

ISTH DIC score		JAAM DIC score		SIC score	
		SIRS criteria		**Total sum SOFA score**	
		0–2	0 points	0	0 points
		≥3	1 point	1	1 point
				≥2	2 points
Platelet count		Platelet count		Platelet count	
>100 × 10⁹/L	0 points	≥120 × 10⁹/L	0 points	≥150 × 10⁹/L	0 points
50–100 × 10⁹/L	1 point	80–120 × 10⁹/L or	1 point	100 to <150 × 10⁹/L	1 point
<50 × 10⁹/L	2 points	>30% decrease in 24 h	3 points	<100 × 10⁹/L	2 points
		<80 × 10⁹/L or >50% decrease in 24 h			
PT (sec prolonged)		PTr (sec, value of patient/normal value)		INR	
≤3	0 points	<1.2	0 points	≤1.2	0 points
3–6	1 point	≥1.2	1 point	>1.2 to 1.4	1 point
>6	2 points			>1.4	2 points
Fibrinogen (g/L)		Fibrin/FDP (mg/L)			
>1	0 points	<10	0 points		
<1	1 point	10–25	1 point		
		≥25	3 points		
FDP/D-dimer					
No change	0 points				
Moderate rise	2 points				
Strong rise	3 points				

14.5 Viscoelastic Tests in the Diagnosis of Inflammation-Induced Coagulopathy

Viscoelastic tests such as rotational thromboelastometry (ROTEM) and thrombo-elastography (TEG) are point-of-care tests that evaluate whole clot formation and degradation, including hypercoagulability. Although limited evidence suggests that viscoelastic tests in sepsis patients may differentiate between patients with a hypo- and hypercoagulable profile [45], current evidence is not sufficient to support the use of viscoelastic testing in these patients since cutoff values that correspond to DIC or hypo- and hypercoagulability remain to be elucidated.

14.6 Clinical Consequences of Inflammation-Induced Coagulopathy

14.6.1 Risk of Bleeding: Incidence and Risk Factors

Inflammation-induced coagulopathy-related bleeding can differ from mild blood loss to spontaneous, massive, and life threatening bleeding [46]. Main bleeding locations include petechiae/ecchymoses or oozing from wounds, sites of intravascular access, mucosal surfaces, and the gastrointestinal tract. Bleeding and thromboembolic events may occur simultaneously, which complicates management. Previous studies report an incidence of major bleeding complications (e.g., intracranial, intrathoracic, intra-abdominal bleeding, or bleeding requiring transfusion) in patients with DIC between 5 and 12% [47, 48]. Although patients with a platelet count $<50 \times 10^9/L$ have a four- to fivefold higher risk for bleeding as compared with patients with a higher platelet count [49–51], risk of bleeding is already increasing in patients with a mildly decreased platelet count, suggesting that a safe platelet "threshold" does not exist [1].

14.6.2 Risk of Thromboembolic Events: Incidence and Risk Factors

Thrombosis in patients with DIC is difficult to diagnose because clot formation primarily involves the microvasculature and therefore often presents as organ failure [37]. Apart from microthrombi, thromboembolic events can also manifest in large arteries and venous vessels, including deep venous thrombosis and pulmonary embolism. In patients with sepsis-associated DIC, microthrombus formation leading to organ failure occurs in up to 70% of patients, while this is a less prominent feature in patients with malignancy-associated DIC [37]. Apart from underlying disease, specific risk factors for (micro)thrombosis have not yet been identified.

14.6.3 Organ Failure

Patients with DIC can have renal, hepatic, and respiratory organ failure, as well as central nervous system (CNS) and cutaneous/skin sequelae. Organ failure, or multiorgan dysfunction syndrome (MODS) in its severest form, during inflammation-induced coagulopathy, is thought to occur both from thrombotic occlusions of small and midsize vessels and by the release of DAMPs and PAMPs during inflammation or injury, which are highly toxic to cells [52]. In line with this, the presence of DIC is an independent and relatively strong predictor of organ dysfunction in critically ill patients [48].

14.6.4 Mortality

DIC occurs secondary to another condition, but it is important to consider that DIC increases the risk of mortality to levels that are higher than those of the initiating disorder. Thereby, DIC is an independent predictor of mortality regardless of the underlying condition [53]. This is illustrated by a study demonstrating that the development of DIC in patients with sepsis increases the risk of death from 27 to 43% [54].

14.7 Prevention of Bleeding in Inflammation-Induced Coagulopathic Patients

Due to prolonged PT and low platelet counts, patients with inflammation-induced coagulopathy quite often receive prophylactic transfusion of plasma or platelets. In general, while managing bleeding risk in patients with inflammation-induced coagulopathy or DIC, the most important issue is to be restrictive with these interventions, as a benefit of liberal use has not been shown and procoagulants *may* confer harm by increasing microthrombus formation in an already procoagulant milieu, contributing to organ failure.

14.7.1 Prophylactic Platelet Transfusion

Thrombocytopenia occurs in 10–30% of ICU patients [34]. Platelet transfusions are commonly used in the ICU; 9–30% of critically ill patients receive a transfusion, approximately 59–68% of which are used to prevent rather than to treat bleeding [55, 56]. Also, risk of bleeding is not merely due to decreased platelet counts, but also due to platelet dysfunction. Currently, due to an absence of tools for reliable assessment of platelet function, guidelines on platelet transfusion often reference isolated tests of platelet count. Based on a trial performed in hematology patients [57], a platelet count of $10–20 \times 10^9$/L is suggested as a trigger for prophylactic platelet transfusions.

14.7.2 Prophylactic Plasma Transfusion

Despite a lack of evidence, an INR of greater than 1.5 is frequently recommended as the threshold for considering FFP transfusion and has been present in (former) guidelines. This cutoff is associated with impending hemostatic failure and represents a fall in the activity of some coagulation factors to less than 50% of normal.

However, an INR of >1.5 does not indicate an increased bleeding risk [58]. Currently, there is no good screening tests for the risk of bleeding.

There is an absence of data indicating benefit of plasma in terms of prevention of bleeding [59, 60]. In addition, plasma does not correct coagulopathy. Naturally, plasma corrects an increased INR because plasma contains factors II, VII, XI, and X. However, there is no effect on thrombin generation [59]. This is also not to be expected, as plasma contains coagulation factors but also anticoagulant proteins. If anything, plasma is associated with increased use of red blood cell transfusion in cardiac surgery patients [60], probably due to dilution. We do not support the use of prophylactic plasma [61].

14.7.3 Tranexamic Acid

A reduction in fibrinolysis is a feature of inflammation-induced coagulopathy in ICU. Thereby, antifibrinolytics should generally be withheld, with the exception of specific situations where hyper-fibrinolysis is present, which can occur in acute promyelocytic leukemia and in some specific solid cancers. Viscoelastic testing can indicate hyperactive fibrinolysis and can help to distinguish in these cases.

14.7.4 Prevention of Bleeding in Coagulopathic Patients Undergoing an Invasive Procedure

In critically ill patients with a coagulopathy, the incidence of major bleeding requiring intervention following placement of central venous catheters is low, with an estimated 0–0.2% [58]. The same numbers are found for chest tube placement or percutaneous tracheotomy. There is no evidence supporting prophylactic administration of plasma [58]. In line with this, correction with plasma is not expected to have any clinical benefits, and our opinion is to abandon the practice of prophylactic plasma transfusion.

For low platelet count, observational data suggest an increase in bleeding risk. For central venous lines, the risk increases at a platelet count of $<20 \times 10^9$/L [62]. For other interventions, there is a paucity of data to support evidence-based practice. However, it is widely accepted that patients requiring surgery or interventional procedures should have a higher platelet transfusion trigger. For the majority of procedures (e.g., laparotomy, drain insertion) in stable, non-bleeding patients, the platelet count should be $>50 \times 10^9$/L. For procedures in critical sites (e.g., brain, eye), the platelet count should be at least 100×10^9/L. We refer to ICU guidelines for further guidance on prophylactic platelet transfusion in specific situations [63].

14.7.5 Treatment of Bleeding in Inflammation-Induced Coagulopathic Patients

Treatment of massive bleeding follows the same principles as in patients without inflammation-induced coagulopathy, aiming at ensuring adequate DO_2 by maintaining Hb levels around 8 g/dL while attempting to correct specific coagulation deficiencies. Of importance, bleeding patients should not be resuscitated with clear fluids in order to avoid dilutional coagulopathy.

Obviously, clinicians should be aware of earlier depletion of factor levels (including fibrinogen) and platelets, as these levels are lower than normal, and thrombin generation is hampered in coagulopathic ICU patients [59]. A recent guideline appeared on the management of bleeding in ICU patients, which was not able to make many recommendations due to the lack of data [64]. Outside the context of massively bleeding trauma patients, the guideline generally suggests to be restrictive with blood products. Concerning antifibrinolytic therapy, tranexamic acid is recommended for patients early after trauma, after obstetric hemorrhage and early after cardiac surgery. In contrast, in patients with a GI bleeding, the guideline suggests to withhold tranexamic acid.

14.8 Clinical Management of Risk of Thrombosis

Critically ill patients have a substantially increased risk of developing a venous thromboembolism (VTE), including deep venous thrombosis and pulmonary embolism, which contribute significantly to patient morbidity and mortality [65].

14.8.1 Pharmacological Thromboprophylaxis

As omission of thromboprophylaxis in the first 24 h after ICU admission is associated with increased mortality, it is advised to start thromboprophylaxis immediately after ICU admission to reduce the occurrence of VTE [66, 67].

Pharmacological thromboprophylactic treatment is also recommended in the presence of DIC and should perhaps only be discontinued in bleeding patients. A policy of discontinuation of thromboprophylaxis in patients with severe thrombocytopenia may appear prudent. However, as outlined, during inflammation, a procoagulant response is ongoing, also in these patients. This is underlined by the finding that patients with mild/moderate thrombocytopenia ($>50 \times 10^9$/L) are not protected against VTE occurrence [68]. In patients with very low platelet counts, the risk of VTE may be lower [69], but the risk is not absent. The risk/benefit of administration of thromboprophylaxis in these patients is not known. Given that ICU patients with inflammation-induced coagulopathy are at risk for thrombosis, that the occurrence of thrombosis requiring full anticoagulation is unwanted in patients with severe thrombocytopenia, and that administration of pharmacological thromboprophylaxis was found to *protect* against the occurrence of thrombocytopenia [1], it is our opinion that ICU patients with inflammation-induced coagulopathy with a very low platelet count should also receive pharmacological thromboprophylaxis.

14.8.2 Type of Pharmacological Thromboprophylaxis

Both unfractionated heparin (UFH) and LMWH, produced by the cleavage of heparin molecules, can be used for thromboprophylaxis. The American Society of

Hematology guidelines recommend that LMWH should be considered over UFH in critically ill patients [66]. In line with this, a recent meta-analysis also demonstrated that the use of LMWH reduced DVT compared to unfractionated heparin [70], without a difference in bleeding complications while occurrence of HITT with LMWH was lower [71].

14.9 Management of Patients with DIC

The cornerstone of DIC treatment remains management of the underlying disorder [72]. Because DIC is characterized by consumption of both the coagulation factors and anticoagulant proteins, possible treatment strategies involving substitution of anticoagulant proteins are also discussed.

14.9.1 Anticoagulant Treatment of (Micro)thrombotic Events

Therapeutic anticoagulation should be administered in the case of an overt thromboembolic event or when organ failure related to clot formation is present (e.g., purpura fulminans) [73].

Therapeutic anticoagulation can be started with either LMWH or UFH considering that to date there are no clinical data to support the choice of one over the other.

In patients with DIC that suffer from both a venous thromboembolism and concomitant bleeding, if possible, it is suggested to discontinue anticoagulation and use a retrievable inferior vena cava filter. When bleeding has ceased, risks and benefits of starting anticoagulation should be assessed on a daily basis [72].

The use of danaparoid sodium and synthetic protease inhibitors such as gabexate mesilate and nafamostat as an anticoagulant therapy in DIC has also been suggested [74], but a beneficial effect on mortality or DIC resolution has not yet been demonstrated in trials. At present, the effect of anti-FXa agents such as fondaparinux or direct oral anticoagulants for anticoagulant treatment in patients with DIC is unclear.

14.9.2 Substitution of Anticoagulant Proteins

Antithrombin (AT) is a protein that inhibits the activity of coagulation factors IIa and Xa, and reduced AT levels in sepsis have been associated with poor outcome [75, 76]. In spite of this, suppletion with AT concentrate failed to improve survival in sepsis patients while increasing bleeding [77]. Of interest, in a subgroup analysis of patients with DIC that did not receive heparin, a remarkable survival benefit was found in the AT concentrate treatment group compared to patients who received placebo [78]. In line with this, both a meta-analysis [79] and an observational multicenter study [80] report a clinical beneficial effect of AT concentrate substitution in septic patients with DIC. However, prospective trials evaluating the effect of AT in patients with sepsis-induced DIC have not yet validated these results.

14

Thrombomodulin is a protein expressed on the surface of endothelial cells that forms a complex with thrombin, thereby inhibiting thrombin activity as well as amplifying the formation of activated protein C. Recombinant human-soluble thrombomodulin (rTM) substitution has been suggested to provide a clinical benefit in patients with DIC [81, 82]. However, a recent RCT investigating the effect of rTM on 28-day mortality in patients with sepsis-associated coagulopathy demonstrated only a nonsignificant mortality reduction of 2.6% in patients treated with rTM compared to patients treated with placebo [83]. Of note, rTM therapy did not provide an increased risk of bleeding. A survival benefit was also reported by a recent meta-analysis that demonstrated a mortality reduction of 13% in patients with a sepsis-induced coagulopathy treated with rTM compared to controls, although also here, statistical significance was not reached [84]. As a result, rTM treatment may provide a potential survival benefit in patients with a sepsis-induced coagulopathy, but findings are uncertain.

Protein C is a proenzyme that is activated by either thrombin, thrombomodulin, or endothelial protein C receptor. Then, activated protein C can inhibit factors Va and VIIIa. Although recombinant activated protein C (rAPC) was initially approved for the treatment of sepsis after promising results in a large-scale RCT [85], rAPC was withdrawn from the market after multiple RCTs failed to demonstrate a survival benefit [86, 87]. There are no RCTs that specifically report on the use of rAPC in patients with DIC.

Tissue factor pathway inhibitor (TFPI) directly inhibits factor Xa as well as the TF/FVII complex, but in spite of positive results in animal studies, a phase 3 trial was not able to show a survival benefit of recombinant TFPI compared to placebo in patients with severe sepsis [88].

In conclusion, prophylactic anticoagulant treatment should be administered in patients with DIC without (a high risk of) bleeding, and therapeutic anticoagulation should be started in case of an overt thrombotic event or when clot-related organ failure is present. Substitution of anticoagulants is not generally recommended as a treatment for DIC but can be considered.

14.10 Treatment of Thrombosis in Inflammation-Induced Coagulopathy

Therapeutic anticoagulation with either unfractionated heparin or LMWH to prevent thrombus propagation is the mainstay of treatment for non-life-threatening thrombosis. For therapeutic purposes, unfractionated heparin remains the most frequently used parenteral therapy. Advantages and disadvantages of UFH and LMWH are listed in ◘ Table 14.3.

In case of a life-threatening thromboembolic event, fibrinolytic therapy with alteplase should be considered. Other pharmacological treatments for therapeutic anticoagulation should only be considered if there are contraindications for UFH or LMWH or if the patient develops a complication from UFH or LMWH treatment and therefore fall out of the scope of this chapter.

◘ Table 14.3 Advantages and disadvantages of UFH vs. LMWH in the critically ill

	Unfractionated heparin (UFH)	Low-molecular-weight heparin (LMWH)
Advantages	Immediate action Continuous administration Short half-life Rapidly reversable No impact on renal function Low cost	Monitoring generally not required Low risk of HITT
Disadvantages	Monitoring required Occurrence of heparin resistance Risk of HITT	Accumulation during renal insufficiency No continuous anticoagulant coverage
Antidote	Protamine	Protamine (but much less effective than in UFH)

Summary

In this chapter, we highlighted the intricate relationship between host response and coagulopathy, arguing that inflammation drives a procoagulant condition with ensuing consumption of factor levels and platelets, resulting in an increased risk of dying, associated with increased bleeding as well as (micro)thrombotic events. Obviously, this condition poses a challenge for optimal management, balancing between pro- and anticoagulation.

There is a clear need for tools to discriminate patients with a high risk of bleeding and vice versa: a need to determine which patients have a high likelihood of benefitting from an anticoagulant intervention.

14

Take-Home Messages

- Inflammation drives a procoagulant condition with ensuing consumption of platelets and coagulation factor levels, resulting in an increased risk of dying, associated with increased bleeding and microthrombotic events.
- The procoagulant response during inflammation is caused by pro-inflammatory mediators that activate platelets, whereas antithrombin and protein C are downregulated leading to a malfunctioning anticoagulant system.
- Coagulation disturbances during critical illness are not an "on or off phenomenon," but a continuum which is demonstrated by the linear relationship between platelet count and mortality.
- Disseminated intravascular coagulation (DIC) is the severest form of inflammation-induced coagulopathy and is defined as a systemic intravascular activation of coagulation leading to access generation of thrombin and deposition of fibrin, with formation of widespread microvascular thrombosis.
- DIC is most frequently caused by sepsis, but solid tumors, hematologic malignancies, obstetrical complications, acute pancreatitis, trauma, severe transfusion reactions, snake venom, and hyperthermia are also risk factors.
- The following three clinical scoring systems can be used for the diagnosis of DIC: firstly, the ISTH DIC score that assesses platelet count, PT, fibrinogen, and fibrinolysis markers; secondly, the JAAM score that assesses SIRS criteria, platelet count, PT ratio, and fibrin; and lastly, the SIC score that assesses SOFA score, platelet count, and INR.
- The cornerstone of DIC treatment remains management of the underlying disorder.
- During inflammation-induced coagulopathy, a platelet count of 10×10^9/L is suggested as the threshold for prophylactic platelet transfusion. Tranexamic acid should generally be withheld, and prophylactic plasma transfusion is not advised.
- Prophylactic anticoagulant treatment should be administered in patients with DIC without (a high risk of) bleeding, and therapeutic anticoagulation should be started in case of an overt thrombotic event or when clot-related organ failure is present.

References

1. Williamson DR, Albert M, Heels-Ansdell D, Arnold DM, Lauzier F, Zarychanski R, et al. Thrombocytopenia in critically ill patients receiving thromboprophylaxis: frequency, risk factors, and outcomes. Chest. 2013;144(4):1207–15.
2. van Hinsbergh VWM. Endothelium—role in regulation of coagulation and inflammation. Semin Immunopathol. 2012;34(1):93–106.
3. Sucker C, Zotz RB. The cell-based coagulation model. In: Marcucci CE, Schoettker P, editors. Perioperative hemostasis: coagulation for anesthesiologists. Berlin: Springer Berlin Heidelberg; 2015. p. 3–11.
4. Perutelli P, Mori PG. Interaction of the von Willebrand factor with platelets and thrombosis. Recenti Prog Med. 1997;88(11):526–9.
5. Heemskerk JWM, Mattheij NJA, Cosemans JMEM. Platelet-based coagulation: different populations, different functions. J Thromb Haemost. 2013;11(1):2–16.

6. Powling MJ, Hardisty RM. Glycoprotein IIb-IIIa complex and Ca2+ influx into stimulated platelets. Blood. 1985;66(3):731–4.
7. Nesbitt WS, Giuliano S, Kulkarni S, Dopheide SM, Harper IS, Jackson SP. Intercellular calcium communication regulates platelet aggregation and thrombus growth. J Cell Biol. 2003;160(7):1151–61.
8. Mackie IJ, Bull HA. Normal haemostasis and its regulation. Blood Rev. 1989;3(4):237–50.
9. Crawley JTB, Zanardelli S, Chion CKNK, Lane DA. The central role of thrombin in hemostasis. J Thromb Haemost. 2007;5(s1):95–101.
10. Ariëns RAS, Lai T-S, Weisel JW, Greenberg CS, Grant PJ. Role of factor XIII in fibrin clot formation and effects of genetic polymorphisms. Blood. 2002;100(3):743–54.
11. Dahlbäck B. Blood coagulation and its regulation by anticoagulant pathways: genetic pathogenesis of bleeding and thrombotic diseases. J Intern Med. 2005;257(3):209–23.
12. Quinsey NS, Greedy AL, Bottomley SP, Whisstock JC, Pike RN. Antithrombin: in control of coagulation. Int J Biochem Cell Biol. 2004;36(3):386–9.
13. Esmon CT. The protein C pathway. Chest. 2003;124(3 Suppl):26s–32s.
14. Esmon CT. The endothelial protein C receptor. Curr Opin Hematol. 2006;13(5):382–5.
15. Hepner M, Karlaftis V. Protein S. Methods Mol Biology (Clifton, NJ). 2013;992:373–81.
16. Mast AE. Tissue factor pathway inhibitor. Arterioscler Thromb Vasc Biol. 2016;36(1):9–14.
17. Collen D, Lijnen HR. The fibrinolytic system in man. Crit Rev Oncol Hematol. 1986;4(3):249–301.
18. Rijken DC, Lijnen HR. New insights into the molecular mechanisms of the fibrinolytic system. J Thromb Haemost. 2009;7(1):4–13.
19. Wenzel C, Kofler J, Locker GJ, Laczika K, Quehenberger P, Frass M, et al. Endothelial cell activation and blood coagulation in critically ill patients with lung injury. Wien Klin Wochenschr. 2002;114(19–20):853–8.
20. Mutch NJ, Thomas L, Moore NR, Lisiak KM, Booth NA. TAFIa, PAI-1 and alpha-antiplasmin: complementary roles in regulating lysis of thrombi and plasma clots. J Thromb Haemost. 2007;5(4):812–7.
21. Sillen M, Declerck PJ. Thrombin activatable fibrinolysis inhibitor (TAFI): an updated narrative review. Int J Mol Sci. 2021;22(7):3670.
22. Esmon CT. The interactions between inflammation and coagulation. Br J Haematol. 2005;131(4):417–30.
23. Levi M, van der Poll T. Inflammation and coagulation. Crit Care Med. 2010;38(2 Suppl):S26–34.
24. Wada T, Shiraishi A, Gando S, Yamakawa K, Fujishima S, Saitoh D, et al. Disseminated intravascular coagulation immediately after trauma predicts a poor prognosis in severely injured patients. Sci Rep. 2021;11(1):11031.
25. Levi M, ten Cate H, van der Poll T, van Deventer SJ. Pathogenesis of disseminated intravascular coagulation in sepsis. JAMA. 1993;270(8):975–9.
26. Levi M, Opal SM. Coagulation abnormalities in critically ill patients. Crit Care. 2006;10(4):222.
27. Engelmann B, Massberg S. Thrombosis as an intravascular effector of innate immunity. Nat Rev Immunol. 2013;13(1):34–45.
28. de Bont CM, Boelens WC, Pruijn GJM. NETosis, complement, and coagulation: a triangular relationship. Cell Mol Immunol. 2019;16(1):19–27.
29. Gautam I, Storad Z, Filipiak L, Huss C, Meikle CK, Worth RG, et al. From classical to unconventional: the immune receptors facilitating platelet responses to infection and inflammation. Biology (Basel). 2020;9(10):343.
30. Foley JH, Conway EM. Cross talk pathways between coagulation and inflammation. Circ Res. 2016;118(9):1392–408.
31. Sørensen OE, Borregaard N. Neutrophil extracellular traps—the dark side of neutrophils. J Clin Invest. 2016;126(5):1612–20.
32. Markiewski MM, Nilsson B, Ekdahl KN, Mollnes TE, Lambris JD. Complement and coagulation: strangers or partners in crime? Trends Immunol. 2007;28(4):184–92.
33. Bernardo A, Ball C, Nolasco L, Moake JF, Dong JF. Effects of inflammatory cytokines on the release and cleavage of the endothelial cell-derived ultralarge von Willebrand factor multimers under flow. Blood. 2004;104(1):100–6.
34. Hui P, Cook DJ, Lim W, Fraser GA, Arnold DM. The frequency and clinical significance of thrombocytopenia complicating critical illness: a systematic review. Chest. 2011;139(2):271–8.

14

35. Lieberman L, Bercovitz RS, Sholapur NS, Heddle NM, Stanworth SJ, Arnold DM. Platelet transfusions for critically ill patients with thrombocytopenia. Blood. 2014;123(8):1146–51; quiz 280.

36. Walsh TS, Stanworth SJ, Prescott RJ, Lee RJ, Watson DM, Wyncoll D. Prevalence, management, and outcomes of critically ill patients with prothrombin time prolongation in United Kingdom intensive care units. Crit Care Med. 2010;38(10):1939–46.

37. Adelborg K, Larsen JB, Hvas AM. Disseminated intravascular coagulation: epidemiology, biomarkers, and management. Br J Haematol. 2021;192(5):803–18.

38. Oren H, Cingöz I, Duman M, Yilmaz S, Irken G. Disseminated intravascular coagulation in pediatric patients: clinical and laboratory features and prognostic factors influencing the survival. Pediatr Hematol Oncol. 2005;22(8):679–88.

39. Carey MJ, Rodgers GM. Disseminated intravascular coagulation: clinical and laboratory aspects. Am J Hematol. 1998;59(1):65–73.

40. Gilbert WM, Danielsen B. Amniotic fluid embolism: decreased mortality in a population-based study. Obstet Gynecol. 1999;93(6):973–7.

41. Goshua G, Pine AB, Meizlish ML, Chang CH, Zhang H, Bahel P, et al. Endotheliopathy in COVID-19-associated coagulopathy: evidence from a single-centre, cross-sectional study. Lancet Haematol. 2020;7(8):e575–82.

42. Stanworth SJ, Davenport R, Curry N, Seeney F, Eaglestone S, Edwards A, et al. Mortality from trauma haemorrhage and opportunities for improvement in transfusion practice. Br J Surg. 2016;103(4):357–65.

43. Kleinveld DJB, Simons DDG, Dekimpe C, Deconinck SJ, Sloos PH, Maas MAW, et al. Plasma and rhADAMTS13 reduce trauma-induced organ failure by restoring the ADAMTS13-VWF axis. Blood Adv. 2021;5(17):3478–91.

44. Bick RL. Disseminated intravascular coagulation: objective clinical and laboratory diagnosis, treatment, and assessment of therapeutic response. Semin Thromb Hemost. 1996;22(1):69–88.

45. Sivula M, Pettilä V, Niemi TT, Varpula M, Kuitunen AH. Thromboelastometry in patients with severe sepsis and disseminated intravascular coagulation. Blood Coagul Fibrinolysis. 2009;20(6):419–26.

46. Levi M, van der Poll T. A short contemporary history of disseminated intravascular coagulation. Semin Thromb Hemost. 2014;40(8):874–80.

47. Bernard GR, Margolis BD, Shanies HM, Ely EW, Wheeler AP, Levy H, et al. Extended evaluation of recombinant human activated protein C United States trial (ENHANCE US): a single-arm, phase 3B, multicenter study of drotrecogin alfa (activated) in severe sepsis. Chest. 2004;125(6):2206–16.

48. Dhainaut JF, Shorr AF, Macias WL, Kollef MJ, Levi M, Reinhart K, et al. Dynamic evolution of coagulopathy in the first day of severe sepsis: relationship with mortality and organ failure. Crit Care Med. 2005;33(2):341–8.

49. Vanderschueren S, De Weerdt A, Malbrain M, Vankersschaever D, Frans E, Wilmer A, et al. Thrombocytopenia and prognosis in intensive care. Crit Care Med. 2000;28(6):1871–6.

50. Strauss R, Wehler M, Mehler K, Kreutzer D, Koebnick C, Hahn EG. Thrombocytopenia in patients in the medical intensive care unit: bleeding prevalence, transfusion requirements, and outcome. Crit Care Med. 2002;30(8):1765–71.

51. Oppenheim-Eden A, Glantz L, Eidelman LA, Sprung CL. Spontaneous intracerebral hemorrhage in critically ill patients: incidence over six years and associated factors. Intensive Care Med. 1999;25(1):63–7.

52. Semeraro N, Ammollo CT, Semeraro F, Colucci M. Sepsis, thrombosis and organ dysfunction. Thromb Res. 2012;129(3):290–5.

53. Cauchie P, Cauchie C, Boudjeltia KZ, Carlier E, Deschepper N, Govaerts D, et al. Diagnosis and prognosis of overt disseminated intravascular coagulation in a general hospital—meaning of the ISTH score system, fibrin monomers, and lipoprotein-C-reactive protein complex formation. Am J Hematol. 2006;81(6):414–9.

54. Dhainaut JF, Yan SB, Joyce DE, Pettilä V, Basson B, Brandt JT, et al. Treatment effects of drotrecogin alfa (activated) in patients with severe sepsis with or without overt disseminated intravascular coagulation. J Thromb Haemost. 2004;2(11):1924–33.

55. Stanworth SJ, Walsh TS, Prescott RJ, Lee RJ, Watson DM, Wyncoll DL. Thrombocytopenia and platelet transfusion in UK critical care: a multicenter observational study. Transfusion. 2013;53(5):1050–8.

56. McIntyre L, Tinmouth AT, Fergusson DA. Blood component transfusion in critically ill patients. Curr Opin Crit Care. 2013;19(4):326–33.

57. Stanworth SJ, Estcourt LJ, Powter G, Kahan BC, Dyer C, Choo L, et al. A no-prophylaxis platelet-transfusion strategy for hematologic cancers. N Engl J Med. 2013;368(19):1771–80.

58. Müller MCA, Stanworth SJ, Coppens M, Juffermans NP. Recognition and management of hemostatic disorders in critically ill patients needing to undergo an invasive procedure. Transfus Med Rev. 2017;31(4):223–9.

59. Muller MC, Straat M, Meijers JC, Klinkspoor JH, de Jonge E, Arbous MS, et al. Fresh frozen plasma transfusion fails to influence the hemostatic balance in critically ill patients with a coagulopathy. J Thromb Haemost. 2015;13(6):989–97.

60. Desborough M, Sandu R, Brunskill SJ, Doree C, Trivella M, Montedori A, et al. Fresh frozen plasma for cardiovascular surgery. Cochrane Database Syst Rev. 2015;2015(7):CD007614.

61. Juffermans NP, Muller MM. Prophylactic plasma: can we finally let go? Transfusion. 2021;61(7):1991–2.

62. Zeidler K, Arn K, Senn O, Schanz U, Stussi G. Optimal preprocedural platelet transfusion threshold for central venous catheter insertions in patients with thrombocytopenia. Transfusion. 2011;51(11):2269–76.

63. Vlaar AP, Oczkowski S, de Bruin S, Wijnberge M, Antonelli M, Aubron C, et al. Transfusion strategies in non-bleeding critically ill adults: a clinical practice guideline from the European Society of Intensive Care Medicine. Intensive Care Med. 2020;46(4):673–96.

64. Vlaar APJ, Dionne JC, de Bruin S, Wijnberge M, Raasveld SJ, van Baarle F, et al. Transfusion strategies in bleeding critically ill adults: a clinical practice guideline from the European Society of Intensive Care Medicine. Intensive Care Med. 2021;47(12):1368–92.

65. Minet C, Potton L, Bonadona A, Hamidfar-Roy R, Somohano CA, Lugosi M, et al. Venous thromboembolism in the ICU: main characteristics, diagnosis and thromboprophylaxis. Crit Care. 2015;19:287.

66. Schünemann HJ, Cushman M, Burnett AE, Kahn SR, Beyer-Westendorf J, Spencer FA, et al. American Society of Hematology 2018 guidelines for management of venous thromboembolism: prophylaxis for hospitalized and nonhospitalized medical patients. Blood Adv. 2018;2(22):3198–225.

67. Ho KM, Chavan S, Pilcher D. Omission of early thromboprophylaxis and mortality in critically ill patients: a multicenter registry study. Chest. 2011;140(6):1436–46.

68. Tufano A, Guida A, Di Minno MN, Prisco D, Cerbone AM, Di Minno G. Prevention of venous thromboembolism in medical patients with thrombocytopenia or with platelet dysfunction: a review of the literature. Semin Thromb Hemost. 2011;37(3):267–74.

69. Baelum JK, Moe EE, Nybo M, Vinholt PJ. Venous thromboembolism in patients with thrombocytopenia: risk factors, treatment, and outcome. Clin Appl Thromb Hemost. 2017;23(4):345–50.

70. Fernando SM, Tran A, Cheng W, Sadeghirad B, Arabi YM, Cook DJ, et al. Venous thromboembolism prophylaxis in critically ill adults: a systematic review and network meta-analysis. Chest. 2022;161(2):418–28.

71. Martel N, Lee J, Wells PS. Risk for heparin-induced thrombocytopenia with unfractionated and low-molecular-weight heparin thromboprophylaxis: a meta-analysis. Blood. 2005;106(8):2710–5.

72. Squizzato A, Hunt BJ, Kinasewitz GT, Wada H, Ten Cate H, Thachil J, et al. Supportive management strategies for disseminated intravascular coagulation. An international consensus. Thromb Haemost. 2016;115(5):896–904.

73. Levi M, Scully M. How I treat disseminated intravascular coagulation. Blood. 2018;131(8):845–54.

74. Wada H, Asakura H, Okamoto K, Iba T, Uchiyama T, Kawasugi K, et al. Expert consensus for the treatment of disseminated intravascular coagulation in Japan. Thromb Res. 2010;125(1):6–11.

75. Fourrier F, Chopin C, Goudemand J, Hendrycx S, Caron C, Rime A, et al. Septic shock, multiple organ failure, and disseminated intravascular coagulation. Compared patterns of antithrombin III, protein C, and protein S deficiencies. Chest. 1992;101(3):816–23.

76. Mesters RM, Mannucci PM, Coppola R, Keller T, Ostermann H, Kienast J. Factor VIIa and antithrombin III activity during severe sepsis and septic shock in neutropenic patients. Blood. 1996;88(3):881–6.

14

77. Warren BL, Eid A, Singer P, Pillay SS, Carl P, Novak I, et al. Caring for the critically ill patient. High-dose antithrombin III in severe sepsis: a randomized controlled trial. JAMA. 2001;286(15):1869–78.

78. Kienast J, Juers M, Wiedermann CJ, Hoffmann JN, Ostermann H, Strauss R, et al. Treatment effects of high-dose antithrombin without concomitant heparin in patients with severe sepsis with or without disseminated intravascular coagulation. J Thromb Haemost. 2006;4(1):90–7.

79. Wiedermann CJ. Antithrombin concentrate use in disseminated intravascular coagulation of sepsis: meta-analyses revisited. J Thromb Haemost. 2018;16(3):455–7.

80. Tanaka K, Takeba J, Matsumoto H, Ohshita M, Annen S, Moriyama N, et al. Anticoagulation therapy using rh-thrombomodulin and/or antithrombin III agent is associated with reduction in in-hospital mortality in septic disseminated intravascular coagulation: a nationwide registry study. Shock. 2019;51(6):713–7.

81. Saito H, Maruyama I, Shimazaki S, Yamamoto Y, Aikawa N, Ohno R, et al. Efficacy and safety of recombinant human soluble thrombomodulin (ART-123) in disseminated intravascular coagulation: results of a phase III, randomized, double-blind clinical trial. J Thromb Haemost. 2007;5(1):31–41.

82. Aikawa N, Shimazaki S, Yamamoto Y, Saito H, Maruyama I, Ohno R, et al. Thrombomodulin alfa in the treatment of infectious patients complicated by disseminated intravascular coagulation: subanalysis from the phase 3 trial. Shock. 2011;35(4):349–54.

83. Vincent JL, Francois B, Zabolotskikh I, Daga MK, Lascarrou JB, Kirov MY, et al. Effect of a recombinant human soluble thrombomodulin on mortality in patients with sepsis-associated coagulopathy: the SCARLET randomized clinical trial. JAMA. 2019;321(20):1993–2002.

84. Yamakawa K, Murao S, Aihara M. Recombinant human soluble thrombomodulin in sepsis-induced coagulopathy: an updated systematic review and meta-analysis. Thromb Haemost. 2019;119(1):56–65.

85. Bernard GR, Vincent JL, Laterre PF, LaRosa SP, Dhainaut JF, Lopez-Rodriguez A, et al. Efficacy and safety of recombinant human activated protein C for severe sepsis. N Engl J Med. 2001;344(10):699–709.

86. Abraham E, Laterre PF, Garg R, Levy H, Talwar D, Trzaskoma BL, et al. Drotrecogin alfa (activated) for adults with severe sepsis and a low risk of death. N Engl J Med. 2005;353(13):1332–41.

87. Ranieri VM, Thompson BT, Barie PS, Dhainaut JF, Douglas IS, Finfer S, et al. Drotrecogin alfa (activated) in adults with septic shock. N Engl J Med. 2012;366(22):2055–64.

88. Abraham E, Reinhart K, Opal S, Demeyer I, Doig C, Rodriguez AL, et al. Efficacy and safety of tifacogin (recombinant tissue factor pathway inhibitor) in severe sepsis: a randomized controlled trial. JAMA. 2003;290(2):238–47.

Dysregulated Immune Response and Organ Dysfunction: The Muscles

Luke Flower, Charlotte Summers, and Zudin Puthucheary

Contents

- To understand the definition and pathophysiology of critical illness-associated muscle wasting and persistent inflammation, immunosuppression, and catabolism syndrome (PICS).
- To understand how muscle metabolism is altered in critical illness.
- To understand how intramuscular inflammation and mitochondrial dysfunction may lead to myocyte necrosis.

15.1 Introduction

Critical care-associated muscle wasting affects 40% of intensive care patients and is associated with significant morbidity and mortality [1–3]. It results from the disruption of the balance between muscle protein synthesis (MPS) and muscle protein breakdown (MPB), which is present in health [1, 3]. The underlying pathology is multi-factorial and yet to be fully defined. It likely results from immune dysfunction, with both systemic vascular and intramuscular inflammation, mitochondrial dysfunction, and immobilisation.

A type of chronic inflammation associated with muscle wasting has been described—the persistent inflammation, immunosuppression, and catabolic syndrome (PICS) [4, 5]. This persistent inflammation has recognised detrimental effects on patient outcomes, predisposing them to nosocomial infections, continued protein catabolism, malnutrition, and poor physical recovery after intensive care unit (ICU) discharge [5]. In this chapter, we outline the muscular changes seen in critical illness and discuss the potential immunological mechanisms underlying them.

15.2 Critical Illness-Associated Muscle Wasting

In health, muscle protein homeostasis is balanced by both intrinsic (old age, chronic disease, low muscle mass) and extrinsic (inflammation, inadequate intake, sedation, and immobilisation) factors [1–3]. In critical illness, this fine balance is disturbed by an excess of extrinsic anti-anabolic factors, for example systemic inflammation, resulting in reduced MPS and a net loss of muscle mass.

The rate of muscle loss is fastest in early disease and in the most critically unwell patients [1, 3]. Muscle loss may reach 3–5% per day, and a net catabolic state may persist for up to 30 days in prolonged critical illness [1, 3]. Both immunological and metabolic mechanisms likely contribute.

15.3 Muscle Metabolism and Mitochondrial Dysfunction in Critical Illness

In health, glucose is the major source of fuel for cellular metabolism and anabolic stimuli, such as spikes in serum amino acid concentration and increase in MPS [6–8]. The Pasteur effect refers to the increase in aerobic respiration and inhibition of

15

anaerobic respiration seen in the presence of oxygen. A mitochondrial PaO_2 of 0.15–0.3 kPa is often quoted as the Pasteur point, below which the Pasteur effect is inhibited in humans. This effect ensures that glucose can enter the citric acid cycle in the form of acetyl-CoA and thereby produce a net gain of 36 molecules of adenosine triphosphate (ATP) for each glucose molecule [9].

In critical illness, inflammation and hypoxic signalling disrupt the Pasteur effect, resulting in anaerobic glucose metabolism, lactate production, and net production of only two ATP molecules for each glucose molecule (Fig. 15.1) [1, 9–11]. Fatty acid metabolism is also disrupted, with impaired beta-oxidation and reduced mitochondrial enzyme concentrations (specifically carnitine palmitoyltransferase-1, medium-chain acyl-CoA dehydrogenase, and 2,4-dienoyl-CoA reductase), leading to a reduction in ATP production. In health, the metabolism of a single 16-carbon atom containing fatty acid can produce 129 ATP molecules, and thus disruption of this efficient process has significant effects on cellular energy supply. These combined effects are associated with decreased mitochondrial biogenesis and a compromised bioenergetic status, contributing to muscle wasting [10, 12, 13]. Adenosine monophosphate-activated protein kinase (AMP-K) is a fuel-sensing enzyme found in all human cells that is activated in ATP-deficient states to stimulate energy production via the inhibition of energy-consuming anabolic pathways (i.e., lipogenesis) and stimulation of energy-releasing catabolic pathways (i.e., fatty acid oxidation) [14]. Skeletal muscle levels of AMP-K are raised in critically ill patients, highlighting the compromised bioenergetic status and the attempts by muscle tissue to counteract this [2].

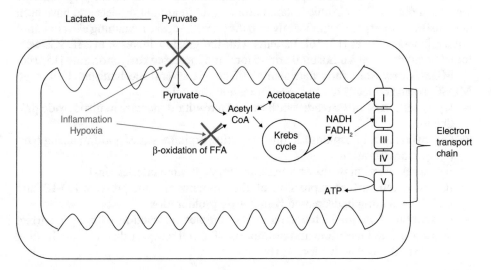

 Fig. 15.1 Mitochondrial dysfunction in critical illness. Inflammation and hypoxia inhibit the Pasteur effect and β-oxidation resulting in increased conversion of pyruvate to lactate, reduced ATP production, and a bioenergetic crisis. *ATP* adenosine triphosphate, *FADH₂* flavin adenine dinucleotide, *FFA* free fatty acids, *NADH* nicotinamide adenine dinucleotide

15.4   Immune Dysfunction in Critical Illness

The initial physiological insult caused by critical illness results from an early innate immune response, which may lead to the systemic inflammatory response syndrome (SIRS), and what has often been termed compensatory anti-inflammatory response syndrome (CARS). The resultant immune dysfunction leads to intramuscular inflammation, a bioenergetic crisis, and myocyte necrosis.

15.4.1   Persistent Inflammation, Immunosuppression, and Catabolism Syndrome

Patients that survive the initial inflammatory insult have two potential outcomes. In some, the aberrant immunological function may recover, but in a subset of patients, it can persist in the form of PICS. In patients admitted for >14 days, persistent critical illness is characterised by inflammation (CRP >50 μg/dL), persistent immunosuppression (lymphocyte count of <0.80 × 10^9/L), and a catabolic state (serum albumin <3.0 g/dL, pre-albumin <10 mg g/dL, creatinine height index <80%, and weight loss of >10%) [4].

The underlying pathology is driven by "emergency myelopoiesis", a process where increased myeloid cell production results in reduced ability for lymphopoiesis and erythropoiesis, leading to immunosuppression and anaemia, and proliferation of inducible immature myeloid cells named myeloid-derived suppressor cells (MDSCs). These MDSCs are immunosuppressive and inflammatory in nature [15]. MDSCs have been observed in chronic inflammatory states in animal models and have been demonstrated to expand significantly in patients with sepsis, remaining elevated until critical illness resolves [15, 16]. Patients with the greatest increase in MDSCs were found to have prolonged hospital admissions and increased early mortality [15, 16].

MDSCs may exert their detrimental effects via several mechanisms. Prolonged MDSC expansion leads to immunosuppression through:

- Upregulation of nitric oxide synthase and a resultant increase in nitric oxide production
- Overexpression of arginase 1, thus depleting arginine stores and impairing lymphocyte proliferation
- Increased secretion of the anti-inflammatory cytokine interleukin-10
- Increased cell surface expression of the immunoadjuvant proteins PD-L1 and CTLA4, resulting in decreased lymphocyte proliferation
- Prevention of major histocompatibility complex interaction with their correct respective T-cell receptors and promotion of T-cell receptor dissociation, leading to impaired T-cell activation [4, 16]

Expanded MDSCs also result in chronic inflammation due to increased secretion of tumour necrosis factor and macrophage inflammatory protein-1β, as well as production of reactive oxygen species. An ongoing anti-angiogenic and pro-inflammatory state may also be induced by a reduction in vascular endothelial growth factor and a raised erythropoietin ratio [4, 16].

15

Whilst in the acute phase the expansion of MDSCs appears to have a protective effect, prolonged elevation of MDSC levels is associated with increased ICU length of stay, nosocomial infection, and limited post-ICU recovery. Patients with persistent inflammatory, immunosupressed, and catabolic states suffer from increased ventilator dependence, compromised rehabilitation, and significant impairment in quality of life (e.g. ability to resume their usual activities) [4].

15.4.2 Intramuscular Inflammation, Mitochondrial Dysfunction, and Myocyte Necrosis

Muscle wasting in critical illness is associated with intramuscular inflammation and myocyte necrosis. Muscle biopsies in critically ill patients demonstrate necrosis to be associated with both neutrophil and macrophage infiltration [3]. The specific mechanisms underlying this remain undefined.

Systemic Inflammation as a Cause for Necrosis

One theory is that local immune dysregulation is precipitated by extrinsic systemic inflammation. This local dysregulation then leads to an increase in local pro-inflammatory cytokines, neutrophil chemotaxis, and macrophage infiltration (◘ Fig. 15.2), with a relative increase in the pro-inflammatory M1 macrophage phenotype. Muscle biopsies from patients with critical illness myopathy have demonstrated initial neutrophil infiltration of the muscle (day 3) followed later by macrophage infiltration (day 7) [3]. The chronology of these findings is likely due to systemically circulating monocytes requiring the presence or orchestration of neutrophils to infiltrate tissue. Once inside the tissues, macrophages clear neutrophils by efferocytosis. We therefore see intramuscular neutrophils in early critical illness myopathy, and intramuscular macrophages later in the disease process. Extrinsic systemic inflammation may therefore act as an anti-anabolic stimulus, reducing MPS and impairing mitochondrial metabolism. A rise in systemic IL-6 and TNF also increases insulin resistance, thus impairing glucose utilisation and causing muscle atrophy. The net effect of the above is necroptosis.

Research in the non-critically ill patient population with systemic chronic inflammatory disease appears to support the above hypothesis, with an increase in serum pro-inflammatory cytokines in diseases such as rheumatoid arthritis (specifically IL-1, IL-6, IFN-γ, and TNF-α) associated with increased muscle wasting.

Patients with COPD are known to suffer from sarcopenia. Several potential mechanisms have been suggested, with a combination of hypoxaemia and elevation of inflammatory factors hypothesised to be the driver. Similarly, muscle wasting is a characteristic finding in patients with rheumatoid arthritis, with the use of IL-1, IL-6, and TNF antagonists associated with clinical improvement and reduced sarcopenia. The inflammatory myopathies also support the hypothesis that systemic and intramuscular inflammation may be the primary driving mechanism: Patients with polymyositis and inclusion body myositis characteristically demonstrate a predominance of T and B cells in their muscles, an overexpression of MHC class I and II, and an association with specific autoantibodies [17].

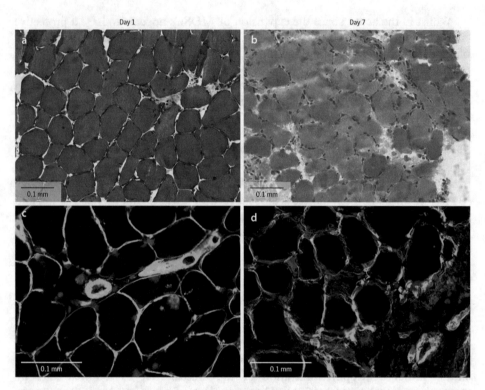

◻ Fig. 15.2 Healthy muscle is seen on day 1 **a**, **c** with necrosis and a cellular infiltrate on day 7 (**b**, **d**. This infiltrate was CD68 positive on immunostaining, indicating macrophage origin (red)). **a**, **b** are haematoxylin and eosin stain, and **c**, **d** show immunostaining, with CD68 for red, laminin (myofiber outline) for green, and 4′,6-diamidino-2-phenylindole (a nuclear marker) for blue. (Reproduced with permission from Puthucheary et al. 2013, JAMA)

Mitochondrial Dysfunction as a Cause of Myocyte Necrosis

A second theory is that, rather than extrinsic systemic inflammation causing muscle cell death, it may be mitochondrial dysfunction and a resultant inadequate supply of ATP that instead drives myocyte necrosis and subsequent intramuscular inflammation. As previously mentioned, critical illness is associated with impaired mitochondrial function, leading to an intrinsic ATP deficiency and a bioenergetic crisis. Evidence to support this hypothesis includes the association between critical illness and mitochondrial swelling, reduced mitochondrial content, and density [18]. Primary mitochondrial disorders with defects in oxidative phosphorylation are associated with significant myopathy. Mitochondrial dysfunction has also been recognised as an early event in cancer-induced muscle wasting and immobilisation-associated muscle wasting [12, 19, 20].

Studies of sepsis survivors with profound muscle weakness at least 1 month after recovery observed abnormal mitochondrial ultrastructure, impaired oxidative phosphorylation, and persistent oxidative damage [21]. These patients demonstrated persistent muscle weakness despite recovery of muscle mass, strongly implying a role in mitochondrial dysfunction beyond muscle wasting [18, 21].

15.4.3 So Which Mechanism Predominates?

Determining the dominate mechanism of muscle wasting in critical illness is challenging. It requires isolation of inflammatory and ATP-deficient states or attempts to extrinsically alter white cell metabolic pathways. In practice, critical illness-associated muscle wasting and PICS likely result from a combination of mechanisms—immune dysfunction, intramuscular inflammation, and a bioenergetic crisis. If the cycle of myocyte necrosis and inflammation persists in muscle tissue, it may itself become a source of persistent inflammation.

Summary

Critical illness-associated muscle wasting is common and associated with significant morbidity and mortality. It likely results from dysregulated immune function and systemic inflammation, impaired mitochondrial function, and a bioenergetic crisis. To date, no specific therapies have been identified—early mobilisation is key, and the use of alternative feeding regimens (such as ketogenic feeds) is currently being investigated.

Take-Home Messages

- Critical illness-associated muscle wasting is a common and significant complication affecting intensive care patients.
- Immune dysfunction likely plays a key role in its development, disrupting the fine balance between muscle protein synthesis and muscle protein breakdown.
- The precise underlying aetiology is unclear, but dysregulated inflammation, mitochondrial dysfunction, and immobilisation all likely contribute.
- No specific treatment strategies have been identified, but early immobilisation appears key, with alternative substrates such as ketones currently being investigated.

References

1. Flower L, Puthucheary Z. Muscle wasting in the critically ill patient: how to minimise subsequent disability. Br J Hosp Med (Lond). 2020;81(4):1–9. https://doi.org/10.12968/hmed.2020.0045.
2. Puthucheary ZA, Astin R, Mcphail MJW, et al. Metabolic phenotype of skeletal muscle in early critical illness. Thorax. 2018;73(10):926–35. https://doi.org/10.1136/thoraxjnl-2017-211073.
3. Puthucheary ZA, Rawal J, McPhail M, et al. Acute skeletal muscle wasting in critical illness [published correction appears in JAMA. 2014 Feb 12;311(6):625. Padhke, Rahul [corrected to Phadke, Rahul]]. JAMA. 2013;310(15):1591–1600. https://doi.org/10.1001/jama.2013.278481.
4. Mira JC, Brakenridge SC, Moldawer LL, Moore FA. Persistent inflammation, immunosuppression and catabolism syndrome. Crit Care Clin. 2017;33(2):245–58. https://doi.org/10.1016/j.ccc.2016.12.001.
5. Griffith DM, Lewis S, Rossi AG, et al. Systemic inflammation after critical illness: relationship with physical recovery and exploration of potential mechanisms. Thorax. 2016;71(9):820–9. https://doi.org/10.1136/thoraxjnl-2015-208114.

6.   McNelly AS, Bear DE, Connolly BA, et al. Effect of intermittent or continuous feed on muscle wasting in critical illness: a phase 2 clinical trial. Chest. 2020;158(1):183–94. https://doi.org/10.1016/j.chest.2020.03.045.

7.   Pitkanen HT, Nykanen T, Knuutinen J, et al. Free amino acid pool and muscle protein balance after resistance exercise. Med Sci Sports Exerc. 2003;35(5):784–92. https://doi.org/10.1249/01.MSS.0000064934.51751.F9.

8.   Bohé J, Low JF, Wolfe RR, Rennie MJ. Latency and duration of stimulation of human muscle protein synthesis during continuous infusion of amino acids. J Physiol. 2001;532(Pt 2):575–9. https://doi.org/10.1111/j.1469-7793.2001.0575f.x.

9.   Barker J, Khan MAA, Solomos T. Mechanism of the Pasteur effect. Nature. 1964;201:1126–7. https://doi.org/10.1038/2011126a0.

10. Spinelli JB, Haigis MC. The multifaceted contributions of mitochondria to cellular metabolism. Nat Cell Biol. 2018;20(7):745–54. https://doi.org/10.1038/s41556-018-0124-1.

11. Hayes K, Holland AE, Pellegrino VA, Mathur S, Hodgson CL. Acute skeletal muscle wasting and relation to physical function in patients requiring extracorporeal membrane oxygenation (ECMO). J Crit Care. 2018;48:1–8. https://doi.org/10.1016/j.jcrc.2018.08.002.

12. Ji LL, Yeo D. Mitochondrial dysregulation and muscle disuse atrophy. F1000Res. 2019;8:F1000 Faculty Rev-1621. Published 2019 Sep 11. https://doi.org/10.12688/f1000research.19139.1.

13. Brealey D, Brand M, Hargreaves I, et al. Association between mitochondrial dysfunction and severity and outcome of septic shock. Lancet. 2002;360(9328):219–23. https://doi.org/10.1016/S0140-6736(02)09459-X.

14. Mihaylova MM, Shaw RJ. The AMPK signalling pathway coordinates cell growth, autophagy and metabolism. Nat Cell Biol. 2011;13(9):1016–23. Published 2011 Sep 2. https://doi.org/10.1038/ncb2329.

15. Mathias B, Delmas AL, Ozrazgat-Baslanti T, et al. Human myeloid-derived suppressor cells are associated with chronic immune suppression after severe sepsis/septic shock. Ann Surg. 2017;265(4):827–34. https://doi.org/10.1097/SLA.0000000000001783.

16. Mira JC, Gentile LF, Mathias BJ, et al. Sepsis pathophysiology, chronic critical illness, and persistent inflammation-immunosuppression and catabolism syndrome. Crit Care Med. 2017;45(2):253–62. https://doi.org/10.1097/CCM.0000000000002074.

17. Londhe P, Guttridge DC. Inflammation induced loss of skeletal muscle. Bone. 2015;80:131–42. https://doi.org/10.1016/j.bone.2015.03.015.

18. Schefold JC, Wollersheim T, Grunow JJ, Luedi MM, Z'Graggen WJ, Weber-Carstens S. Muscular weakness and muscle wasting in the critically ill. J Cachexia Sarcopenia Muscle. 2020;11(6):1399–412. https://doi.org/10.1002/jcsm.12620.

19. Argilés JM, López-Soriano FJ, Busquets S. Muscle wasting in cancer: the role of mitochondria. Curr Opin Clin Nutr Metab Care. 2015;18(3):221–5. https://doi.org/10.1097/MCO.0000000000000164.

20. Hyatt H, Deminice R, Yoshihara T, Powers SK. Mitochondrial dysfunction induces muscle atrophy during prolonged inactivity: a review of the causes and effects. Arch Biochem Biophys. 2019;662:49–60. https://doi.org/10.1016/j.abb.2018.11.005.

21. Owen AM, Patel SP, Smith JD, et al. Chronic muscle weakness and mitochondrial dysfunction in the absence of sustained atrophy in a preclinical sepsis model. Elife. 2019;8:e49920. Published 2019 Dec 3. https://doi.org/10.7554/eLife.49920.

Modulating the Immune Response

Contents

The Role of Steroids

Nicholas Heming and Djillali Annane

Contents

> **Learning Objectives**
> - To understand the mechanisms underlying sepsis that are relevant to corticosteroids
> - To understand the mechanisms of action of corticosteroids that are relevant to the management of sepsis
> - To know how to identify patients with sepsis, community-acquired pneumonia, ARDS, or COVID-19 who should be treated with corticosteroids
> - To know how to give corticosteroids in these patients, including type of molecule, dose, and duration of treatment
> - To know the risks associated with corticosteroids and how to prevent them

16.1 Introduction

A number of conditions in intensive care units are associated with dysregulated immune responses. Among these diseases, sepsis is a model of dysregulated immune response in the critically ill. Sepsis is characterized by life-threatening organ dysfunction caused by a dysregulated host response to infection. It affects more than 44 million people annually, causing approximately 11 million fatalities [1, 2]. The incidence of sepsis increases steadily in industrialized countries, due to an ageing and frailer population [3]. Approximately half of all sepsis survivors will suffer physical and psychological sequelae, which may significantly alter their subsequent quality of life [4]. Septic shock is the most severe subtype of sepsis associating metabolic, cellular, immune, and circulatory abnormalities and a significant risk of death [1]. Treatment of septic shock is based on antimicrobial therapy, source control, and symptomatic organ support [5]. Over the years, a large number of experimental interventions have been investigated in the management of patients with sepsis, mostly unsuccessfully [6]. Corticosteroids are the only treatment to reduce mortality in septic shock [7–9], and this treatment should probably be part of routine management of septic shock [5]. In this review, we will briefly describe the pathophysiology of septic shock and describe when and how to administer corticosteroids. More recently, corticosteroids were shown to significantly reduce coronavirus disease (COVID-19)-related mortality paving the way for a broader use of corticosteroids in severe respiratory infections.

16.2 Pathophysiology of Sepsis Relevant to Corticosteroids

Sepsis results from the interaction between a host and a pathogen [10]. Septic shock results from imbalanced inflammatory response and corticotrope insufficiency, leading to organ failure [11]. During septic shock, the initial inflammatory response is described as exaggerated and is partially compounded by activation of anti-inflammatory pathways [12]. The initial inflammatory response arises through the interaction between pathogen-associated molecular patterns (PAMPs, such as lipopolysaccharide (LPS), flagellin, or bacterial DNA) and the innate immune system. PAMPs are recognized by receptors bound to the membrane of immune cells (Toll-like receptors, NOD-like receptors, mannose-binding lectin, or receptor for advanced glycation end products (RAGE) [13]. The interaction between PAMPS and their specific receptor leads to the activation of cell signaling pathways. These signaling pathways subsequently induce the activation and translocation of the nuclear transcription factor (NF)-κB into the cell nucleus, leading to the transcription of pro-inflammatory cytokines such as tumor necrosis factor (TNF)-α, interleukin (IL)-1β, or IL-6 [13].

Glucocorticoids exhibit anti-inflammatory effects by upregulating the production of anti-inflammatory mediators (▣ Table 16.1). Glucocorticoids act on a cellular level by binding to the glucocorticoid receptor (GR), a member of the nuclear receptor superfamily. Glucocorticoids bound to the GR subsequently translocate from the cytoplasm to the nucleus. Within the nucleus, the GR interacts with specific DNA sequences, downregulating the expression of pro-inflammatory cytokines [14]. Glucocorticoids also exhibit an anti-inflammatory activity via non-genomic mechanisms of action; that is, this effect is not mediated by an interaction with cellular DNA [14].

Septic shock is also characterized by an inappropriate hormonal response [10]. At baseline, adrenal biosynthesis of glucocorticoids and mineralocorticoids is stimulated by the adrenocorticotropic hormone (ACTH). ACTH production is in turn dependent on corticotropin-releasing hormone (CRH) production. Cortisol is secreted following a circadian rhythm; a morning peak in cortisol concentration is followed by a gradual decrease over the day. The hypothalamic-pituitary-adrenal (HPA) axis may dysfunction in sepsis due to irreversible neuroendocrine cellular damage, impaired ACTH/CRH synthesis, impaired corticoid biosynthesis, and peripheral steroid resistance [15]. A maladaptive HPA axis response is observed in 60% of septic shock patients [10]. This maladaptive response of the hypothalamic-pituitary-adrenal axis is coined critical illness-related corticosteroid insufficiency [10]. Taken together, all of these mechanisms may contribute to hemodynamic failure during sepsis.

☐ **Table 16.1** Main immune effects of glucocorticoids in sepsis

Species	Effects
Rodent	– Improves survival [1]
Dog	– Improves survival [2]
Man	– Lowers plasma concentration of TNF-α [3] – Lowers plasma concentration of soluble E-selectin [4] – Lowers plasma concentration of plasma nitrite/nitrate, IL-6, IL-8, MIF, as well as markers of activation of neutrophiles (CD11b, CD64) [4] – Lowers the plasma concentration of phospholipase A [5] – Lowers the number of circulating eosinophils [6] – Lowers membrane expression of mHLA-DR [4] – Improves survival [7]

Adapted from [14]

16.3 Should Glucocorticoids Be Used in Sepsis?

Five large randomized trials studied the role of glucocorticoids in septic shock. The Ger-Inf-05 trial was the first phase 3 trial to assess the combination of low-dose hydrocortisone and fludrocortisone in septic shock patients that were nonresponsive to an ACTH test. The trial found that glucocorticoids had a significant benefit on survival (HR, 0.67; 95% CI, 0.47–0.95; $P = 0.02$) and on reducing vasopressor dependence (HR, 1.91; 95% CI, 1.29–2.84; $P = 0.001$) in patients with septic shock and CIRCI [7]. The CORTICUS trial did not demonstrate a similar impact of hydrocortisone on survival in septic shock with CIRCI (D28 mortality in patients nonresponsive to an ACTH test treated by hydrocortisone 39.2% vs. 36.1% treated by placebo, $P = 0.69$) while confirming the beneficial effect of hydrocortisone on vasopressor dependency [16]. In the VANISH trial, hydrocortisone did not significantly alter D28 mortality in septic shock (30.8% in the hydrocortisone group versus 27.5% in the placebo group; absolute difference, 3.3% [95% CI, −5.5 to 12.1%]) [17].

More recently, the ADRENAL study compared a continuous intravenous administration of 200 mg of hydrocortisone per day for 7 days vs. placebo in 3800 septic shock patients. The primary endpoint was all-cause mortality at D90. At D90, 511 patients (27.9%) in the hydrocortisone group and 526 (28.8%) in the placebo group had died (odds ratio, 0.95; CI 95%, 0.82–1.10; $P = 0.50$). However, in the hydrocortisone group, vasopressors were weaned faster than in the placebo group (median time, 3 days [quartiles, 2–5] vs. 4 days [quartiles, 2–9]; HR, 1.32; CI 95%, 1.23–1.41; $P < 0.001$), and hydrocortisone-treated patients required less blood transfusion (37% vs. 41.7%; odds ratio, 0.82; CI 95%, 0.72–0.94; $P = 0.004$) [18].

The APPROCCHSS trial compared a discontinuous intravenous administration of 200 mg hydrocortisone per day for 7 days plus 50 μg enteral fludrocortisone vs. placebo in 1241 patients with septic shock. The primary endpoint was also mortality at D90. At D90, 264 patients (43%) in the hydrocortisone plus fludrocortisone group had died vs. 308 (49.1%) in the placebo group ($P = 0.03$) (relative risk 0.88 95% CI 0.78–0.99; $P = 0.03$). The number of days alive free of vasopressors, as well as the number of days alive free of organ failure, was also significantly higher in the hydrocortisone and fludrocortisone group than in the placebo group, without increased incidence of side effects [9].

ADRENAL and APPROCCHSS differed in several ways (◧ Table 16.2) [19, 20]. At baseline, the population included in APPROCCHSS accounted for more cases of pulmonary sepsis, and patients were more severe and required higher doses of vasopressors. Additionally, although daily administered doses of hydrocortisone were identical (200 mg/day), modalities of administration differed; in ADRENAL, the administration was continuous, while in APPROCCHSS the administration was discontinuous and combined with enteral fludrocortisone. A recent meta-analysis including 61 clinical trials and 12,192 participants confirmed that low-dose hydrocortisone had a beneficial effect on mortality in septic shock [8].

Table 16.2 Main clinical trials assessing corticosteroids in septic shock

Variable	Annane et al. [9]	Sprung et al. [10]	Gordon et al. [11]	Venkatesh et al. [12]	Annane et al. [13]
Effect on D28 mortality (% absolute value)	−6	+2.8	+3.3		−6
Effect on D90 mortality (% absolute value)				−1	−6
Steroid	Hydrocortisone / Fludrocortisone	Hydrocortisone	Hydrocortisone	Hydrocortisone	Hydrocortisone / Fludrocortisone
Administration	IV bolus every 6 h / Enteral administration every 24 h	IV bolus every 6 h	IV bolus every 6 h	Continuous IV administration over 24 h	IV bolus every 6 h / Enteral administration every 24 h
Daily dose	200 mg / 50 µg	200 mg	200 mg	200 mg	200 mg / 50 µg
Duration of treatment (day)	7 / 7	5 days + 6 days of tapering	5 days + 6 days of tapering	7	7 / 7
Tapering off at the end of the treatment	No	Yes	Yes	No	No

Adapted from [19]

16.4 When and How to Administer Glucocorticoids in Septic Shock

16.4.1 When Should Steroids Be Administrated in Septic Shock?

Early administration of glucocorticoids is unlikely to benefit patients with sepsis without shock. The HYPRESS trial [21] demonstrated that hydrocortisone in sepsis did not prevent a subsequent occurrence of shock. Recent guidelines recommend the administration of hydrocortisone in septic shock [5]. Data provided by a recent meta-analysis suggest that in sepsis, glucocorticoids reduce D28 mortality (relative risk (RR) 0.91, 95% CI 0.84–0.99) and in-hospital mortality (RR 0.90, 95% CI 0.82–0.99), without any significant long-term effect on mortality (RR 0.97, 95% CI 0.91–1.03) [8]. Glucocorticoids, in sepsis, also reduce ICU length of stay (mean difference −1.07 days, 95% CI −1.95 to −0.19) and hospital length of stay (mean difference-1.63 days, 95% CI −2.93 to −0.33) [8]. Common side effects include increased risk of muscle weakness, hyperglycemia, and hypernatremia without any increased risk of superinfection [8]. We propose that corticosteroids be administered in septic shock when vasopressors are required to achieve MAP ≥65 mmHg for 6 h or more. Several types of synthetic glucocorticoids are available; however, not all glucocorticoids exhibit the same anti-inflammatory potency [14]. Similarly, not all steroids exhibit non-genomic effects; for instance, neither betamethasone nor fludrocortisone exhibit non-genomic effect. There is however no evidence that a particular glucocorticoid is more efficient for treating sepsis. In sepsis, since hydrocortisone is by far the most studied compound, we recommend the use of hydrocortisone for treating septic shock.

16.4.2 What Dose of Steroids Should Be Administered?

High-dose steroids do not reduce mortality in sepsis at D28 (RR 0.96; 95% CI 0.80–1.16) [8], contrary to low-dose steroids (RR 0.91; 95% CI 0.86–0.97). Therefore, in septic shock, low doses (200 mg/day) of hydrocortisone (or equivalent) are preferred. The daily administration of 100 mg hydrocortisone was associated with a reduced incidence of hyperglycemia compared to 200 mg hydrocortisone [22]. Alternatively, in septic shock, 300 mg/day of hydrocortisone was not associated with reduced mortality at D28 [23]. We therefore recommend administrating 200 mg/day of hydrocortisone in septic shock.

16.4.3 Should Fludrocortisone Be Associated with Hydrocortisone?

Fludrocortisone is a far more potent mineralocorticoid agonist than hydrocortisone. Binding to the same mineralocorticoid receptor of either aldosterone (or fludrocortisone) or cortisol (or hydrocortisone) induces distinct intracellular signals. Cortisol acts either as an agonist or as an antagonist for the mineralocorticoid receptor. During septic shock, both mineralocorticoid receptor expression

Modulating the Immune Response

Contents

The Role of Steroids

Nicholas Heming and Djillali Annane

Contents

⊜ **Learning Objectives**

- To understand the mechanisms underlying sepsis that are relevant to corticosteroids
- To understand the mechanisms of action of corticosteroids that are relevant to the management of sepsis
- To know how to identify patients with sepsis, community-acquired pneumonia, ARDS, or COVID-19 who should be treated with corticosteroids
- To know how to give corticosteroids in these patients, including type of molecule, dose, and duration of treatment
- To know the risks associated with corticosteroids and how to prevent them

16.1 Introduction

A number of conditions in intensive care units are associated with dysregulated immune responses. Among these diseases, sepsis is a model of dysregulated immune response in the critically ill. Sepsis is characterized by life-threatening organ dysfunction caused by a dysregulated host response to infection. It affects more than 44 million people annually, causing approximately 11 million fatalities [1, 2]. The incidence of sepsis increases steadily in industrialized countries, due to an ageing and frailer population [3]. Approximately half of all sepsis survivors will suffer physical and psychological sequelae, which may significantly alter their subsequent quality of life [4]. Septic shock is the most severe subtype of sepsis associating metabolic, cellular, immune, and circulatory abnormalities and a significant risk of death [1]. Treatment of septic shock is based on antimicrobial therapy, source control, and symptomatic organ support [5]. Over the years, a large number of experimental interventions have been investigated in the management of patients with sepsis, mostly unsuccessfully [6]. Corticosteroids are the only treatment to reduce mortality in septic shock [7–9], and this treatment should probably be part of routine management of septic shock [5]. In this review, we will briefly describe the pathophysiology of septic shock and describe when and how to administer corticosteroids. More recently, corticosteroids were shown to significantly reduce coronavirus disease (COVID-19)-related mortality paving the way for a broader use of corticosteroids in severe respiratory infections.

16

16.2 Pathophysiology of Sepsis Relevant to Corticosteroids

Sepsis results from the interaction between a host and a pathogen [10]. Septic shock results from imbalanced inflammatory response and corticotrope insufficiency, leading to organ failure [11]. During septic shock, the initial inflammatory response is described as exaggerated and is partially compounded by activation of anti-inflammatory pathways [12]. The initial inflammatory response arises through the interaction between pathogen-associated molecular patterns (PAMPs, such as lipopolysaccharide (LPS), flagellin, or bacterial DNA) and the innate immune system. PAMPs are recognized by receptors bound to the membrane of immune cells (Toll-

like receptors, NOD-like receptors, mannose-binding lectin, or receptor for advanced glycation end products (RAGE) [13]). The interaction between PAMPS and their specific receptor leads to the activation of cell signaling pathways. These signaling pathways subsequently induce the activation and translocation of the nuclear transcription factor (NF)-κB into the cell nucleus, leading to the transcription of pro-inflammatory cytokines such as tumor necrosis factor (TNF)-α, interleukin (IL)-1β, or IL-6 [13].

Glucocorticoids exhibit anti-inflammatory effects by upregulating the production of anti-inflammatory mediators (◻ Table 16.1). Glucocorticoids act on a cellular level by binding to the glucocorticoid receptor (GR), a member of the nuclear receptor superfamily. Glucocorticoids bound to the GR subsequently translocate from the cytoplasm to the nucleus. Within the nucleus, the GR interacts with specific DNA sequences, downregulating the expression of pro-inflammatory cytokines [14]. Glucocorticoids also exhibit an anti-inflammatory activity via non-genomic mechanisms of action; that is, this effect is not mediated by an interaction with cellular DNA [14].

Septic shock is also characterized by an inappropriate hormonal response [10]. At baseline, adrenal biosynthesis of glucocorticoids and mineralocorticoids is stimulated by the adrenocorticotropic hormone (ACTH). ACTH production is in turn dependent on corticotropin-releasing hormone (CRH) production. Cortisol is secreted following a circadian rhythm; a morning peak in cortisol concentration is followed by a gradual decrease over the day. The hypothalamic-pituitary-adrenal (HPA) axis may dysfunction in sepsis due to irreversible neuroendocrine cellular damage, impaired ACTH/CRH synthesis, impaired corticoid biosynthesis, and peripheral steroid resistance [15]. A maladaptive HPA axis response is observed in 60% of septic shock patients [10]. This maladaptive response of the hypothalamic-pituitary-adrenal axis is coined critical illness-related corticosteroid insufficiency [10]. Taken together, all of these mechanisms may contribute to hemodynamic failure during sepsis.

◻ **Table 16.1** Main immune effects of glucocorticoids in sepsis

Species	Effects
Rodent	– Improves survival [1]
Dog	– Improves survival [2]
Man	– Lowers plasma concentration of TNF-α [3] – Lowers plasma concentration of soluble E-selectin [4] – Lowers plasma concentration of plasma nitrite/nitrate, IL-6, IL-8, MIF, as well as markers of activation of neutrophiles (CD11b, CD64) [4] – Lowers the plasma concentration of phospholipase A [5] – Lowers the number of circulating eosinophils [6] – Lowers membrane expression of mHLA-DR [4] – Improves survival [7]

Adapted from [14]

16.3 Should Glucocorticoids Be Used in Sepsis?

Five large randomized trials studied the role of glucocorticoids in septic shock. The Ger-Inf-05 trial was the first phase 3 trial to assess the combination of low-dose hydrocortisone and fludrocortisone in septic shock patients that were nonresponsive to an ACTH test. The trial found that glucocorticoids had a significant benefit on survival (HR, 0.67; 95% CI, 0.47–0.95; $P = 0.02$) and on reducing vasopressor dependence (HR, 1.91; 95% CI, 1.29–2.84; $P = 0.001$) in patients with septic shock and CIRCI [7]. The CORTICUS trial did not demonstrate a similar impact of hydrocortisone on survival in septic shock with CIRCI (D28 mortality in patients nonresponsive to an ACTH test treated by hydrocortisone 39.2% vs. 36.1% treated by placebo, $P = 0.69$) while confirming the beneficial effect of hydrocortisone on vasopressor dependency [16]. In the VANISH trial, hydrocortisone did not significantly alter D28 mortality in septic shock (30.8% in the hydrocortisone group versus 27.5% in the placebo group; absolute difference, 3.3% [95% CI, −5.5 to 12.1%]) [17].

More recently, the ADRENAL study compared a continuous intravenous administration of 200 mg of hydrocortisone per day for 7 days vs. placebo in 3800 septic shock patients. The primary endpoint was all-cause mortality at D90. At D90, 511 patients (27.9%) in the hydrocortisone group and 526 (28.8%) in the placebo group had died (odds ratio, 0.95; CI 95%, 0.82–1.10; $P = 0.50$). However, in the hydrocortisone group, vasopressors were weaned faster than in the placebo group (median time, 3 days [quartiles, 2–5] vs. 4 days [quartiles, 2–9]; HR, 1.32; CI 95%, 1.23–1.41; $P < 0.001$), and hydrocortisone-treated patients required less blood transfusion (37% vs. 41.7%; odds ratio, 0.82; CI 95%, 0.72–0.94; $P = 0.004$) [18].

The APPROCCHSS trial compared a discontinuous intravenous administration of 200 mg hydrocortisone per day for 7 days plus 50 µg enteral fludrocortisone vs. placebo in 1241 patients with septic shock. The primary endpoint was also mortality at D90. At D90, 264 patients (43%) in the hydrocortisone plus fludrocortisone group had died vs. 308 (49.1%) in the placebo group ($P = 0.03$) (relative risk 0.88 95% CI 0.78–0.99; $P = 0.03$). The number of days alive free of vasopressors, as well as the number of days alive free of organ failure, was also significantly higher in the hydrocortisone and fludrocortisone group than in the placebo group, without increased incidence of side effects [9].

ADRENAL and APPROCCHSS differed in several ways (◻ Table 16.2) [19, 20]. At baseline, the population included in APPROCCHSS accounted for more cases of pulmonary sepsis, and patients were more severe and required higher doses of vasopressors. Additionally, although daily administered doses of hydrocortisone were identical (200 mg/day), modalities of administration differed; in ADRENAL, the administration was continuous, while in APPROCCHSS the administration was discontinuous and combined with enteral fludrocortisone. A recent meta-analysis including 61 clinical trials and 12,192 participants confirmed that low-dose hydrocortisone had a beneficial effect on mortality in septic shock [8].

■ **Table 16.2** Main clinical trials assessing corticosteroids in septic shock

Variable	Annane et al. [9]	Sprung et al. [10]	Gordon et al. [11]	Venkatesh et al. [12]	Annane et al. [13]
Effect on D28 mortality (% absolute value)	−6	+2.8	+3.3		−6
Effect on D90 mortality (% absolute value)				−1	−6
Steroid	Hydrocortisone / Fludrocortisone	Hydrocortisone	Hydrocortisone	Hydrocortisone	Hydrocortisone / Fludrocortisone
Administration	IV bolus every 6 h / Enteral administration every 24 h	IV bolus every 6 h	IV bolus every 6 h	Continuous IV administration over 24 h	IV bolus every 6 h / Enteral administration every 24 h
Daily dose	200 mg / 50 µg	200 mg	200 mg	200 mg	200 mg / 50 µg
Duration of treatment (day)	7 / 7	5 days + 6 days of tapering	5 days + 6 days of tapering	7	7 / 7
Tapering off at the end of the treatment	No	Yes	Yes	No	No

Adapted from [19]

16.4 When and How to Administer Glucocorticoids in Septic Shock

16.4.1 When Should Steroids Be Administrated in Septic Shock?

Early administration of glucocorticoids is unlikely to benefit patients with sepsis without shock. The HYPRESS trial [21] demonstrated that hydrocortisone in sepsis did not prevent a subsequent occurrence of shock. Recent guidelines recommend the administration of hydrocortisone in septic shock [5]. Data provided by a recent meta-analysis suggest that in sepsis, glucocorticoids reduce D28 mortality (relative risk (RR) 0.91, 95% CI 0.84–0.99) and in-hospital mortality (RR 0.90, 95% CI 0.82–0.99), without any significant long-term effect on mortality (RR 0.97, 95% CI 0.91–1.03) [8]. Glucocorticoids, in sepsis, also reduce ICU length of stay (mean difference −1.07 days, 95% CI −1.95 to −0.19) and hospital length of stay (mean difference −1.63 days, 95% CI −2.93 to −0.33) [8]. Common side effects include increased risk of muscle weakness, hyperglycemia, and hypernatremia without any increased risk of superinfection [8]. We propose that corticosteroids be administered in septic shock when vasopressors are required to achieve MAP ≥65 mmHg for 6 h or more. Several types of synthetic glucocorticoids are available; however, not all glucocorticoids exhibit the same anti-inflammatory potency [14]. Similarly, not all steroids exhibit non-genomic effects; for instance, neither betamethasone nor fludrocortisone exhibit non-genomic effect. There is however no evidence that a particular glucocorticoid is more efficient for treating sepsis. In sepsis, since hydrocortisone is by far the most studied compound, we recommend the use of hydrocortisone for treating septic shock.

16.4.2 What Dose of Steroids Should Be Administered?

High-dose steroids do not reduce mortality in sepsis at D28 (RR 0.96; 95% CI 0.80–1.16) [8], contrary to low-dose steroids (RR 0.91; 95% CI 0.86–0.97). Therefore, in septic shock, low doses (200 mg/day) of hydrocortisone (or equivalent) are preferred. The daily administration of 100 mg hydrocortisone was associated with a reduced incidence of hyperglycemia compared to 200 mg hydrocortisone [22]. Alternatively, in septic shock, 300 mg/day of hydrocortisone was not associated with reduced mortality at D28 [23]. We therefore recommend administrating 200 mg/day of hydrocortisone in septic shock.

16.4.3 Should Fludrocortisone Be Associated with Hydrocortisone?

Fludrocortisone is a far more potent mineralocorticoid agonist than hydrocortisone. Binding to the same mineralocorticoid receptor of either aldosterone (or fludrocortisone) or cortisol (or hydrocortisone) induces distinct intracellular signals. Cortisol acts either as an agonist or as an antagonist for the mineralocorticoid receptor. During septic shock, both mineralocorticoid receptor expression

and plasma concentration of aldosterone decrease [24, 25]. Animal studies showed that mineralocorticoids have a beneficial effect on survival in septic shock, an effect mainly driven through the restoration of vascular α-adrenoceptors [24, 26]. Fludrocortisone appears to have an additive effect to that of hydrocortisone on the cardiovascular system in septic shock [27, 28]. There is no intravenous formulation of fludrocortisone, meaning that poor digestive absorption during shock may become an issue. A pharmacokinetic study of enteral fludrocortisone in septic shock did however confirm its rapid absorption [29]. Two distinct trials assessing the efficacy of hydrocortisone and fludrocortisone found survival benefits in sepsis from this combination of drugs [7, 9]. An open-label trial involving 500 participants compared the administration of hydrocortisone and fludrocortisone vs. hydrocortisone alone in septic shock. The primary objective of this 2×2 factorial trial was to assess the effect of intensive insulin therapy in glucocorticoid-treated septic shock. In this trial, hydrocortisone combined with fludrocortisone was associated with a trend towards reduced in-hospital mortality (primary endpoint) of approximately 3%, compared to hydrocortisone alone [30]. We suggest adding 50 µg of fludrocortisone to hydrocortisone in the routine management of patients with septic shock.

16.4.4 What Is the Optimal Duration of Glucocorticoid Administration?

Prolonged treatment with moderate to low doses of glucocorticoids ($\geq$3 days) is associated with a shorter duration of shock and reduced mortality [8]. Nevertheless, no study has formally compared a fixed-duration corticosteroid regimen with a shorter, clinical endpoint-guided regimen. We suggest administrating steroids for a fixed duration of 7 days.

16.4.5 Should Glucocorticoids Be Tapered Off?

A possible rebound effect following the abrupt discontinuation of steroids has been hypothesized. No study has formally compared tapering versus abrupt discontinuation of steroids. An indirect comparison of discontinuation methods found that the risk of mortality was reduced (RR 0.87, 95% CI 0.78–0.98) when steroid discontinuation was abrupt [8]. We suggest that steroids be interrupted without tapering.

16.4.6 What Are the Main Side Effects of Steroids?

The main side effects of steroids are metabolic and mainly include hyperglycemia and hypernatremia. An increased risk of muscle weakness has also been reported (RR 1.21, 95% CI 1.01–1.44) [8]. The administration of glucocorticoids in septic shock was not associated with an increased incidence of superinfections (RR 1.06, 95% CI 0.95–1.19) or with cardiovascular and cerebrovascular adverse events, or gastrointestinal bleeding [8].

16.4.7 Should Other Conditions Be Treated by Glucocorticoids in the ICU?

Community-acquired pneumonia is associated with systemic inflammation, and therefore these patients may benefit from glucocorticoids. Thirteen trials (total $n = 2005$) assessed the impact of glucocorticoid therapy in community-acquired pneumonia, using various types and doses of corticosteroids. Twelve trials found that glucocorticoids had a favorable impact on mortality, with a marked effect on the sickest patients [15, 31]. Corticosteroids may reduce the length of hospital stay and the need of invasive mechanical ventilation and may prevent acute respiratory distress syndrome (ARDS) [15, 31].

Glucocorticoids may also be of benefit to patients with ARDS [32]. Nine trials have assessed the effects of glucocorticoids in patients with ARDS, mainly in the early ARDS [8]. Glucocorticoids reduced lung and systemic inflammation, duration of mechanical ventilation, and possibly mortality [32]. Methylprednisolone may be the corticosteroid of choice to treat patients with ARDS owing to rapid, marked, and long-lasting diffusion into lung tissues. Owing to a possible increased risk of superinfection, rigorous screening is therefore mandatory to detect and treat any nosocomial infections without delay. Finally, corticosteroids are the standard of care of patients with oxygen-dependent COVID [33]. Indeed, systematic review with meta-analysis of trials demonstrated that glucocorticoids are associated with reduced mortality (OR 0.66 [95% CI, 0.53–0.82]; $P < 0.001$ fixed-effect meta-analysis) [34]. The favorable effects of corticosteroids is a class effect and did not vary with age, gender, time from onset of symptoms, or dose [34, 35]. Treatment should be given at the daily dose of 6 mg of dexamethasone (or equivalent) for 5–10 days [33].

16.4.8 Can Glucocorticoid Treatment Be Personalized in Sepsis?

The positive impact of personalized treatments has been effectively demonstrated notably in the field of oncology [36]. Given the diverse pathophysiological mechanisms and clinical phenotypes in sepsis, optimizing the selection of septic shock patients who may benefit from glucocorticoids is of the utmost importance. Indeed, personalizing corticosteroid treatment in septic shock would prevent the unnecessary exposure of patients who are likely to be harmed by this therapy. There are several approaches to select patients that are candidates for corticosteroids. First, CIRCI may affect up to 60% of septic shock patients [37]. CIRCI is identified by means of an ACTH test or a random cortisol assay [15]. In a septic shock trial, in nonresponders to the ACTH test, mortality was 63% in the placebo arm and 53% in the corticosteroid arm (hazard ratio, 0.67; 95% CI, 0.47–0.95; $P = 0.02$) [7]. However, these findings were not replicated in subsequent studies [16]. These conflicting findings may be explained in part by significant variations in cortisol measurements [38]. Current researches are investigating omics-derived or cellular derived biomarkers to guide corticotherapy. In a recent study, patients with an immunocompetent transcriptomic signature may have increased odds of dying when receiving corticosteroids [39]. In another study, lymphopenia and increased monocyte distribution width were associated with resistance to hydrocortisone in a large cohort of patients with sepsis [40].

Summary

Glucocorticoids may benefit patients with septic shock, community-acquired pneumonia, ARDS, or COVID-19. Corticosteroid-related improved survival was associated with improvement in organ function and reduction in the need and length of life-supportive therapies. Fludrocortisone, a mineralocorticoid receptor agonist, may be added to hydrocortisone in patients with septic shock. In these patients, we suggest a duration of corticotherapy of 7 days without tapering off. Novel biomarker-guided personalized corticotherapy is a promising approach to the management of patients with sepsis, community-acquired pneumonia, ARDS, or COVID-19.

Take-Home Messages

- Dysregulated endocrine host response to infection, with inappropriate endogenous corticosteroid activity, is the hallmark of about half of patients with sepsis.
- Corticosteroids modulate innate and adaptative immunity through non-genomic and genomic effects, thereby contributing to restoring immune homeostasis in patients with sepsis.
- Evidence from clinical trials and systematic reviews suggested that corticosteroids may probably reduce mortality from septic shock, community-acquired pneumonia, ARDS, and COVID-19.
- There is strong heterogeneity in response to corticosteroids, suggesting that patients may benefit from individualized approach based on biomarkers of sensitivity/resistance to corticosteroids.

? Questions

1. Is measurement of serum cortisol required to guide corticotherapy in sepsis or ARDS?
2. What is the optimal dose of corticosteroids in patients with septic shock?
3. Are high-dose corticosteroids required in COVID-19-related ARDS?

✓ Answers

1. Measurement of cortisol level is not mandatory in the management of patients with sepsis or ARDS. CIRCI may be recognized by serum cortisol of less than 10 μg/dL or a cortisol increase post-Synacthen of less than 9 μg/dL.
2. In patients with septic shock, corticosteroids should probably be given as intravenous bolus of 50 mg hydrocortisone (or equivalent) q6 for 7 days without taper off.
3. In COVID-19 ARDS, corticosteroids should be given at a dose of 6 mg per day of dexamethasone (or equivalent) intravenously or enterally, for 5–10 days.

References

1. Singer M, Deutschman CS, Seymour CW, et al. The third international consensus definitions for sepsis and septic shock (Sepsis-3). JAMA. 2016;315:801–10. https://doi.org/10.1001/jama.2016.0287.
2. Fleischmann C, Scherag A, Adhikari NKJ, et al. Assessment of global incidence and mortality of hospital-treated sepsis. Current estimates and limitations. Am J Respir Crit Care Med. 2016;193:259–72. https://doi.org/10.1164/rccm.201504-0781OC.
3. Gaieski DF, Edwards JM, Kallan MJ, Carr BG. Benchmarking the incidence and mortality of severe sepsis in the United States. Crit Care Med. 2013;41:1167–74. https://doi.org/10.1097/CCM.0b013e31827c09f8.
4. Annane D, Sharshar T. Cognitive decline after sepsis. Lancet Respir Med. 2015;3:61–9. https://doi.org/10.1016/S2213-2600(14)70246-2.
5. Evans L, Rhodes A, Alhazzani W, et al. Surviving sepsis campaign: international guidelines for management of sepsis and septic shock 2021. Intensive Care Med. 2021;47:1181–247. https://doi.org/10.1007/s00134-021-06506-y.
6. Marshall JC. Why have clinical trials in sepsis failed? Trends Mol Med. 2014;20:195–203. https://doi.org/10.1016/j.molmed.2014.01.007.
7. Annane D, Sébille V, Charpentier C, et al. Effect of treatment with low doses of hydrocortisone and fludrocortisone on mortality in patients with septic shock. JAMA. 2002;288:862–71.
8. Annane D, Bellissant E, Bollaert PE, et al. Corticosteroids for treating sepsis in children and adults. Cochrane Database Syst Rev. 2019;12:CD002243. https://doi.org/10.1002/14651858.CD002243.pub4.
9. Annane D, Renault A, Brun-Buisson C, et al. Hydrocortisone plus fludrocortisone for adults with septic shock. N Engl J Med. 2018;378:809–18. https://doi.org/10.1056/NEJMoa1705716.
10. Annane D, Pastores SM, Arlt W, et al. Critical illness-related corticosteroid insufficiency (CIRCI): a narrative review from a Multispecialty Task Force of the Society of Critical Care Medicine (SCCM) and the European Society of Intensive Care Medicine (ESICM). Intensive Care Med. 2017;43:1781–92. https://doi.org/10.1007/s00134-017-4914-x.
11. Angus DC, van der Poll T. Severe sepsis and septic shock. N Engl J Med. 2013;369:840–51. https://doi.org/10.1056/NEJMra1208623.
12. Hotchkiss RS, Monneret G, Payen D. Immunosuppression in sepsis: a novel understanding of the disorder and a new therapeutic approach. Lancet Infect Dis. 2013;13:260–8. https://doi.org/10.1016/S1473-3099(13)70001-X.
13. Gay NJ, Symmons MF, Gangloff M, Bryant CE. Assembly and localization of Toll-like receptor signalling complexes. Nat Rev Immunol. 2014;14:546–58. https://doi.org/10.1038/nri3713.
14. Heming N, Sivanandamoorthy S, Meng P, et al. Immune effects of corticosteroids in sepsis. Front Immunol. 2018;9:1736. https://doi.org/10.3389/fimmu.2018.01736.
15. Annane D, Pastores SM, Rochwerg B, et al. Guidelines for the diagnosis and management of critical illness-related corticosteroid insufficiency (CIRCI) in critically ill patients (part I): Society of Critical Care Medicine (SCCM) and European Society of Intensive Care Medicine (ESICM) 2017. Intensive Care Med. 2017;43:1751–63. https://doi.org/10.1007/s00134-017-4919-5.
16. Sprung CL, Annane D, Keh D, et al. Hydrocortisone therapy for patients with septic shock. N Engl J Med. 2008;358:111–24. https://doi.org/10.1056/NEJMoa071366.
17. Gordon AC, Mason AJ, Thirunavukkarasu N, et al. Effect of early vasopressin vs norepinephrine on kidney failure in patients with septic shock: the VANISH randomized clinical trial. JAMA. 2016;316:509–18. https://doi.org/10.1001/jama.2016.10485.
18. Venkatesh B, Finfer S, Cohen J, et al. Adjunctive glucocorticoid therapy in patients with septic shock. N Engl J Med. 2018;378:797–808. https://doi.org/10.1056/NEJMoa1705835.
19. Annane D. Why my steroid trials in septic shock were "positive"? Crit Care Med. 2019;47(12):1789–93. https://doi.org/10.1097/CCM.0000000000003889.
20. Venkatesh B, Cohen J. Why the adjunctive corticosteroid treatment in critically ill patients with septic shock (ADRENAL) trial did not show a difference in mortality? Crit Care Med. 2019;47(12):1785–8. https://doi.org/10.1097/CCM.0000000000003834.
21. Keh D, Trips E, Marx G, et al. Effect of hydrocortisone on development of shock among patients with severe sepsis: the HYPRESS randomized clinical trial. JAMA. 2016;316:1775. https://doi.org/10.1001/jama.2016.14799.

16

22. Ngaosuwan K, Ounchokdee K, Chalermchai T. Clinical outcomes of minimized hydrocortisone dosage of 100 mg/day on lower occurrence of hyperglycemia in septic shock patients. Shock. 2018;50:280–5. https://doi.org/10.1097/SHK.0000000000001061.

23. Hyvernat H, Barel R, Gentilhomme A, et al. Effects of increasing hydrocortisone to 300 mg per day in the treatment of septic shock: a pilot study. Shock. 2016;46:498–505. https://doi.org/10.1097/SHK.0000000000000665.

24. Fadel F, André-Grégoire G, Gravez B, et al. Aldosterone and vascular mineralocorticoid receptors in murine endotoxic and human septic shock. Crit Care Med. 2017;45:e954–62. https://doi.org/10.1097/CCM.0000000000002462.

25. du Cheyron D, Lesage A, Daubin C, et al. Hyperreninemic hypoaldosteronism: a possible etiological factor of septic shock-induced acute renal failure. Intensive Care Med. 2003;29:1703–9. https://doi.org/10.1007/s00134-003-1986-6.

26. Laviolle B, Annane D, Fougerou C, Bellissant E. Gluco- and mineralocorticoid biological effects of a 7-day treatment with low doses of hydrocortisone and fludrocortisone in septic shock. Intensive Care Med. 2012;38:1306–14. https://doi.org/10.1007/s00134-012-2585-1.

27. Hicks CW, Sweeney DA, Danner RL, et al. Efficacy of selective mineralocorticoid and glucocorticoid agonists in canine septic shock. Crit Care Med. 2012;40:199–207. https://doi.org/10.1097/CCM.0b013e31822efa14.

28. Hebbar KB, Stockwell JA, Fortenberry JD. Clinical effects of adding fludrocortisone to a hydrocortisone-based shock protocol in hypotensive critically ill children. Intensive Care Med. 2011;37:518–24. https://doi.org/10.1007/s00134-010-2090-3.

29. Polito A, Hamitouche N, Ribot M, et al. Pharmacokinetics of oral fludrocortisone in septic shock. Br J Clin Pharmacol. 2016;82:1509–16. https://doi.org/10.1111/bcp.13065.

30. COIITSS Study Investigators. Corticosteroid treatment and intensive insulin therapy for septic shock in adults: a randomized controlled trial. JAMA. 2010;303:341–8. https://doi.org/10.1001/jama.2010.2.

31. Pastores SM, Annane D, Rochwerg B, Corticosteroid Guideline Task Force of SCCM and ESICM. Guidelines for the diagnosis and management of critical illness-related corticosteroid insufficiency (CIRCI) in critically ill patients (part II): Society of Critical Care Medicine (SCCM) and European Society of Intensive Care Medicine (ESICM) 2017. Intensive Care Med. 2018;44:474–7. https://doi.org/10.1007/s00134-017-4951-5.

32. Meduri GU, Bridges L, Shih M-C, et al. Prolonged glucocorticoid treatment is associated with improved ARDS outcomes: analysis of individual patients' data from four randomized trials and trial-level meta-analysis of the updated literature. Intensive Care Med. 2016;42:829–40. https://doi.org/10.1007/s00134-015-4095-4.

33. Rochwerg B, Agarwal A, Siemieniuk RA, et al. A living WHO guideline on drugs for covid-19. BMJ. 2020;370:m3379. https://doi.org/10.1136/bmj.m3379. Update in: BMJ. 2020 Nov 19;371:m4475. Update in: BMJ. 2021 Mar 31;372:n860. Update in: BMJ. 2021 Jul 6;374:n1703. Update in: BMJ 2021 Sep 23;374:n2219.

34. WHO Rapid Evidence Appraisal for COVID-19 Therapies (REACT) Working Group. Association between administration of systemic corticosteroids and mortality among critically ill patients with COVID-19: a meta-analysis. JAMA. 2020;324(13):1330–41. https://doi.org/10.1001/jama.2020.17023.

35. COVID STEROID 2 Trial Group. Effect of 12 mg vs 6 mg of dexamethasone on the number of days alive without life support in adults with COVID-19 and severe hypoxemia: the COVID STEROID 2 randomized trial. JAMA. 2021;326(18):1807–17. https://doi.org/10.1001/jama.2021.18295. PMID: 34673895; PMCID: PMC8532039.

36. Marini JJ, Vincent J-L, Annane D. Critical care evidence—new directions. JAMA. 2015;313:893–4. https://doi.org/10.1001/jama.2014.18484.

37. Marik PE, Pastores SM, Annane D, et al. Recommendations for the diagnosis and management of corticosteroid insufficiency in critically ill adult patients: consensus statements from an international task force by the American College of Critical Care Medicine. Crit Care Med. 2008;36:1937–49. https://doi.org/10.1097/CCM.0b013e31817603ba.

38. Briegel J, Sprung CL, Annane D, et al. Multicenter comparison of cortisol as measured by different methods in samples of patients with septic shock. Intensive Care Med. 2009;35:2151–6. https://doi.org/10.1007/s00134-009-1627-9.

39. Antcliffe DB, Burnham KL, Al-Beidh F, et al. Transcriptomic signatures in sepsis and a differential response to steroids. From the VANISH randomized trial. Am J Respir Crit Care Med. 2019;199:980–6. https://doi.org/10.1164/rccm.201807-1419OC.

40. MOCORSEP Study Group. Monocyte distribution width as a biomarker of resistance to corticosteroids in patients with sepsis: the MOCORSEP observational study. Intensive Care Med. 2021;47:1161–4. https://doi.org/10.1007/s00134-021-06478-z.

Anti-cytokine Therapy in Critical Illness: Is There a Role?

John C. Marshall

Contents

Learning Objectives

After reading this chapter, students will be able to describe the complexities of the cytokine response, identify illnesses where it has been found to be an effective therapeutic target, and discuss the challenges associated with applying this strategy to critically ill patients with sepsis.

17.1 Introduction

The word "cytokine," from Greek words for "cell" and "motion," describes a group of low-molecular-weight proteins that play a pivotal role in signaling between cells during an acute response to an injurious or infectious stimulus. Transcribed and released in response to an exogenous stimulus such as microbial antigens or products of injured cells, cytokines signal to immune cells to activate the appropriate defense responses and to other cells to modify normal cellular function.

Interventions that target specific cytokines—either monoclonal antibodies or recombinant proteins—or the signal transduction cascades activated following their interactions with target cells (typically small-molecule inhibitors) have found a therapeutic role in diseases as diverse as cancer, arthritis, and inflammatory bowel disease. Yet although studies into the biology of life-threatening inflammation have been central to our understanding of cytokines, and although the COVID-19 pandemic has demonstrated a role for cytokine manipulation in the treatment of viral illness [1], the strategy has yet to show unequivocal evidence of efficacy in treating life-threatening acute illness.

17.2 Cytokines in the Regulation of a Systemic Response to Danger: A Historical Perspective

17.2.1 Cytokines and Hormones: How Do They Differ?

Coordination of function at the whole-organism level is mediated either through signals delivered from the central nervous system to peripheral tissues or through the activity of circulating host-derived mediators that bind to specific target cells and elicit a discrete response.

Ernest Starling in 1905 coined the word "hormone" (from the Greek *hormon* "that which sets in motion") to describe "the chemical messengers which speeding from cell to cell along the bloodstream may coordinate the activities and growth of different parts of the body" [2]. The concept fueled a search for other soluble effectors of cell function, particularly endocrine cell function, and rapidly led to the identification of insulin, thyroid hormone, cortisol, and adrenergic hormones amongst others. The identification of hormones also gave rise to a new biologic and medical discipline—endocrinology [3]—the study of the regulation of physiologic function by the secretion of products from endocrine glands [4].

Cytokines share features with hormones, and the distinction between these two groups of endogenous signaling molecule may be more a function of historical precedent than inherent biology. As a general principle, hormone levels are regulated centrally through the release of hormone-releasing factors, whereas cytokine release is induced peripherally through the activity of the innate immune system. Hormones exert their effects on target cells in endocrine glands, whereas cytokines bind to a promiscuous group of receptors that are expressed on immune cells, but also on epithelial and endothelial cells. Circulating levels of hormones tend to be higher and less volatile than cytokine levels, and hormones often have readily identified counter-hormones. Perhaps the greatest difference, however, is that hormones represent a smaller and more constrained group of molecules with more clearly identifiable biologic functions, and so a conceptual model of their activity is more readily within reach.

17.2.2 Cytokines: An Evolving Understanding

The first evidence that endogenous factors generated by a response to infection could impact outcome came from the work of William Coley in the late nineteenth century [5]. Building on the empiric observation that patients who developed infection following malignant tumor resection seemed to have better outcomes [6], Coley hypothesized that soluble factors generated during infection could inhibit the growth of malignant tumors. He championed the injection of a combination of killed *Serratia marcescens* and *Streptococcus pyogenes* into solid tumors and showed some striking, if anecdotal, responses (◘ Fig. 17.1) [7].

However, it was not until 60 years later that the first evidence emerged that the systemic effects of infection are mediated not by products of the infecting organism,

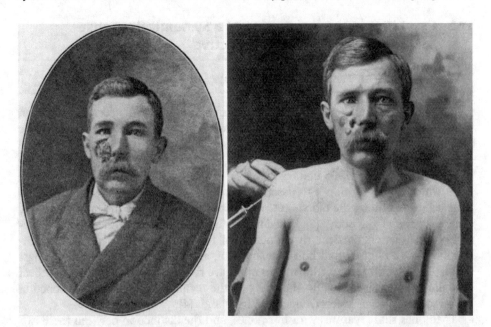

◘ **Fig. 17.1** A veterinarian with an inoperable round-cell sarcoma of the jaw, treated with systemic Coley's adjuvant and assessed after 63 treatments (left) and a full course of 103 injections (right). He remained alive and disease-free 6 years later. (From [7])

17

but by molecules released by the infected host. Atkins and colleagues in 1955 studied the pathogenesis of fever induced by typhoid vaccine. They reported,

》 *With the use of a passive transfer method and pyrogen-tolerant recipients, the biological properties of this substance have been differentiated from those of the uncleared vaccine in the circulation. The newly identified factor resembles leucocytic pyrogen in the rapidity with which it produces fever and in its failure to exhibit cross-tolerance with bacterial pyrogen. This striking similarity of properties suggests that the circulating factor is of endogenous origin and may arise from cell injury* [8].

The work was pivotal. It identified the host as the cause of the sequelae of infection and suggested that the response was not unique to infection, but rather a response to cell injury. Both of these concepts have yet to be fully integrated into our understanding of sepsis and its contribution to the pathogenesis of acute illness.

Endogenous pyrogen was ultimately isolated, sequenced, and designated as interleukin-1 [9], a designation signaling that mediated communication between white blood cells, and was the first such protein identified. Subsequent naming of interleukins reflects only the temporal sequence of their discovery, and not shared biology. The most recently identified member of this diverse family of proteins is interleukin-41, isolated from the synovial fluid of patients with rheumatoid arthritis [10]. Not only are there more than 40 named interleukins, but also multiple isoforms of individual proteins have been identified. The interleukin-1 family, for example, includes IL-1α and IL-1β as well as the inhibitory IL-1 receptor antagonist that binds the IL-1 receptor but does not transmit a signal [11].

Interleukins have multiple effects on signaling between immune cells, influencing the function of cells of both the innate and adaptive immune systems. These effects have been considered broadly pro- and anti-inflammatory, based on the consequences of their manipulation in models of acute inflammation. The distinction is overly simplistic, and the function of any given interleukin is often redundant, or contingent upon the concomitant effects of other cytokines.

To make matters more complex, multiple other circulating immunoregulatory proteins have been described. Their naming has been even more chaotic, based on the initial biologic activity originally identified, rather than on their dominant role in cellular homeostasis. Tumor necrosis factor (TNF), for example, was so named based on the identification of a protein with tumoricidal activity in the cultures of endotoxin-treated macrophages, a putative candidate for Coley's toxin [12]; the same protein was called cachectin based on its ability to induce wasting [13]. It was a decade before its seminal role as a mediator of endotoxin activity was identified [14]. Its lytic activity arises from its capacity to induce apoptosis, a biologic process that was only dimly recognized at the time of its naming. Some cytokines are named as growth factors—granulocyte-macrophage colony-stimulating factor, for example— or proteins that otherwise support or inhibit cell growth—leukemia inhibitory factor, pre-B-cell colony-enhancing factor, and adiponectin, for example.

Cytokines, therefore, are proteins that mediate communications between cells and so support an acute host response to a potential threat to homeostasis. They share features with hormones and with other proteins that are known to play a role in the response to infection—for example, coagulation factors, complement proteins, and acute-phase reactants.

◘ **Table 17.1** Diverse cellular responses triggered by cytokines

Biologic process	Examples
Activation of innate host defenses	*Priming of NADPH oxidase assembly*: IL-1ß, TNF, platelet-derived growth factor, thrombin, PBEF/Nampt *Activation of nitric oxide synthase*: IL-1ß, TNF, interferon-γ
Cell growth	*Myeloid cell growth*: G-CSF, GM-CSF *Erythroid cell growth*: erythropoietin *Epithelial cell growth*: EGF *Vascular cell growth*: platelet-derived growth factor, VEGF
Tissue repair	*Induction of fibrosis:* transforming growth factor-ß
Regulation of adaptive immunity	*Lymphocyte proliferation*: IL-2, IL-4, IL-7 *Lymphocyte differentiation*: IL-4, IL-5, IL-17 *Induction of HLA-DR expression*: IFN-γ
Alteration of cellular metabolism	*Induction of aerobic glycolysis*: IL-2 IL-3, IL-7
Programmed cell death	*Apoptosis*: TNF, Fas ligand *Necroptosis*: TNFα

A large number of individual proteins have been found to be implicated by virtue of their capacity to alter mortality in murine models of acute inflammation—typically either endotoxin challenge or the more complex infectious model, cecal ligation and puncture (CLP). ◘ Table 17.1 summarizes some of these; it will be apparent that the effects of intervention are model dependent and that both excess and inadequate expression may improve survival, depending on the experimental circumstances [15].

17.2.3 How Do Cytokines Alter Cellular Functioning?

Cytokines are not inherently cytotoxic, but rather exert their effects by altering cellular function. The consequences may be either beneficial or detrimental and arise through evolutionary pressure to sustain life in the face of an acute threat and to restore homeostasis once that threat has been addressed. Cytokines in the extracellular environment typically bind to a dedicated receptor on a target cell. Receptor engagement, in turn, results in a topological change of the receptor that facilitates interactions with key associated intracellular adapter proteins to form a signaling complex at the cell membrane. Posttranslational modifications in these adapter proteins, such as phosphorylation on key amino acid residues, facilitate the assembly of these signaling complexes and result in the activation of intracellular transcription factors that promote differential gene transcription in the cell (◘ Fig. 17.2).

Cytokines exert multiple effects on cellular function. The diversity of these responses, the number of different types of cells impacted, and the number of individual cytokines identified have made it difficult to develop functional classification systems. From the perspective of the host response to infection and injury, cytokines orchestrate a number of key responses (◘ Table 17.1)—priming and activation of

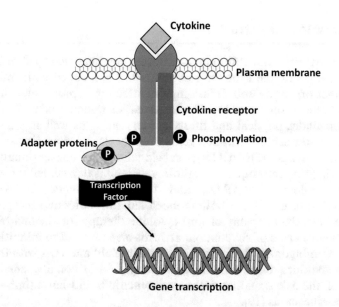

Fig. 17.2 Signaling through a cytokine receptor. Cytokines released locally by other immune cells or from the systemic circulation bind to specific receptors on their target cells. Binding typically results in the aggregation of several receptors. Posttranslational changes in the intracellular portion of the receptor, particularly the phosphorylation of tyrosine, serine, or threonine residues, facilitate interactions with intracellular adapter proteins. This complex of cytokine receptor and adapter proteins, in turn, activates transcription factors in the cytoplasm, enabling them to translocate to the nucleus where they induce changes in gene transcription

innate host defense mechanisms such as coagulation or generation of reactive oxygen species or nitric oxide, promotion of cell proliferation, activation or suppression of an adaptive immune response, alteration of cellular metabolism, and induction of programmed cell death. The examples in ☐ Table 17.1 are far from comprehensive; they reflect both the scope and the redundancy of cytokine activity. They further underline the complexity of this network of inducible proteins, released at nanomolar levels, that orchestrate an integrated host response to danger. In this lies the naïveté of the assumption that targeting a single protein mediator that is either over- or under-expressed during a complex and dynamic disease process might sufficiently alter the course of that process that its victims would be more likely to be alive at its conclusion.

Yet treatments targeting the cytokine response have shown benefit in a number of diseases.

17.3 Cytokine-Targeted Therapy in Chronic Inflammatory Diseases

While the complex networks that comprise the cytokine response have largely been identified through the study of models of acute illness, treatments targeting individual mediators have shown the greatest evidence of benefit in chronic disease—either inflammatory or malignant.

17.3.1 Rheumatoid Arthritis

Rheumatoid arthritis is an autoimmune disorder characterized by chronic destructive inflammation of the synovium of joints but associated with inflammatory injury to other organs as well. It is common, affecting approximately 0.6% of the population at any given time [16]. The treatment of rheumatoid arthritis is multimodal and includes physical and lifestyle intervention as well as pharmacologic therapy. The latter centers around agents broadly classified as disease-modifying antirheumatic drugs (DMARDs), subclassified as conventional synthetic DMARDs (hydroxychloroquine, methotrexate, sulfasalazine, leflunomide, corticosteroids), biologic DMARDs, and targeted synthetic DMARDs [17]. Interventions to target TNF—both monoclonal antibodies and receptor antagonists—have been the mainstay of anti-cytokine therapy for rheumatoid arthritis [18]. More severe cases of rheumatoid arthritis also respond to inhibition of IL-6 with receptor antagonists (tocilizumab and sarilumab) and IL-1 with the receptor antagonist anakinra or monoclonal antibodies. Additionally, small-molecule inhibitors of the Jak signaling pathway—tofacitinib and baricitinib—have also shown to be efficacious [19].

17.3.2 Other Autoimmune Disorders

Cytokine-targeted therapies have found a role in the treatment of a number of other autoimmune disorders that share similarities with rheumatoid arthritis. TNF inhibition is effective in ankylosing spondylitis, a disorder that primarily affects the spine [20]. Antibodies to the T cell product, IL-17, have also been approved for use in patients with ankylosing spondylitis [21]. Targeting IL-17 and IL-23 has also proven efficacious in patients with psoriasis and psoriatic arthritis [22]. B cell-activating factor (BAFF), a TNF family member that binds one of the three receptors of the TNF receptor family, promotes B cell survival, and is over-expressed in systemic lupus erythematosus (SLE); its neutralization with a monoclonal antibody attenuates the symptoms of SLE [23].

17.3.3 Inflammatory Bowel Disease

Anti-TNF therapy has become a mainstay of the treatment of inflammatory bowel disease, and particularly in the management of fistulizing Crohn's disease [24]. A variety of TNF inhibitors have been shown to induce remission in patients with Crohn's disease, as has treatment with a monoclonal antibody to IL-23 [25] and an antibody to integrin α4ß7 [26]. Anti-cytokine strategies effective in patients with ulcerative colitis include these same agents, as well as an antibody to IL-12 and tofacitinib [27].

17

17.3.4 **Oncology**

Oncology has been at the forefront in harnessing the therapeutic potential of cytokine-dependent therapies. TNF likely made its first biologic appearance as the active factor in Coley's adjuvant; however, its evolving role in the management of malignancies has been limited to the regional control of sarcomas and melanoma [28]. But, underlining the complexity of the immune response, TNF inhibition has also demonstrated efficacy in the management of cancer.

17.3.5 **Other Diseases**

Canakinumab, an antibody against IL-1ß, has been shown to reduce the risk of cardiovascular complications when given to patients who have sustained a myocardial infarction [29]. The anti-TNF antibody, adalimumab, has also been approved for the treatment of hidradenitis suppurativa [30]. Treatments targeting interleukin-5 have shown efficacy in the treatment of asthma [31].

17.4 **Targeting Cytokines in Acute Inflammatory Diseases**

17.4.1 **Preclinical Insights**

It has proven remarkably easy to protect a mouse from a variety of different acute experimental inflammatory insults by blocking the activity of some cytokines or, conversely, by administering others. This dichotomy—that some cytokines are harmful in excess, whereas for others, a deficiency drives disease—has led to the overly simplistic classification of their effects as either pro- or anti-inflammatory (◘ Table 17.2).

Small animal models are of necessity reductionist. They do not so much model human illness, as replicate in vitro studies in a living organism where compensatory physiologic changes can occur and where the readout for biologic activity is visible illness or death. The conclusions of studies in murine models are also model dependent and may vary with the timing of treatment (prior to, synchronous with, or after the experimental insult), the nature of the insult, the provision of resuscitation and support, and the age and strain of the animals used [32]. Understanding the strengths and limitations of these models is useful in evaluating the results obtained and may provide insight into sources of heterogeneity in human illness.

Preclinical studies of the role of TNF in experimental infection illustrate the extent to which conclusions of efficacy are model dependent [15]. The potential for TNF as an adjuvant treatment for sepsis emerged from studies in models of endotoxemia [14] or bacteremia with Gram-positive [33] or Gram-negative [34] organisms, in which TNF was neutralized prior to the experimental insult. When TNF was neutralized in a cecal ligation and puncture model, there was no signal for benefit, whereas its neutralization in challenge models using *S. pneumoniae*, *Listeria*, *Candida*, or *M. tuberculosis* resulted in increased lethality (◘ Fig. 17.3) [15].

◻ **Table 17.2**   In vivo consequences of cytokine activity in murine endotoxemia

Increase lethality (neutralization improves survival)	Decrease lethality (neutralization worsens survival)
Interleukin-1	Interleukin-1α
Interleukin-12	Interleukin-1 receptor antagonist (IL-1ra)
Interleukin-17	Interleukin-4
Interleukin-18	Interleukin-10
Interleukin-25	Interleukin-13
Interleukin-33	C-reactive protein
Tumor necrosis factor	Interferon-β
Interferon-α	Bactericidal permeability increasing protein
Interferon regulatory factor-2 (IRF2)	(BPI)
Granulocyte colony-stimulating factor (G-CSF)	Very-low-density lipoprotein (VLDL)
Macrophage inflammatory protein-1α (MIP-1α)	Orexin
Macrophage migration inhibitory factor (MIF)	Apolipoprotein A1
Leukemia inhibitory factor (LIF)	Apolipoprotein E
Leptin	Hepatocyte growth factor (HGF)
Activin A	Leukemia inhibitory factor (LIF)
Ghrelin	Monocyte chemoattractant protein-1 (MCP1)
Triggering receptor expressed on myeloid cells-1	Cationic antimicrobial protein-18 (CAP-18)
(TREM 1)	TNF-stimulated gene-14 (TSG-14)
Vascular endothelial growth factor (VEGF)	Vasoactive intestinal peptide (VIP)
High mobility group box-1 (HMGB-1)	Protein C
Vasoactive intestinal peptide (VIP)	Lipocalin-2
Fetuin A	Follistatin
S100A8	Soluble fms-like tyrosine kinase-1 (sflt-1)
Adrenomedullin	Park7/DJ-1
Calcitonin gene-related peptide (CGRP)	Platelet-derived growth factor β
Heat-shock factor-1 (HSF1)	Erythropoietin
Parathyroid hormone-releasing protein	Ang 1–7
Lipopolysaccharide-binding protein (LBP)	Annexin V
	Thymosin-α
	Triggering receptor expressed on myeloid cells-2 (TREM2)
	Adrenomedullin

17.4.2   Insights from Clinical Trials in COVID-19

The COVID-19 pandemic has provided an exceptional opportunity to test the cytokine hypothesis in life-threatening infection and has confirmed that some patients with viral sepsis benefit from interventions that target the innate immune response.

The first insight to emerge from the hundreds of clinical trials evaluating the treatment of severe COVID-19 was that corticosteroids—either dexamethasone [35] or hydrocortisone [36]—improved the survival of the sickest COVID-19 patients [37]. Whether this effect is a consequence of the endocrine action of corticosteroids or a result of modulation of the cytokine response is uncertain.

Early reports suggested increased levels of circulating IL-6 in patients with severe disease, and trials in which IL-6 was blocked with one of the two antibodies that

17

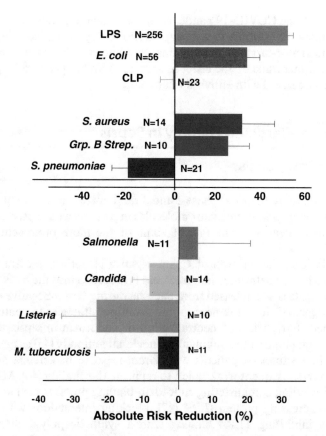

□ **Fig. 17.3** A systematic review of 480 published manuscripts describing the effects of neutralization of TNF in animal models of sepsis. In studies involving eight separate species, TNF neutralization improved survival in models of endotoxemia and Gram-negative bacteremia, but not in a complex infectious challenge model such as cecal ligation and puncture. In contrast, TNF neutralization increased the lethality of models of pneumococcal infection, and following experimental challenge with *Candida*, *Listeria*, or *M. tuberculosis*. (From [15])

block the IL-6 receptor—tocilizumab or sarilumab—showed that IL-6 antagonism increased patient survival [1]. On the other hand, the effects of antagonism of IL-1 have been disappointing, although a European trial in which SUPAR levels were used to identify a subset of patients more likely to benefit from treatment did show a mortality reduction [38]. Pooled data from studies in which patients received anti-TNF therapies for unrelated reasons showed benefit for TNF neutralization [39]; however, data from definitive trials are limited.

Finally, small-molecule inhibitors of the Jak/stat signal transduction pathway—baricitinib and tofacitinib—have also been shown to improve survival in patients with COVID-19 [40, 41].

COVID-19 is associated with a significant risk of intravascular coagulation, and consequently the effects of heparin on disease progression have been assessed. Clinical trials suggest a benefit for heparin anticoagulation in moderate [42], but not severe [43], disease.

Insights from the COVID-19 pandemic are still emerging; however, two observations are striking. In contrast to a disappointing legacy of clinical trials for sepsis, efficacy for mediator-targeted therapy has been shown for a variety of strategies. Moreover, the magnitude of the effect is impressive and appears to be greater than what has been observed with antiviral treatments.

17.5 Cytokine-Targeted Therapy in Sepsis

17.5.1 The Story So Far

There have been more than 100 phase 2 and 3 randomized trials testing novel therapies that target endogenous mediator molecules in patients with sepsis; none of these is licensed for clinical use. The fate of some of the more prominent of these is summarized below.

Endotoxin from the cell wall of Gram-negative bacteria is present in health in large amounts in the gastrointestinal tract and is absorbed into the body in a number of disease states. It is also released from bacteria during Gram-negative infections. It is a potent trigger of the cytokine response. Multiple strategies to neutralize it have been evaluated. Early trials of neutralization of endotoxin in sepsis with either a polyclonal serum [44] or a recombinant monoclonal antibody [45] suggested benefit, particularly in a subset of patients with Gram-negative bacteremia and/or septic shock; however, subsequent work failed to replicate this finding [46]. Multiple other approaches including administering endotoxin-binding proteins such as bactericidal permeability-increasing protein (BPI) [47], blocking interactions with CD14 [48], competitively inhibiting TLR4 binding with a synthetic polysaccharide [49], or removing circulating endotoxin with a polymyxin-containing filter [50] have all yielded disappointing results.

Circulating TNF in patients with sepsis has been targeted with specific monoclonal and polyclonal antibodies as well as with recombinant soluble TNF receptor proteins. The impact has been modest. A single trial of a monoclonal antibody showed benefit for patients with elevated baseline levels of IL-6 [51], whereas another study of a soluble receptor antagonist suggested harm [52]. Pooled data from more than 8000 studied patients does reveal a significant reduction in mortality [53]; however, the effect size is small, and anti-TNF therapies have not been licensed for the treatment of sepsis.

Interleukin-1 has been inhibited by the use of a recombinant interleukin-1 receptor antagonist. Pooled data from three trials do show a reduction in mortality for treated patients [54], but the small and inconsistent effect has precluded licensure of the agent for the treatment of sepsis.

An alternate concept to that of blunting a pro-inflammatory cytokine response has been to target the procoagulant state that accompanies the activation of inflammation. In truth, the distinction between inflammation and coagulation is arbitrary: the induction of coagulation is a key host antibacterial mechanism, and there is substantial overlap between the two processes [55]. Protein C is an endogenous anticoagulant that exerts both anticoagulant and anti-inflammatory activities, the latter through interactions with a dedicated cell receptor, the endothelial protein C receptor (EPCR). It is activated by interactions with thrombomodulin and EPCR, and recombinant activated protein C has been evaluated as a treatment for sepsis. Initial work showed a significant impact on mortality in sepsis [56], and the drug was briefly licensed for clinical use. However, this signal was not replicated in subsequent trials [57], and rhAPC is no longer available as a therapeutic. Other endogenous anticoagulants including antithrombin [58], tissue factor pathway inhibitor [59], and soluble thrombomodulin [60] have yielded similarly disappointing results.

The biologic rationale for anti-cytokine therapy is strong, and preclinical studies have revealed a wealth of potentially promising strategies. The concept has shown efficacy in chronic inflammatory diseases and, more recently, in the treatment of severe viral illness caused by SARS-CoV-2. The lack of efficacy in sepsis is, therefore, puzzling, and it is instructive to look at some of the reasons for this failure. They provide a road map for future studies and, ultimately, for a new class of treatments for severe acute inflammatory diseases.

17.6 Why Have Clinical Trials of Anti-cytokine Therapy for Sepsis Been So Disappointing?

The shortcomings of our current approach to sepsis trials are many and have been the subject of a number of reviews and commentaries [61]. Eight core themes are explored further here.

17.6.1 Sepsis Is Intrinsically Heterogeneous

The current construct of sepsis as organ dysfunction resulted from a dysregulated host response to infection [62] and identifies a highly heterogeneous population of acutely ill patients. Entry criteria for trials are almost uniformly based on a combination of evidence of infection and nonspecific physiologic derangements. As a consequence, a trial may enroll a 33-year-old patient with fulminant pneumococcal pneumonia, but also include a middle-aged patient with an exacerbation of chronic lung disease or an elderly nursing home resident with a urinary tract infection: the probability of a similar response to treatment seems unlikely.

Heterogeneity in sepsis occurs at multiple levels. Patients differ in the site and bacteriology of their inciting infection; the presence of microbial products such as endotoxin is variable and correlates poorly with the nature of the underlying infection [63]. Approaches to the treatment of the infection vary, and the probability of successful anti-infectious therapy may vary with the resistance profile of the infecting organisms or the potential for achieving adequate source control. Patients themselves vary with respect to age, frailty, and comorbidities, factors that may impact both overall prognosis and responsiveness to treatment. They also differ in their philosophies of care, and so decisions to continue or withdraw support may differ from patient to patient. Finally, resources and clinical expertise vary widely around the world, and even within an individual healthcare system, so that the prognosis for affected patients also differs.

Genetic factors contribute substantially to variability in sepsis outcomes. A classic Scandinavian study of children adopted in infancy revealed an almost sixfold greater risk of infectious death in the biologic offspring of parents who had died of infectious causes before the age of 50 [64]. Common single nucleotide polymorphisms in innate immune response genes appear to underlie this variability [65], underlining the critical role that infection has played in shaping the human genome over evolutionary time.

Biologic heterogeneity amongst patients recruited to sepsis clinical trials, arising from the combined effects of these sources of variability, can be striking. A trial of a monoclonal antibody to TNF which stratified patients on the basis of their IL-6 levels showed an 8000-fold difference in circulating levels of TNF and a 200,000-fold difference in levels of IL-6 [51].

17.6.2 The Innate Immune Response Is Vital to Effective Anti-infectious Host Defense

The innate immune response that mediates tissue injury in sepsis is complex and conserved precisely because it favors the survival of the host during an acute infection. Genetic studies demonstrate the selection of certain genetic variants because of the evolutionary advantage they provide in the face of specific threats. Perhaps the best known of these are the SNPs in the hemoglobin gene responsible for sickle cell disease, thalassemia, and G6PD deficiency that emerged in areas where malaria is endemic [66].

While manipulation of the innate immune response may be rational in circumstances in which the inciting infection has been controlled using antibiotics and source control measures, it might be detrimental if infection is not adequately controlled. Moreover, the response to cytokine manipulation in experimental models varies with the infecting organism [15] (◘ Fig. 17.3), a variable that is not usually incorporated into trial inclusion and exclusion criteria. Microorganisms or their products appear to play a role in the anti-infectious response. A clinical trial of eritoran, a synthetic inhibitor of the interaction of endotoxin with TLR4, showed no evidence of benefit for patients with Gram-negative infection, but a signal for harm in patients with Gram-positive infections [49], a counterintuitive finding that has been seen in other trials of endotoxin antagonism [46]. The phagocytosis of a microorganism induces the apoptosis of a phagocytosing neutrophil, and experimental studies have shown that lung injury following ischemia/reperfusion injury can be attenuated, and survival improved, by the intratracheal instillation of killed bacteria [67]. The interaction between host and microorganism is not only complex but nuanced, and concepts and study design need to acknowledge these nuances. It is, perhaps, unsurprising that cytokine manipulation has shown its initial efficacy in the management of noninfectious causes of inflammation, where the imperative to control an infectious threat is not present.

17.6.3 The Host Innate Immune Response Is Biologically Redundant

Beyond the heterogeneity inherent in populations of patients with sepsis, the innate host response is effected through the release of dozens, if not hundreds, of molecular species that can trigger or inhibit the release of others and whose activity can be reproduced by multiple mediators. Endotoxin, for example, can trigger the release of both IL-1β and TNF, and both can activate downstream effects such as the induction of expression of nitric oxide synthase [68]. Targeting any one of these agents, particularly after a response has been activated, may be inadequate to blunt the ongoing response.

Interventions that modulate the expression of multiple cytokines by altering intracellular signal transduction pathways may theoretically overcome this limitation, and efficacy has been shown, for example, in targeting Jak signaling in COVID-19; however, this strategy has not been evaluated in bacterial sepsis.

17.6.4 Preliminary Evaluation of Potential Strategies Is Often Inadequate

Given the complexity of the biologic challenge, and the well-established pattern of disappointment in phase 3 clinical trials, a much more cautious investigative approach based on a well-developed portfolio of preclinical and early clinical work seems prudent. Yet, phase 3 trials are repeatedly driven by a combination of inadequate preparation, unrealistic expectations, and a desire to generate immediate returns on what is perceived to be a lucrative opportunity. Preclinical models emphasize potential efficacy, whereas their more important role may be in identifying circumstances where lack of efficacy or harm might be anticipated. Generic study inclusion criteria based on early formulations of sepsis syndrome [69] or systemic inflammatory response syndrome (SIRS) [70] are used to identify patients for therapy, despite their repeated failures to show that they reliably do so. Early-phase clinical studies fail to explore enrichment strategies or to identify potential biomarkers to enhance the selection of patients most likely to benefit. The net result is that trials of interventions that are biologically diverse adopt designs that are indistinguishable from each other, and the results of these trials are consistently disappointing.

17.6.5 Mortality Endpoints Are Insensitive to Potential Benefits

Sepsis trials have generally used 28-day all-cause mortality as a measure of the effectiveness of treatment. A mortality endpoint is intuitively attractive for studies of a condition that carries a significant risk of death; it is definitive and easy to capture and integrates the net benefits and harms of treatment [71]. But it may be insensitive to signals that not only reflect benefit for the individual patient, but also provide insight into how best to target specific treatments. The risk of death in sepsis is impacted by multiple factors, many of which may not be susceptible to therapeutic manipulation. Patients with sepsis characteristically have comorbid conditions that independently affect their outcomes, and present for care at varying times after the onset of illness when complications of the illness have already developed. Patient preferences and values influence the extent to which aggressive support is deemed desirable. And that support brings additional risks of adverse outcome, even as it defers the immediate risk of dying. The inherent heterogeneity of sepsis implies that a particular treatment may benefit some patients but not others and may even harm some who are treated. When these divergent effects are combined in a single mortality metric, both benefits and harms may be underestimated. Finally, a 28-day time horizon may not be sufficiently long to evaluate the full impact of treatment.

While the prospect that anti-cytokine therapy might save lives is attractive and even plausible, the expectation that this effect is likely to be large and readily demonstrable in a heterogeneous population of patients has proven naïve, and other metrics of benefit are needed. Indeed, cytokine-directed does not impact the survival of rheumatoid arthritis, despite its salutary effects on inflammatory symptoms, and a richer understanding of what interventions might achieve when given to septic patients could provide important insight into their potential therapeutic roles.

17.6.6 Timing, Dose, and Duration of Treatment Are Poorly Understood

Sepsis trials typically assess a single dose and duration of therapy and proceed from the assumption that early intervention is likely to be better. These assumptions are unproven and largely untested. They are likely to be important in a dynamic and variable process such as sepsis. A trial of nitric oxide inhibition in septic shock, for example, reported overall harm, but benefit for patients treated with a lower dose of the agent [72]. Titration of dose based on levels of a biomarker or on response to therapy has not been assessed, although this approach is standard in the use of other ICU interventions such as oxygen, vasopressors, or insulin.

There is also evidence suggesting that some agents studied have lacked in vivo biologic activity. A clinical trial of an antibody to TNF found that the agent, while detectable in the circulation, failed to inhibit TNF bioactivity [73].

17.6.7 The Study Model Is Ill-Adapted to Understand the Reasons for Failure

Sepsis trials are conducted primarily to demonstrate a treatment effect that will translate into a marketable therapeutic. But understanding why interventions do not work is, from a scientific perspective, equally important, for it provides the field with the insights that can inform future work and increase the likelihood of success. Pharma trials are reluctant to restrict the scope of a study cohort because doing so will reduce the size of the potential market if the trial is successful. They emphasize speed in obtaining results because a longer study time equates to a shorter period of patent protection. They provide generous per-patient reimbursements, and incentives for rapid recruitment, but doing so may dilute the study result through the inclusion of patients for whom treatment would otherwise not have been contemplated—the patient with cholangitis who is likely to respond well to bile duct drainage or the patient with advanced dementia for whom comfort measures alone may be preferable.

The large number of unsuccessful trials of cytokine-directed therapy has left a rich legacy of data that could provide invaluable insights into how to modify research approaches in the future. Sadly, this resource is not readily available for analysis, and few such secondary assessments have been conducted.

17.6.8 Sepsis Lacks Effective Systems for Staging and Stratification

Effective multimodal therapy in oncology has been made possible through the development of staging systems such as the tumor, node, metastasis (TNM) system [74]. The TNM system stratifies malignancy by anatomic site and cell type and further by the extent of spread at the time of diagnosis. This method of stratification also guides treatment decisions. Tumors that have not spread beyond the site of origin are typically amenable to treatment with surgery alone, whereas adjuvant chemotherapy is most effective when there is evidence of lymph node spread, without distant metastases. Biologic therapies are reserved for cancers that are more advanced and, in particular, for cancers that express specific markers that predict a better probability of response to a particular treatment. For women with breast cancer, for example, lumpectomy with or without local radiotherapy may be adequate for a cancer localized to the breast, while the presence of estrogen receptors or Her2 expression in the tumor predicts potential responsiveness to antiestrogens such as tamoxifen or the antibody trastuzumab, respectively.

Staging systems for sepsis or other forms of acute illness have been proposed, but work is at a very early stage. The PIRO (predisposition, insult, response, organ dysfunction) model is one such proposed model [75], and stratification based on each of the component variables can be associated with differential prognosis and treatment responsiveness [76]. However, a functional model has not been evaluated in the context of a trial. Retrospective analyses of completed trials have suggested that stratification on the basis of clinical features or biomarkers may increase a therapeutic signal [77, 78]; however, prospective validation is lacking.

Summary

Cytokines represent a biologically diverse family of soluble factors that mediate communications between cells and, in doing so, alter cellular function dynamically and reversibly. They play an important, though poorly understood, role in shaping an innate immune response, and so are an attractive therapeutic target in disorders such as sepsis. That they have not yet achieved that promise is a reflection of the complexity of the process, rather than an indictment of the concept.

> **Take-Home Messages**
>
> - Cytokines comprise a family of more than 100 proteins that are released during an innate immune response and that alter cell function both locally and systemically.
> - Their functions are diverse, overlapping, and even redundant, and as a consequence, we lack a useful taxonomy that can group them with regard to their in vivo activity.
> - While they are often described as pro- or anti-inflammatory, this dichotomy is overly simplistic.
> - Targeting individual cytokines has proven disappointing as a therapeutic strategy in sepsis; however, it has become a standard approach in the management of chronic inflammatory diseases and has shown promise in COVID-19.
> - Success in adapting the strategy to treat critically ill patients requires more sophisticated models of staging and stratification, analogous to those used to guide therapy in oncology.

References

1. The REMAP-CAP Investigators. Interleukin-6 receptor antagonists in critically ill patients with Covid-19. N Engl J Med. 2021;384:1491–502.
2. Tata JR. One hundred years of hormones. EMBO Rep. 2005;6:490–6.
3. Eknoyan G. Emergence of the concept of endocrine function and endocrinology. Adv Chronic Kidney Dis. 2004;11:371–6.
4. Bahadoran Z, Mirmiran P, Azizi F, Ghasemi A. A brief history of modern endocrinology and definitions of a true hormone. Endocr Metab Immune Disord Drug Targets. 2019;19:1116–21.
5. Wiemann B, Starnes CO. Coley's toxins, tumor necrosis factor and cancer research: a historical perspective. Pharmacol Ther. 1994;64:529–64.
6. Kucerova P, Cervinkova M. Spontaneous regression of tumour and the role of microbial infection—possibilities for cancer treatment. Anticancer Drugs. 2016;27:269–77.
7. Coley WB. The treatment of inoperable sarcoma by bacterial toxins (the mixed toxins of the Streptococcus erysipelas and the Bacillus prodigiosus). Proc R Soc Med. 1910;3:1–48.
8. Atkins E, Wood WBJ. Studies on the pathogenesis of fever. II. Identification of an endogenous pyrogen in the blood stream following the injection of typhoid vaccine. J Exp Med. 1955;102:499–516.
9. Dinarello CA. Interleukin-1. Rev Infect Dis. 1984;6:51–95.
10. Loda M, et al. Induction of hepatic protein synthesis by a peptide in blood plasma of patients with sepsis and trauma. Surgery. 1984;96:204–13.
11. Dinarello CA. Overview of the IL-1 family in innate inflammation and acquired immunity. Immunol Rev. 2018;281:8–27.
12. Carswell EA, et al. An endotoxin-induced serum factor that causes necrosis of tumors. Proc Natl Acad Sci U S A. 1975;72:3666–70.
13. Beutler B, Cerami A. Cachectin: more than a tumor necrosis factor. N Engl J Med. 1987;316:379–85.
14. Beutler B, Milsark IW, Cerami AC. Passive immunization against cachectin tumor necrosis factor protects mice from lethal effect of endotoxin. Science. 1985;229:869–71.
15. Lorente JA, Marshall JC. Neutralization of tumor necrosis factor (TNF) in pre-clinical models of sepsis. Shock. 2005;24:107–19.
16. Almutairi KB, Nossent JC, Preen DB, Keen HI, Inderjeeth CA. The prevalence of rheumatoid arthritis: a systematic review of population-based studies. J Rheumatol. 2021;48:669–76.
17. Fraenkel L, et al. 2021 American College of Rheumatology guideline for the treatment of rheumatoid arthritis. Arthritis Care Res (Hoboken). 2021;73:924–39.

18. Feldmann M. Development of anti-TNF therapy for rheumatoid arthritis. Nat Rev Immunol. 2002;2:364–71.

19. Taylor PC. Clinical efficacy of launched JAK inhibitors in rheumatoid arthritis. Rheumatology (Oxford). 2019;58:i17–26.

20. Taurog JD, Chhabra A, Colbert RA. Ankylosing spondylitis and axial spondyloarthritis. N Engl J Med. 2016;374:2563–74.

21. Dubash S, Bridgewood C, McGonagle D, Marzo-Ortega H. The advent of IL-17A blockade in ankylosing spondylitis: secukinumab, ixekizumab and beyond. Expert Rev Clin Immunol. 2019;15:123–34.

22. Erichsen CY, Jensen P, Kofoed K. Biologic therapies targeting the interleukin (IL)-23/IL-17 immune axis for the treatment of moderate-to-severe plaque psoriasis: a systematic review and meta-analysis. J Eur Acad Dermatol Venereol. 2020;34:30–8.

23. Mockel T, Basta F, Weinmann-Menke J, Schwarting A. B cell activating factor (BAFF): structure, functions, autoimmunity and clinical implications in systemic lupus erythematosus (SLE). Autoimmun Rev. 2021;20:102736.

24. Townsend CM, et al. Adalimumab for maintenance of remission in Crohn's disease. Cochrane Database Syst Rev. 2020;5:CD012877.

25. Singh S, et al. Comparative efficacy and safety of biologic therapies for moderate-to-severe Crohn's disease: a systematic review and network meta-analysis. Lancet Gastroenterol Hepatol. 2021;6:1002–14.

26. Ben-Horin S, et al. Efficacy of biologic drugs in short-duration versus long-duration inflammatory bowel disease: a systematic review and an individual-patient data meta-analysis of randomized controlled trials. Gastroenterology. 2022;162(2):482–94.

27. Raine T, Verstockt B, De Cruz P. Immune therapies in ulcerative colitis: are we beyond anti-TNF yet? Lancet Gastroenterol Hepatol. 2020;5:794–6.

28. van Horssen R, Ten Hagen TL, Eggermont AM. TNF-alpha in cancer treatment: molecular insights, antitumor effects, and clinical utility. Oncologist. 2006;11:397–408.

29. Ridker PM. Anticytokine agents: targeting interleukin signaling pathways for the treatment of atherothrombosis. Circ Res. 2019;124:437–50.

30. Ingram JR. Interventions for hidradenitis suppurativa: updated summary of an original cochrane review. JAMA Dermatol. 2017;153:458–9.

31. Brusselle GG, Koppelman GH. Biologic therapies for severe asthma. N Engl J Med. 2022;386:157–71.

32. Marshall JC, et al. Pre-clinical models of sepsis: what can they tell us? Shock. 2005;24:107–19.

33. Hinshaw LB, et al. Survival of primates in LD100 septic shock following therapy with antibody to tumor necrosis factor (TNF alpha). Circ Shock. 1990;30:279–92.

34. Tracey KJ, et al. Anti-cachectin/TNF monoclonal antibodies prevent septic shock during lethal bacteraemia. Nature. 1987;330:662–4.

35. The RECOVERY Collaborative Group. Dexamethasone in hospitalized patients with Covid-19—preliminary report. N Engl J Med. 2021;384:693–704.

36. Writing Committee for the REMAP-CAP Investigators, et al. Effect of hydrocortisone on mortality and organ support in patients with severe COVID-19: the REMAP-CAP COVID-19 corticosteroid domain randomized clinical trial. JAMA. 2020;324(13):1317–29.

37. WHO Rapid Evidence Appraisal for COVID-19 Therapies (REACT) Working Group, et al. Association between administration of systemic corticosteroids and mortality among critically ill patients with COVID-19: a meta-analysis. JAMA. 2020;324(13):1330–41.

38. Kyriazopoulou E, et al. Early treatment of COVID-19 with anakinra guided by soluble urokinase plasminogen receptor plasma levels: a double-blind, randomized controlled phase 3 trial. Nat Med. 2021;27:1752–60.

39. Kokkotis G, et al. Systematic review with meta-analysis: COVID-19 outcomes in patients receiving anti-TNF treatments. Aliment Pharmacol Ther. 2022;55:154–67.

40. Kalil AC, et al. Baricitinib plus remdesivir for hospitalized adults with Covid-19. N Engl J Med. 2021;384:795–807.

41. Guimaraes PO, et al. Tofacitinib in patients hospitalized with Covid-19 pneumonia. N Engl J Med. 2021;385:406–15.

42. The ATTACC, ACTIV-4a, and REMAP-CAP Investigators, et al. Therapeutic anticoagulation with heparin in noncritically ill patients with Covid-19. N Engl J Med. 2021;385:790–802.

43. The REMAP-CAP, ACTIV-4a, and ATTACC Investigators, et al. Therapeutic anticoagulation with heparin in critically ill patients with Covid-19. N Engl J Med. 2021;385:777–89.
44. Ziegler EJ, et al. Treatment of gram-negative bacteremia and shock with human antiserum to a mutant Escherichia coli. N Engl J Med. 1982;307:1225–30.
45. Ziegler EJ, et al. Treatment of gram-negative bacteremia and septic shock with HA-1A human monoclonal antibody against endotoxin. N Engl J Med. 1991;324:429–36.
46. McCloskey RV, et al. Treatment of septic shock with human monoclonal antibody HA-1A. Ann Intern Med. 1994;121:1–5.
47. Levin M, et al. Recombinant bactericidal/permeability-increasing protein (rBPI21) as adjunctive treatment for children with severe meningococcal sepsis: a randomised trial. Lancet. 2000;356:961–7.
48. Axtelle T, Pribble J. IC14, a CD14 specific monoclonal antibody, is a potential treatment for patients with severe sepsis. J Endotoxin Res. 2001;7:310–4.
49. Opal SM, et al. Effect of eritoran, an antagonist of MD2-TLR4, on mortality in patients with severe sepsis: the ACCESS randomized trial. JAMA. 2013;309:1154–62.
50. Dellinger RP, et al. Effect of targeted polymyxin B hemoperfusion on 28-day mortality in patients with septic shock and elevated endotoxin level: the EUPHRATES randomized clinical trial. JAMA. 2018;320:1455–63.
51. Panacek EA, et al. Efficacy and safety of the monoclonal anti-TNF antibody F(ab')2 fragment in patients with severe sepsis stratified by IL-6 level. Crit Care Med. 2004;32:2173–82.
52. Fisher, C.J., Jr. et al. Treatment of septic shock with the tumor necrosis factor receptor:Fc fusion protein. N Engl J Med 334, 1697–1702 (1996).
53. Qiu P, et al. Antitumor necrosis factor therapy is associated with improved survival in clinical sepsis trials: a meta-analysis. Crit Care Med. 2013;41:2419–29.
54. Marshall JC. Such stuff as dreams are made on: mediator-targeted therapy in sepsis. Nat Rev Drug Discov. 2003;2:391–405.
55. Marshall JC. Inflammation, coagulopathy, and the pathogenesis of the multiple organ dysfunction syndrome. Crit Care Med. 2001;29(Suppl):S106.
56. Bernard GR, et al. Efficacy and safety of recombinant human activated protein C for severe sepsis. N Engl J Med. 2001;344:699–709.
57. Ranieri VM, et al. Drotrecogin alfa (activated) in adults with septic shock. N Engl J Med. 2012;366:2055–64.
58. Warren BL, et al. High-dose antithrombin III in severe sepsis: a randomized, controlled trial. JAMA. 2001;286:1869–78.
59. Abraham E, et al. Efficacy and safety of tifacogin (recombinant tissue factor pathway inhibitor) in severe sepsis: a randomized controlled trial. JAMA. 2003;290:238–47.
60. Vincent JL, et al. Effect of a recombinant human soluble thrombomodulin on mortality in patients with sepsis-associated coagulopathy: the SCARLET randomized clinical trial. JAMA. 2019;321:1993–2002.
61. Marshall JC. Why have clinical trials in sepsis failed? Trends Mol Med. 2014;20:195–203.
62. Singer M, et al. The third international consensus definitions for sepsis and septic shock (Sepsis-3). JAMA. 2016;315:801–10.
63. Marshall JC, et al. Diagnostic and prognostic implications of endotoxemia in critical illness: results of the MEDIC study. J Infect Dis. 2004;190:527–34.
64. Sorenson TI, Nielsen GG, Andersen PK, Teasdale PW. Genetic and environmental influences on premature death in adult adoptees. N Engl J Med. 1988;318:727–32.
65. Khor CC, et al. A Mal functional variant is associated with protection against invasive pneumococcal disease, bacteremia, malaria and tuberculosis. Nat Genet. 2007;39:523–8.
66. Kwiatkowski DP. How malaria has affected the human genome and what human genetics can teach us about malaria. Am J Hum Genet. 2005;77:171–92.
67. Sookhai S, et al. A novel therapeutic strategy for attenuating neutrophil-mediated lung injury in vivo. Ann Surg. 2002;235:285–91.
68. Green SJ, et al. Nitric oxide: cytokine-regulation of nitric oxide in host resistance to intracellular pathogens. Immunol Lett. 1994;43:87–94.
69. Bone RC, et al. Sepsis syndrome: a valid clinical entity. Crit Care Med. 1989;17:389–93.
70. Bone RC, et al. Definitions for sepsis and organ failure and guidelines for the use of innovative therapies in sepsis. Chest. 1992;101:1644–55.

17

71. Petros AJ, Marshall JC, van Saene HKF. Is mortality an appropriate endpoint for clinical trials in critical illness? Lancet. 1995;345:369–71.

72. Lopez A, et al. Multiple-center, randomized, placebo-controlled, double-blind study of the nitric oxide synthase inhibitor 546C88: effect on survival in patients with septic shock. Crit Care Med. 2004;32:21–30.

73. Abraham E, et al. Double-blind randomised controlled trial of monoclonal antibody to human tumour necrosis factor in treatment of septic shock. Lancet. 1998;351:929–33.

74. Gospodarowicz M, et al. History and international developments in cancer staging. Cancer Prev Control. 1998;2:262–8.

75. Levy MM, et al. 2001 SCCM/ESICM/ACCP/ATS/SIS international sepsis definitions conference. Crit Care Med. 2003;34:1250–6.

76. Marshall JC. The PIRO (Predisposition, Insult, Response, Organ Dysfunction) model: towards a staging system for acute illness. Virulence. 2014;5:27–5.

77. Shakoory B, et al. Interleukin-1 receptor blockade is associated with reduced mortality in sepsis patients with features of macrophage activation syndrome: reanalysis of a prior phase III trial. Crit Care Med. 2016;44:275–81.

78. Calfee CS, et al. Acute respiratory distress syndrome subphenotypes and differential response to simvastatin: secondary analysis of a randomised controlled trial. Lancet Respir Med. 2018;6:691–8.

Extracorporeal Cytokine Removal

Christopher Rugg and Zsolt Molnar

Contents

Learning Objectives

After reading this chapter, you will be able
- To understand the rationale behind extracorporeal cytokine removal
- To describe different techniques used
- To identify potentials and limitations of techniques used

18.1 Introduction

Inflammation plays a key role in the pathophysiology of organ dysfunction in the critically ill. Regardless of the origin of the initiating injury, multiorgan dysfunction is triggered by an overwhelming host response resulting in the overproduction of various cytokines [1]. Pathogen- or damage-associated molecular patterns (PAMPs, DAMPs) activate neutrophils, stimulate hypercytokinemia, and subsequently have the potential to cause cell death and further release of DAMPs [2]. This vicious circle has been given the name "cytokine storm." Depending on various factors, possible trajectories range from fulminant death to rapid recovery but can also include disease states most appropriately described as persistent inflammation, immunosuppression, and catabolism syndrome [3].

Accordingly, the attenuation of this maladaptive response has been recognized as a potential cornerstone of therapy. By regaining immune homeostasis, potential damage caused by the dysregulated immune response is hoped to be reduced (◘ Fig. 18.1). Given the broad variety of involved cytokines and the high redundancy of the human immune system [4], the broad removal of cytokines may seem

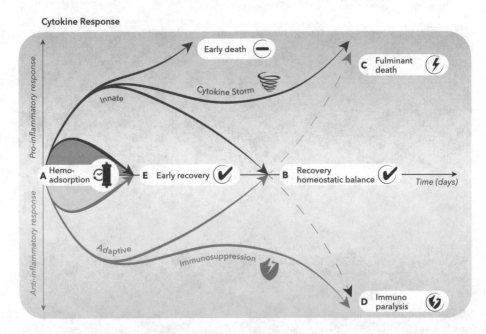

◘ **Fig. 18.1** Cytokine response after an (infectious) insult. **a** Baseline. **b** Recovery to homeostatic balance. **c** Fulminant death. **d** Immunoparalysis as seen in persistent inflammatory immunosuppression and catabolism syndrome. **e** Attenuation of the inflammatory response resulting in early recovery

more promising in hyperinflammatory states than the mere blockage of single pathways (◻ Fig. 18.2). To that effect, extracorporeal cytokine removal, also known as blood purification therapy, has gained increasing attention. The theory behind its beneficial effects mainly relies on a combination between the peak concentration and the cytokinetic hypothesis. The former is based on a cytotoxic theory, where high peak concentrations are declared to be the main noxious stimulus; hence, their attenuation could prove beneficial [5–8]. The latter is based on the restoration of an intact

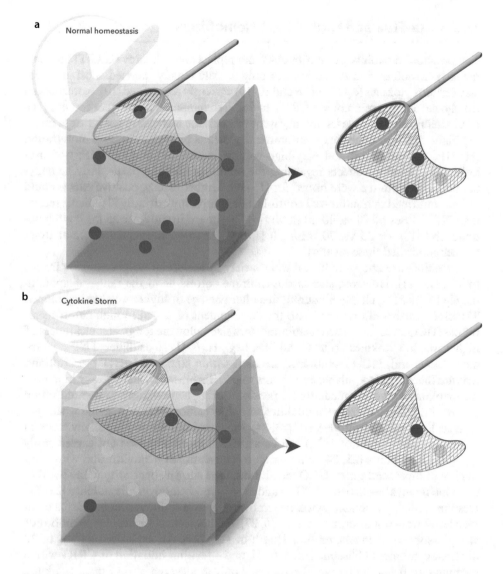

◻ **Fig. 18.2** The rationale behind broad cytokine removal. Hemoadsorption takes place in a concentration-dependent manner. During normal homeostasis **a** with balanced pro- and anti-inflammatory mediators, adsorption also takes place at similar rates. During cytokine storm with immuno-dysbalance **b**, abundant cytokines are also removed at proportionally higher rates. Thus, hemoadsorption may help regain homeostatic balance

cytokine gradient between bloodstream and tissues by removing cytokines from the blood compartment, therefore allowing appropriate leukocyte trafficking [9].

Different techniques for extracorporeal cytokine removal have evolved over the years including high-volume and high-cutoff hemofiltration, use of hemofilters with adsorptive properties, dedicated hemoadsorption columns, and lastly combined plasma filtration and adsorption or therapeutic plasma exchange. In the following, these techniques are meant to be overviewed in the light of current literature.

18.2   High-Flux and High-Cutoff Hemofilters

The principal capability of continuous renal replacement therapy (CRRT) and particularly hemofiltration to remove not only usually renally excreted substances but also certain cytokines (e.g., TNF-α and IL-1β) was early recognized [10]. Nevertheless, the clinical efficacy of common CRRT in doing so remained rather questionable [11]. First attempts to improve its potency went towards the increase in CRRT dose utilizing high- and superhigh-flux membranes. By means of high-volume hemofiltration (HVHF; >35 mL/kg/h) and very-high-volume hemofiltration (VHVHF; >45 mL/kg/h) [12], beneficial effects regarding the course of disease, particularly hemodynamics and mortality, were hoped for [13–16]. Unfortunately, positive effects could not be confirmed in randomized control trials comparing critically ill patients receiving CRRT doses of 20 vs. 40 mL/kg/h [17], 20 (intermittently) vs. 35 mL/kg/h (continuously) [18], or 35 vs. 70 mL/kg/h [19]. Coherently, subsequent meta-analyses further confirmed these results [20].

Cytokines are known to have a wide variety of molecular weight, ranging from 6 to 70 kDa [21]. However, standard membrane cutoffs lie in the range of approximately 15–20 kDa, clearly hindering free filter passage of higher weighted cytokines. Therefore, further efforts went into the development of so-called high-cutoff membranes (HCO) with increased membrane pore sizes allowing for greater clearances of higher weight cytokines up to 45–60 kDa (e.g., IL-6, IL-10 as dimer, TNF-α as trimer). In general, HCO membranes are used within standard CRRT prescriptions, making them widely available and simple to use. Technically, their efficacy in removing cytokines and other mediators is possible during hemodialysis or hemofiltration but maximized in convective modalities, and thus hemofiltration [22], and when synergistically combined with HVHF [23, 24]. Increased protein and especially albumin loss (molecular weight 66 kDa) can be an issue but usually does not exceed easily replaceable amounts [23, 24]. Compared to conventional hemofiltration with standard high-flux membranes, HCO membranes have shown superiority with regard to cytokine removal—particularly IL-6 and IL-8—and hemodynamic stability [25–28]. Despite verifiably increased cytokine removal, significant differences in plasma cytokine levels were not always achieved [26, 27], neither were clear benefits in mortality, vasopressor requirements, or ICU length of stay [29]. An extensive analysis of 12 different cytokines at baseline and 1, 6, 24, and 48 h after initiation of CRRT with a medium-cutoff hemofilter (45 kDa) showed only modest removal of most cytokines and suggested that changes in plasma cytokine concentrations during therapy may not solely be influenced by extracorporeal removal [30].

18.3 Adsorptive Hemofilters

The development of synthetic polymeric membranes not only increased the biocompatibility of CRRT—as is the case for the now commonly used polysulfone membranes—but also allowed for additional membrane properties to arise. Polyacrylonitrile and polymethylmethacrylate (PMMA) membranes exert adsorptive properties, additionally clearing molecules sized above the membrane cutoff by surface adhesion. In a canine model of endotoxic shock, polyacrylonitrile membranes demonstrated superior effects regarding cytokine removal and subsequent hemodynamic stability compared to polysulfone membranes [31].

Further development in polyacrylonitrile membranes led to AN69ST membranes consisting of copolymers of acrylonitrile (AN) and sodium methallyl sulfonate. Additional surface treatment (hence the ST) with a polycationic polyethyleneimine (PEI) layer adds a hydrogel structure with additional adsorptive capacity, which is then complemented with a thin layer of—biologically not active—heparin [32]. The mechanisms of adsorption seem to involve ionic binding for the electronegative AN69ST and hydrophobic binding for the PMMA hemofilters [33]. Where convective and diffusive removal of molecules is principally restricted to effluent flow, adsorption is theoretically rather restricted to blood flow. In vitro experiments showed that PMMA and AN69ST but not polysulfone membranes were well capable of clearing TNF-α, IL-6, IL-8, and high-mobility group box 1 protein (HMGB-1) at rates far exceeding effluent flow rates [33, 34]. A prospective, multicenter trial evaluating the AN69ST membrane further confirmed these findings for TNF-α, IL-1β, IL-6, IL-8, IL-10, and HMGB-1 removal [35]. HMGB-1 release is stimulated among others by endotoxin, and as an upstream mediator, it subsequently induces the release of numerous cytokines; its removal from circulation is therefore thought to be highly beneficial. Nevertheless, only low-level evidence exists on possible outcome benefits [36, 37]. Importantly, as adsorption takes place by surface adhesion, total surface area limits this process by saturation. However, it has been shown that in addition to true surface adhesion, adsorption also takes place within the bulk of the membrane, therefore increasing potential surface area and time to saturation [38, 39].

PMMA membranes have been shown to feature larger pore sizes than AN69ST, therefore better clearing larger weighted cytokines as IL-6 [34, 40]. Contrarily, when compared to AN69ST, HMGB-1 clearance is reduced though [34]. In a cohort study on 43 patients with septic shock and elevated IL-6 levels, early PMMA hemofiltration was associated with hemodynamic improvement and reduction in lactate levels and organ failure [41]. Furthermore, very effective endotoxin binding properties have also been shown for the PMMA membrane [42]. Chemically speaking, endotoxins are lipopolysaccharides (LPS) found in the outer membrane of gram-negative bacteria. As mentioned earlier, they can likely induce a cytokine storm, partially via HMGB-1. Their removal from circulation can certainly indirectly reduce hypercytokinemia, which is why endotoxin-adsorbing membranes shall also be mentioned here.

One such membrane is the so-called AN69-Oxiris membrane (Baxter, Illinois, USA), which originated by further modifying the AN69ST membrane. A threefold higher concentrated PEI layer and a third layer of tenfold higher concentrated and therefore biologically active heparin were added [32, 43]. Due to the enhanced PEI layer, membrane surface polarity was modified, and increased cytokine and particularly effective endotoxin adsorption was made possible; the enhanced heparin layer serves as local anticoagulation [44]. Compared to AN69ST, AN69-Oxiris led to decreased shock severity in a porcine model of septic shock [44] and higher reductions in IL-6, lactate, and endotoxin concentrations in a randomized, crossover, double-blind pilot study [45]. Furthermore, vasopressor requirements were reduced as well. As literature—apart from the already mentioned studies—on the use of AN69-Oxiris is scarce and mainly limited to case reports or series, a prospective national registry named oXirisNet (Italy) has been established [46].

Highly selective endotoxin removal can be accomplished by polymyxin B-immobilized fiber columns (PMX). The mode of operation is hemoperfusion for these columns; thus, an additional CRRT membrane is required for conventional hemofiltration. Regarding patients suffering from gram-negative sepsis and assured endotoxemia, from three multicenter randomized control trials, two were able to show improvements in organ failure, one a general reduction in mortality and one a reduction in mortality after post hoc analysis for patients with high endotoxin activity levels [47–50].

18.4 Dedicated Hemoadsorption Columns

Hemoadsorption columns are cartridges designed for hemoperfusion, commonly used pre- or post-filter during CRRT, incorporated in an ECMO circuit or as a stand-alone device. Apart from endotoxin-selective adsorption columns (PMX), the unselective columns contain hydrophobic, styrene-divinylbenzene beads in a diameter of 300–800 μm [51]. These biocompatible polymer beads are highly porous, with pore diameters ranging from 0.8 to 50 nm [52]. Basically speaking, adsorption takes place within the pores, where pore diameter determines the adsorption cutoff. The most common and investigated hemoadsorption device in Europe is the CytoSorb column (CytoSorbents Corporation, New Jersey, USA). Total surface area amounts to as much as 40,000 m^2, and with an adsorption cutoff of approximately 60 kDa, the adsorption capacity and efficacy seem ideal, particularly with regard to the molecular weight of the aimed cytokines. However, it must be noted that, with a molecular weight of approximately 100 kDa, endotoxin is not removed efficiently. In general, adsorption takes place in a concentration-dependent manner, meaning that highly concentrated molecules are cleared more effectively while lower concentrated molecules are removed to a lesser extent [53]. In fact, it was shown that CytoSorb reduced the levels of a broad spectrum of cytokines, PAMPs and DAMPs alike, by more than 50% in an in vitro whole-blood experiment [54]. In direct comparison with the PMMA and a middle-cutoff hemofilter (45 kDa), CytoSorb presented with 1.5- to 3-fold higher clearance rates for IL-1β, IL-6, IL-8, and TNF-α in an experimental study running 1 L of spiked human plasma through a hemofiltration machine [55]. Another in vitro hemoperfusion study with spiked human plasma comparing CytoSorb with AN69-Oxiris and PMX showed missing endotoxin removal for CytoSorb and comparable removal rates for a bulk of pro- and anti-inflammatory mediators between AN69-Oxiris and CytoSorb [56]. As expected, apart from endotoxin, the removal rates of PMX for other cytokines were significantly lower. Animal models of sepsis and burn injury were able to confirm a potent reduction of TNF-α, IL-1β, IL-6, IL-10, NF-κB, CXCL-1, and CCL2 through hemoadsorption with CytoSorb [57–60]. A feasibility study in brain-dead humans showed significant removal of IL-6 (28%) and TNF-α (8.5%) but not IL-10 after the first hour of therapy [61]. Interestingly, the mentioned cytokines then increased again over time until they actually surpassed baseline after 4 h of therapy. In a randomized control trial on 100 patients with severe sepsis or septic shock, efficient IL-6 removal by hemoperfusion was detected but no significant differences in plasma IL-6 levels [62]. Similarly, a propensity score matching analysis including patients with IL-6 levels above 10,000 pg/mL (regardless of origin) could not detect differences in IL-6 reduction with or without the use of CytoSorb [63].

Obviously, cytokine removal with hemoadsorption columns takes place at high rates, but whether removal translates into lower plasma levels or not highly depends on timing and duration (i.e.: dosing) of therapy [53] and probably even more on intrinsic factors influencing cytokine production (e.g., adequacy of source control, choice and dosing of antibiotics, general origin of cytokine storm). If the triggering insult is not controlled and cytokine (over)production is therefore ongoing, then short-term cytokine removal is likely to remain fruitless. Presumably for the same reasons, results on survival benefits regarding CytoSorb treatment differ as well. Compared to predicted mortality, reduced mortality rates prevail [64–66]. Compared to controls (matched or randomized), mortality has been described as reduced [64, 65, 67], equal [62, 63], or even increased [68] in previous trials. To date, large multi-center trials confirming the one or the other are missing.

The most consistent finding regarding CytoSorb treatment seems to be its effect on hemodynamic stabilization. Including 33 studies reporting on vasopressor doses before and after CytoSorb treatment, a meta-analysis detected a significant decrease in median norepinephrine requirements from 0.55 to 0.09 µg/kg/min [69]. Furthermore, analysis of four studies with control cohorts [64, 70–72] showed a large pooled effect size regarding vasopressor decline.

An interesting approach would be the combination of different methods with different targets of action. The literature is very scarce on this topic, consisting only of case reports and a pilot study at present [73–75]. Nevertheless, the authors suggest that combining hemoadsorption with endotoxin removal may prove beneficial, a concept that has to be tested in the future.

A further hemoadsorption column to mention is the HA-330 cartridge (Jafron Biomedical Co., Guangdong, China). Mode of action is similar but not identical to CytoSorb [76], and specific literature is scarce. Two small randomized controlled trials did however describe effectful reduction in cytokine levels and improvement in hemodynamics and mortality [77, 78].

18.5 Combined Plasma Filtration and Adsorption or Therapeutic Plasma Exchange

Combined plasma filtration and adsorption (CPFA) relies on sorbent adsorption as well, differing from conventional hemoadsorption by the preceding separation of plasma from the cellular components of blood. The purified plasma is then reinfused into the circuit and then passed on to an ordinary hemofilter to provide CRRT. By the absence of direct contact between cellular components of blood and adsorption column, biocompatibility is theoretically improved but major problems potentially arise due to increased clotting of the circuit [79]. The effectiveness is dose dependent, requiring over 0.18 L/kg/day of plasma cleared [79]. Two large, randomized controlled trials were performed up to date [79, 80]. Both trials were stopped prematurely due to futility.

Therapeutic plasma exchange (TPE), also known as plasmapheresis, can be provided membrane or centrifugal based and is theoretically highly effective regarding cytokine removal. Basically, plasma is separated in a hemoperfusion device and replaced by donor plasma or albumin. It is commonly used to remove circulating immunoglobulins in order to treat a variety of (autoimmune) diseases (e.g., thrombotic thrombocytopenic purpura, myasthenia gravis, Guillain-Barré syndrome, and many more). Besides a highly effective removal of potentially injurious molecules, a potential replacement of consumed beneficial molecules (e.g., ADAMTS13, angiopoietin-1, antithrombin III) may take place when "healthy" donor plasma is replaced [81, 82]. A prospective pilot trial on early TPE in septic shock detected rapid hemodynamic improvement and a favorable change in cytokine profiles [83]. A meta-analysis on TPE in septic shock reported a mortality benefit, but as none of the studies were powered for survival, they concluded that insufficient evidence exists to recommend TPE at the time [84]. Noteworthy, potential side effects of (high volume) donor plasma transfusion are not to be ignored.

18.6 Summary

The interest in extracorporeal cytokine removal techniques is rapidly growing as it is acknowledged that various disease states originate from or are accompanied by an overwhelming cytokine storm. Due to the multitude of involved pro- and importantly also anti-inflammatory mediators, broad removal seems more tempting than blockage of singular pathways. Cytokine removal can be accomplished by various methods, differing in their efficacy and feasibility. Most feasible is certainly the use of high-flux, high-cutoff, and/or adsorptive hemofilters as the mode of action basically does not differ from conventional CRRT. However, most effective cytokine removal takes place via therapeutic plasma exchange, dedicated hemoadsorption columns, and enhanced adsorptive hemofilters. Regarding clinically relevant outcomes, evidence is often contradictory possibly due to extrinsic (timing and dose of therapy) but also intrinsic factors (uncontrolled trigger). This can only be leveled out in large multicenter trials, which are missing to date. The highest level of evidence is present for hemoadsorption columns but is still not high enough for general recommendations on its use. Yet, in the author's opinion, in patients refractory to the best standard care, the additional use as an adjuvant therapy attempt in hyperinflammatory states seems reasonable.

18

┌─ **Take-Home Messages** ─────────────────────────────────────

- In critically ill patients, multiorgan dysfunction is triggered by an overwhelming overproduction of various cytokines (cytokine storm).
- Due to the multitude of released pro- and anti-inflammatory mediators as well as cytokine redundancy, the broad removal of cytokines seems more promising than the mere blockage of singular pathways.
- Extracorporeal cytokine removal—also known as blood purification therapy— can be performed with the aid of hemofilters (high flux, high cutoff, adsorptive), hemoadsorption columns, therapeutical plasma exchange, or combined plasma filtration and adsorption therapy.
- Regarding feasibility, high-flux, high-cutoff, and/or adsorptive hemofilters are superior as the mode of action does not differ from conventional CRRT.
- Regarding efficacy, therapeutical plasma exchange, enhanced adsorptive hemofilters, and dedicated hemoadsorption columns are superior as removal rates are clearly increased.
- Whether cytokine removal translates into reduced plasma levels or not depends on the amount removed, and hence the efficacy, timing, and dosing of therapy, but also on intrinsic factors influencing ongoing cytokine (over)production (e.g., adequacy of source control, choice and dosing of antibiotics, general origin of cytokine storm).
- Evidence regarding clinically relevant outcome parameters is often contradictory, and large multicenter trials are still missing.
- The highest level of evidence is present for dedicated hemoadsorption columns, where fairly consistent effects on hemodynamic stabilization but inconsistent survival benefits are described.
- There are no general recommendations for extracorporeal cytokine removal, but its additional use as an adjuvant therapy in hyperinflammatory disease states seems reasonable.

└──

References

1. Pinsky MR, Vincent J-L, Deviere J, Alegre M, Kahn RJ, Dupont E. Serum cytokine levels in human septic shock relation to multiple-system organ failure and mortality. Chest. 1993;103(2): 565–75.
2. Moriyama K, Nishida O. Targeting cytokines, pathogen-associated molecular patterns, and damage-associated molecular patterns in sepsis via blood purification. Int J Mol Sci. 2021;22(16):8882.
3. Mira JC, Brakenridge SC, Moldawer LL, Moore FA. Persistent inflammation, immunosuppression and catabolism syndrome. Crit Care Clin. 2017;33:245–58.
4. Kelso A. The enigma of cytokine redundancy. Immunol Cell Biol. 1994;72(1):97–101.
5. Ronco C, Tetta C, Mariano F, Wratten ML, Bonello M, Bordoni V, et al. Interpreting the mechanisms of continuous renal replacement therapy in sepsis: the peak concentration hypothesis. Artif Organs. 2003;27(9):792–801.
6. van der Poll T, van de Veerdonk FL, Scicluna BP, Netea MG. The immunopathology of sepsis and potential therapeutic targets. Nat Rev Immunol. 2017;17(7):407–20.
7. Honoré PM, Matson JR. Extracorporeal removal for sepsis: acting at the tissue level—the beginning of a new era for this treatment modality in septic shock. Crit Care Med. 2004;32(3):896–7.

8. Carlo JVD, Alexander SR. Hemofiltration for cytokine-driven illnesses: the mediator delivery hypothesis. Int J Artif Organs. 2005;28(8):777–86.

9. Peng Z-Y, Bishop JV, Wen X-Y, Elder MM, Zhou F, Chuasuwan A, et al. Modulation of chemokine gradients by apheresis redirects leukocyte trafficking to different compartments during sepsis, studies in a rat model. Crit Care. 2014;18(4):R141.

10. Bellomo R, Tipping P, Boyce N. Continuous veno-venous hemofiltration with dialysis removes cytokines from the circulation of septic patients. Crit Care Med. 1993;21(4):522–6.

11. Vriese ASD, Vanholder RC, Pascual M, Lameire NH, Colardyn FA. Can inflammatory cytokines be removed efficiently by continuous renal replacement therapies? Intensive Care Med. 1999;25(9):903–10.

12. Villa G, Neri M, Bellomo R, Cerda J, Gaudio ARD, Rosa SD, et al. Nomenclature for renal replacement therapy and blood purification techniques in critically ill patients: practical applications. Crit Care. 2016;20(1):283.

13. Cornejo R, Downey P, Castro R, Romero C, Regueira T, Vega J, et al. High-volume hemofiltration as salvage therapy in severe hyperdynamic septic shock. Intensive Care Med. 2006;32(5):713–22.

14. Cole L, Bellomo R, Journois D, Davenport P, Baldwin I, Tipping P. High-volume haemofiltration in human septic shock. Intensive Care Med. 2001;27(6):978–86.

15. Boussekey N, Chiche A, Faure K, Devos P, Guery B, d'Escrivan T, et al. A pilot randomized study comparing high and low volume hemofiltration on vasopressor use in septic shock. Intensive Care Med. 2008;34(9):1646–53.

16. Joannes-Boyau O, Rapaport S, Bazin R, Fleureau C, Janvier G. Impact of high volume hemofiltration on hemodynamic disturbance and outcome during septic shock. ASAIO J. 2004;50(1):102–9.

17. RENAL Replacement Therapy Study Investigators, Bellomo R, Cass A, Cole L, Finfer S, Gallagher M, et al. Intensity of continuous renal-replacement therapy in critically ill patients. N Engl J Med. 2009;361(17):1627–38.

18. VA/NIH Acute Renal Failure Trial Network, Palevsky PM, Zhang JH, O'Connor TZ, Chertow GM, Crowley ST, et al. Intensity of renal support in critically ill patients with acute kidney injury. N Engl J Med. 2008;359(1):7–20.

19. Joannes-Boyau O, Honoré PM, Perez P, Bagshaw SM, Grand H, Canivet J-L, et al. High-volume versus standard-volume haemofiltration for septic shock patients with acute kidney injury (IVOIRE study): a multicentre randomized controlled trial. Intensive Care Med. 2013;39(9):1535–46.

20. Borthwick EM, Hill CJ, Rabindranath KS, Maxwell AP, McAuley DF, Blackwood B. High-volume haemofiltration for sepsis in adults. Cochrane Database Syst Rev. 2017;1(1):CD008075.

21. Stenken JA, Poschenrieder AJ. Bioanalytical chemistry of cytokines—a review. Anal Chim Acta. 2015;853:95–115.

22. Morgera S, Slowinski T, Melzer C, Sobottke V, Vargas-Hein O, Volk T, et al. Renal replacement therapy with high-cutoff hemofilters: impact of convection and diffusion on cytokine clearances and protein status. Am J Kidney Dis. 2004;43(3):444–53.

23. Lee WCR, Uchino S, Fealy N, Baldwin I, Panagiotopoulos S, Goehl H, et al. Super high flux Hemodialysis at high dialysate flows: an ex vivo assessment. Int J Artif Organs. 2004;27(1):24–8.

24. Naka T, Haase M, Bellomo R. 'Super high-flux' or 'high cut-off' hemofiltration and hemodialysis. Contrib Nephrol. 2010;166:181–9.

25. Morgera S, Haase M, Kuss T, Vargas-Hein O, Zuckermann-Becker H, Melzer C, et al. Pilot study on the effects of high cutoff hemofiltration on the need for norepinephrine in septic patients with acute renal failure. Crit Care Med. 2006;34(8):2099–104.

26. Eichhorn T, Hartmann J, Harm S, Linsberger I, König F, Valicek G, et al. Clearance of selected plasma cytokines with continuous veno-venous hemodialysis using Ultraflux EMiC2 versus Ultraflux AV1000S. Blood Purif. 2017;44(4):260–6.

27. Atari R, Peck L, Visvanathan K, Skinner N, Eastwood G, Bellomo R, et al. High cut-off hemofiltration versus standard hemofiltration: effect on plasma cytokines. Int J Artif Organs. 2016;39(9):479–86.

28. Kade G, Lubas A, Rzeszotarska A, Korsak J, Niemczyk S. Effectiveness of high cut-off hemofilters in the removal of selected cytokines in patients during septic shock accompanied by acute kidney injury-preliminary study. Med Sci Monit. 2016;22:4338–44.

18

29. Honoré P, Clark W. Novel therapeutical concepts for extracorporeal treatment of hyperinflammation and sepsis: immunomodulation. approach with a novel high Cut-OFF membrane: the SepteX membrane. Proceedings of 10th Congress of World Federation of CCU (WFSICCM). Florence, Italy; 2009.

30. Lumlertgul N, Hall A, Camporota L, Crichton S, Ostermann M. Clearance of inflammatory cytokines in patients with septic acute kidney injury during renal replacement therapy using the EMiC2 filter (Clic-AKI study). Crit Care. 2021;25(1):39.

31. Rogiers P, Zhang H, Pauwels D, Vincent J-L. Comparison of polyacrylonitrile (AN69) and polysulphone membrane during hemofiltration in canine endotoxic shock. Crit Care Med. 2003;31(4):1219–25.

32. Thomas M, Moriyama K, Ledebo I. AN69: evolution of the world's first high permeability membrane. Contrib Nephrol. 2011;173:119–29.

33. Moriyama K, Kato Y, Hasegawa D, Kurimoto Y, Kawaji T, Nakamura T, et al. Involvement of ionic interactions in cytokine adsorption of polyethyleneimine-coated polyacrylonitrile and polymethyl methacrylate membranes in vitro. J Artif Organs. 2020;23(3):240–6.

34. Yumoto M, Nishida O, Moriyama K, Shimomura Y, Nakamura T, Kuriyama N, et al. In vitro evaluation of high mobility group box 1 protein removal with various membranes for continuous hemofiltration. Ther Apher Dial. 2011;15(4):385–93.

35. Shiga H, Hirasawa H, Nishida O, Oda S, Nakamura M, Mashiko K, et al. Continuous hemodiafiltration with a cytokine-adsorbing Hemofilter in patients with septic shock: a preliminary report. Blood Purif. 2015;38(3–4):211–8.

36. Doi K, Iwagami M, Yoshida E, Marshall MR. Associations of polyethylenimine-coated AN69ST membrane in continuous renal replacement therapy with the intensive care outcomes: observations from a claims database from Japan. Blood Purif. 2017;44(3):184–92.

37. Kobashi S, Maruhashi T, Nakamura T, Hatabayashi E, Kon A. The 28-day survival rates of two cytokine-adsorbing hemofilters for continuous renal replacement therapy: a single-center retrospective comparative study. Acute Med Surg. 2019;6(1):60–7.

38. Nakamura T, Moriyama K, Shimomura Y, Kato Y, Kuriyama N, Hara Y, et al. Adsorption kinetics of high mobility group box 1 protein in a polyacrylonitrile hemofiltration membrane. Ther Apher Dial. 2021;25(1):66–72.

39. Feri M. "In vitro comparison of the adsorption of inflammatory mediators by blood purification devices": a misleading article for clinical practice? Intensive Care Med Exp. 2019;7(1):5.

40. Suzuki S, Moriyama K, Hara Y, Hinoue T, Kato Y, Hasegawa D, et al. Comparison of myoglobin clearance in three types of blood purification modalities. Ther Apher Dial. 2021;25(4):401–6.

41. Nakada T, Oda S, Matsuda K, Sadahiro T, Nakamura M, Abe R, et al. Continuous hemodiafiltration with PMMA Hemofilter in the treatment of patients with septic shock. Mol Med. 2008;14(5–6):257–63.

42. Hirasawa H. Indications for blood purification in critical care. Contrib Nephrol. 2010;166:21–30.

43. Honore PM, Jacobs R, Joannes-Boyau O, Regt JD, Waele ED, van Gorp V, et al. Newly designed CRRT membranes for sepsis and SIRS—A pragmatic approach for bedside intensivists summarizing the more recent advances. ASAIO J. 2013;59(2):99–106.

44. Rimmelé T, Assadi A, Cattenoz M, Desebbe O, Lambert C, Boselli E, et al. High-volume haemofiltration with a new haemofiltration membrane having enhanced adsorption properties in septic pigs. Nephrol Dial Transplant. 2009;24(2):421–7.

45. Broman ME, Hansson F, Vincent J-L, Bodelsson M. Endotoxin and cytokine reducing properties of the oXiris membrane in patients with septic shock: a randomized crossover double-blind study. PLoS One. 2019;14(8):e0220444.

46. Villa G, Rosa SD, Samoni S, Neri M, Chelazzi C, Romagnoli S, et al. oXirisNet registry: a prospective, National Registry on the oXiris membrane. Blood Purif. 2019;47(Suppl 3):16–22.

47. Cruz DN, Antonelli M, Fumagalli R, Foltran F, Brienza N, Donati A, et al. Early use of polymyxin B hemoperfusion in abdominal septic shock: the EUPHAS randomized controlled trial. JAMA. 2009;301(23):2445–52.

48. Payen DM, Guilhot J, Launey Y, Lukaszewicz AC, Kaaki M, et al.; ABDOMIX Group. Early use of polymyxin B hemoperfusion in patients with septic shock due to peritonitis: a multicenter randomized control trial. Intensive Care Med. 2015;41(6):975–984.

49. Dellinger RP, Bagshaw SM, Antonelli M, Foster DM, Klein DJ, Marshall JC, et al. Effect of targeted polymyxin B hemoperfusion on 28-day mortality in patients with septic shock and elevated endotoxin level: the EUPHRATES randomized clinical trial. JAMA. 2018;320(14):1455.

50. Klein DJ, Foster D, Walker PM, Bagshaw SM, Mekonnen H, Antonelli M. Polymyxin B hemoperfusion in endotoxemic septic shock patients without extreme endotoxemia: a post hoc analysis of the EUPHRATES trial. Intensive Care Med. 2018;44(12):2205–12.

51. Song M, Winchester J, Albright RL, Capponi VJ, Choquette MD, Kellum JA. Cytokine removal with a novel adsorbent polymer. Blood Purif. 2004;22(5):428–34.

52. Chen J, Han W, Chen J, Zong W, Wang W, Wang Y, et al. High performance of a unique mesoporous polystyrene-based adsorbent for blood purification. Regen Biomater. 2017;4(1):31–7.

53. Honore PM, Hoste E, Molnár Z, Jacobs R, Joannes-Boyau O, Malbrain MLNG, et al. Cytokine removal in human septic shock: where are we and where are we going? Ann Intensive Care. 2019;9(1):56.

54. Gruda MC, Ruggeberg K-G, O'Sullivan P, Guliashvili T, Scheirer AR, Golobish TD, et al. Broad adsorption of sepsis-related PAMP and DAMP molecules, mycotoxins, and cytokines from whole blood using CytoSorb® sorbent porous polymer beads. PLoS One. 2018;13(1):e0191676.

55. Harm S, Schildböck C, Hartmann J. Cytokine removal in extracorporeal blood purification: an in vitro study. Blood Purif. 2020;49(1–2):33–43.

56. Malard B, Lambert C, Kellum JA. In vitro comparison of the adsorption of inflammatory mediators by blood purification devices. Intensive Care Med Exp. 2018;6(1):12.

57. Kellum JA, Song M, Venkataraman R. Hemoadsorption removes tumor necrosis factor, interleukin-6, and interleukin-10, reduces nuclear factor-kappaB DNA binding, and improves short-term survival in lethal endotoxemia. Crit Care Med. 2004;32(3):801–5.

58. Namas RA, Namas R, Lagoa C, Barclay D, Mi Q, Zamora R, et al. Hemoadsorption reprograms inflammation in experimental gram-negative septic peritonitis: insights from in vivo and in silico studies. Mol Med. 2012;18(10):1366–74.

59. Peng Z-Y, Carter MJ, Kellum JA. Effects of hemoadsorption on cytokine removal and short-term survival in septic rats. Crit Care Med. 2008;36(5):1573–7.

60. Linden K, Scaravilli V, Kreyer SFX, Belenkiy SM, Stewart IJ, Chung KK, et al. Evaluation of the Cytosorb™ hemoadsorptive column in a PIG model of severe smoke and burn injury. Shock. 2015;44(5):487–95.

61. Kellum JA, Venkataraman R, Powner D, Elder M, Hergenroeder G, Carter M. Feasibility study of cytokine removal by hemoadsorption in brain-dead humans. Crit Care Med. 2008;36(1):268–72.

62. Schädler D, Pausch C, Heise D, Meier-Hellmann A, Brederlau J, Weiler N, et al. The effect of a novel extracorporeal cytokine hemoadsorption device on IL-6 elimination in septic patients: a randomized controlled trial. PLoS One. 2017;12(10):e0187015.

63. Scharf C, Schroeder I, Paal M, Winkels M, Irlbeck M, Zoller M, et al. Can the cytokine adsorber CytoSorb® help to mitigate cytokine storm and reduce mortality in critically ill patients? A propensity score matching analysis. Ann Intensive Care. 2021;11(1):115.

64. Rugg C, Klose R, Hornung R, Innerhofer N, Bachler M, Schmid S, et al. Hemoadsorption with CytoSorb in septic shock reduces catecholamine requirements and in-hospital mortality: a single-center retrospective 'genetic' matched analysis. Biomedicines. 2020;8(12):539.

65. Brouwer WP, Duran S, Kuijper M, Ince C. Hemoadsorption with CytoSorb shows a decreased observed versus expected 28-day all-cause mortality in ICU patients with septic shock: a propensity-score-weighted retrospective study. Crit Care. 2019;23(1):317.

66. Friesecke S, Träger K, Schittek GA, Molnar Z, Bach F, Kogelmann K, et al. International registry on the use of the CytoSorb® adsorber in ICU patients. Med Klin Intensivmed Notfmed. 2019;114(8):699–707.

67. Zhou F, Peng Z, Murugan R, Kellum JA. Blood purification and mortality in sepsis. Crit Care Med. 2013;41(9):2209–20.

68. Supady A, Weber E, Rieder M, Lother A, Niklaus T, Zahn T, et al. Cytokine adsorption in patients with severe COVID-19 pneumonia requiring extracorporeal membrane oxygenation (CYCOV): a single centre, open-label, randomised, controlled trial. Lancet Respir Med. 2021;9(7):755–62.

69. Hawchar F, Rao C, Akil A, Mehta Y, Rugg C, Scheier J, et al. The potential role of extracorporeal cytokine removal in hemodynamic stabilization in hyperinflammatory shock. Biomedicines. 2021;9(7):768.

70. Mehta Y, Singh A, Singh A, Gupta A, Bhan A. Modulating the inflammatory response with hemadsorption (CytoSorb®) in patients undergoing major aortic surgery. J Cardiothorac Vasc Anesth. 2020;35(2):673–5.
71. Hawchar F, László I, Öveges N, Trásy D, Ondrik Z, Molnar Z. Extracorporeal cytokine adsorption in septic shock: a proof of concept randomized, controlled pilot study. J Crit Care. 2018;49:172–8.
72. Akil A, Ziegeler S, Reichelt J, Rehers S, Abdalla O, Semik M, et al. Combined use of CytoSorb and ECMO in patients with severe pneumogenic sepsis. Thorac Cardiovasc Surg. 2020;69(3):246–51.
73. Yaroustovsky M, Abramyan M, Rogalskaya E, Komardina E. Selective polymyxin hemoperfusion in complex therapy of sepsis in children after cardiac surgery. Blood Purif. 2021;50(2):222–9.
74. Rossetti E, Guzzo I, Ricci Z, Bianchi R, Picardo S. Double extracorporeal blood purification in refractory pediatric septic shock. Pediatr Anesth. 2019;29(9):966–7.
75. Ruiz-Rodríguez JC, Chiscano-Camón L, Palmada C, Ruiz-Sanmartin A, Pérez-Carrasco M, Larrosa N, et al. Endotoxin and cytokine sequential hemoadsorption in septic shock and multiorgan failure. Blood Purif. 2022;51(7):630–3.
76. Ronco C, Reis T. Continuous renal replacement therapy and extended indications. Semin Dial. 2021;34(6):550–60.
77. Huang Z, Wang S, Su W, Liu J. Removal of humoral mediators and the effect on the survival of septic patients by hemoperfusion with neutral microporous resin column. Ther Apher Dial. 2010;14(6):596–602.
78. Huang Z, Wang S, Yang Z, Liu J. Effect on extrapulmonary sepsis-induced acute lung injury by hemoperfusion with neutral microporous resin column. Ther Apher Dial. 2013;17(4):454–61.
79. Livigni S, Bertolini G, Rossi C, Ferrari F, Giardino M, Pozzato M, et al. Efficacy of coupled plasma filtration adsorption (CPFA) in patients with septic shock: a multicenter randomised controlled clinical trial. BMJ Open. 2014;4(1):e003536.
80. Giménez-Esparza C, Portillo-Requena C, Colomina-Climent F, Allegue-Gallego JM, Galindo-Martínez M, Mollà-Jiménez C, et al. The premature closure of ROMPA clinical trial: mortality reduction in septic shock by plasma adsorption. BMJ Open. 2019;9(12):e030139.
81. David S, Stahl K. To remove and replace—a role for plasma exchange in counterbalancing the host response in sepsis. Crit Care. 2019;23(1):14.
82. Lopez E, Peng Z, Kozar RA, Cao Y, Ko TC, Wade CE, et al. Antithrombin III contributes to the protective effects of fresh frozen plasma following hemorrhagic shock by preventing Syndecan-1 shedding and endothelial barrier disruption. Shock. 2020;53(2):156–63.
83. Knaup H, Stahl K, Schmidt BMW, Idowu TO, Busch M, Wiesner O, et al. Early therapeutic plasma exchange in septic shock: a prospective open-label nonrandomized pilot study focusing on safety, hemodynamics, vascular barrier function, and biologic markers. Crit Care. 2018;22(1):285.
84. Rimmer E, Houston BL, Kumar A, Abou-Setta AM, Friesen C, Marshall JC, et al. The efficacy and safety of plasma exchange in patients with sepsis and septic shock: a systematic review and meta-analysis. Crit Care. 2014;18(6):699.

Printed in the United States
by Baker & Taylor Publisher Services